T0255015

Register Now for Online Access to Your Book!

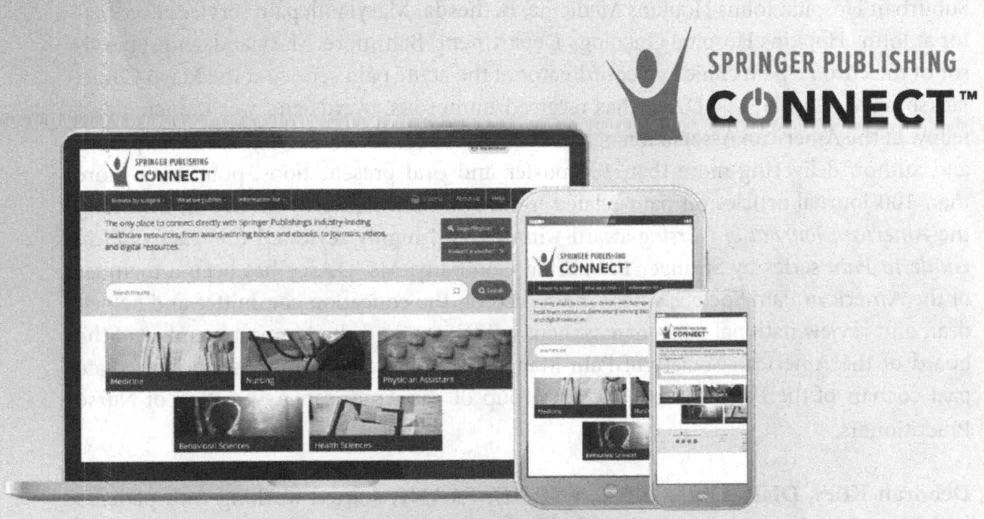

Your print purchase of *Pain Management in Primary Care* **includes online access to the contents of your book—** increasing accessibility, portability, and searchability!

Access today at:
http://connect.springerpub.com/content/book/978-0-8261-4734-9
or scan the QR code at the right with your smartphone and enter the access code below.

JKF117TV

Scan here for quick access.

If you are experiencing problems accessing the digital component of this product, please contact our customer service department at cs@springerpub.com

The online access with your print purchase is available at the publisher's discretion and may be removed at any time without notice.

Publisher's Note: New and used products purchased from third-party sellers are not guaranteed for quality, authenticity, or access to any included digital components.

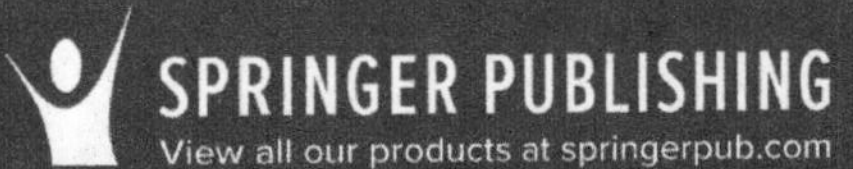

Yvonne D'Arcy, MS, APRN, CNS, FAANP, is an expert pain management and palliative care nurse practitioner and consultant. She has extensive clinical experience in various roles, including leading a nurse practitioner pain-management consulting service at Suburban Hospital Johns Hopkins Medicine, Bethesda, Maryland; pain service coordinator at Johns Hopkins Hospital Oncology Department, Baltimore, Maryland; and supervisor of the chronic pain clinic and coordinator of the acute pain service at the Mayo Clinic, Jacksonville, Florida. Ms. D'Arcy has received numerous awards and was inducted as a fellow of the American Association of Nurse Practitioners in 2016. She is a prolific speaker and author, delivering more than 100 poster and oral presentations, publishing more than 100 journal articles on pain-related topics, and authoring seven books, including the *American Journal of Nursing*-award-winning and highly reviewed *Compact Clinical Guide to Pain* series by Springer Publishing Company. Ms. D'Arcy has been a member of the American Pain Society, where she served on the education committee and helped draft and review national pain-management guidelines; and she is a past member of the board of the American Society of Pain Management Nurses, as well as the immediate past cochair of the Pain Special Practice Group of the American Association of Nurse Practitioners.

Deborah Kiley, DNP, APRN, NP-C, FNP-BC, FAANP, started working with patients with chronic pain as a new graduate family nurse practitioner (FNP) in 1983. She has extensive pain-management experience in primary, specialty, and integrative care practice settings. She uses functional and integrative medicine therapies in combination with prescription medications and other Western pain interventions. A nurse practitioner at the Alaska Center for Pain Relief and the founder of Fearless Wellness LLC, Dr. Kiley addresses the cause of disease when working with patients to identify their best path to improved health. She earned her master's degree at UCLA; received her doctor of nursing practice degree at Rush College of Nursing, Chicago, Illinois; and mastered health behavior coaching at Duke Center for Integrative Medicine, Durham, North Carolina, where she earned certification as an integrative health coach. Dr. Kiley lectures nationally on pain and integrative therapies and has an active social media presence. As a fellow of the American Association of Nurse Practitioners, she continues to mentor nurse practitioners and students in professional development, leadership, patient-centered care, and personal wellness.

PAIN MANAGEMENT IN PRIMARY CARE

Essential Knowledge for APRNs and PAs

Yvonne D'Arcy, MS, APRN, CNS, FAANP

Deborah Kiley, DNP, APRN, NP-C, FNP-BC, FAANP

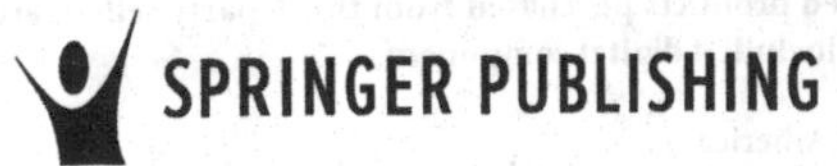

Springer Publishing Company, LLC
11 West 42nd Street, New York, NY 10036
www.springerpub.com
connect.springerpub.com/

Acquisitions Editor: Adrianne Brigido
Compositor: Exeter Premedia Services Private Ltd.

ISBN: 978-0-8261-4733-2
ebook ISBN: 978-0-8261-4734-9
DOI: 10.1891/9780826147349

20 21 22 23 24 / 5 4 3 2 1

The author and the publisher of this Work have made every effort to use sources believed to be reliable to provide information that is accurate and compatible with the standards generally accepted at the time of publication. Because medical science is continually advancing, our knowledge base continues to expand. Therefore, as new information becomes available, changes in procedures become necessary. We recommend that the reader always consult current research and specific institutional policies before performing any clinical procedure or delivering any medication. The author and the publisher shall not be liable for any special, consequential, or exemplary damages resulting, in whole or in part, from the readers' use of, or reliance on, the information contained in this book. The publisher has no responsibility for the persistence or accuracy of URLs for external or third-party Internet websites referred to in this publication and does not guarantee that any content on such websites is, or will remain, accurate or appropriate.

Library of Congress Cataloging-in-Publication Data

Names: D'Arcy, Yvonne M., author. | Kiley, Deborah, author.
Title: Pain management in primary care : essential knowledge for APRNs and PAs / Yvonne D'Arcy, Deborah Kiley.
Description: New York, NY : Springer Publishing Company, [2021] | Includes bibliographical references and index.
Identifiers: LCCN 2020013391 (print) | LCCN 2020013392 (ebook) | ISBN 9780826147332 (paperback) | ISBN 9780826147349 (ebook)
Subjects: MESH: Pain Management—nursing | Primary Care Nursing—methods | Nurse Practitioners | Physician Assistants | Case Reports
Classification: LCC RB127 (print) | LCC RB127 (ebook) | NLM WY 101 | DDC 616/.0472—dc23
LC record available at https://lccn.loc.gov/2020013391
LC ebook record available at https://lccn.loc.gov/2020013392

Publisher's Note: **New and used products purchased from third-party sellers are not guaranteed for quality, authenticity, or access to any included digital components.**

Printed in the United States of America.

I dedicate this book to my family and friends
who supported me during many months of writing.
I also dedicate this book to those frontline
healthcare providers in primary care who are caring for the
many thousands of patients who are in pain and need their help.
We appreciate you for all you do.

—Yvonne D'Arcy

To Dan, Matt, and Steve, who, year after year, adapted
when I had "one more thing to do."

—Deborah Kiley

CONTENTS

FOREWORD

As primary care providers struggle with when and how to manage pain for patients with both acute and chronic pain, this book offers much-needed guidance; it is an essential tool for nurse practitioners and all primary care providers. With substance abuse disorders on the minds of both providers and patients, information on the best practices to use for pain management with medication as well as other treatment modalities is vital to providing patient-centered care. As pain clinics move to more intervention therapies, such as spinal injections, patients with limited access to pain clinics, lack of resources, or the fear of/lack of desire for an injection push pain management to primary care.

The content of this book is relevant for any provider engaged in caring for patients in the primary care setting. Yvonne D'Arcy and Deborah Kiley are not only pain experts, but also clinicians who provide holistic patient-centered, patient-directed care. The methods used to make an accurate pain diagnosis as well as safe prescribing habits are essential for providers to review and consider when treating multiple problems. In light of the opioid epidemic, the authors reveal safe prescribing methods, inclusion of the patient in the decision-making process, and ways to monitor opioid use. In addition, topics that are often not covered, such as opioid withdrawal, working in systems with pain management, and when to refer to a pain clinic, are covered. More importantly, information on what the clinician and the patient should expect from such a referral is provided.

The part of this book that I appreciate the most as a nurse practitioner is the section on integrative and interventional therapies. As pain has many facets that are not treatable by medication alone, this information offers valuable and contemporary alternatives to the treatment of pain that can be used in other areas of practice besides pain management.

As a primary care provider who cares for many patients with pain, as a wife who has a spouse with chronic pain, and as a care provider for a veteran whose pain is more than just physical, I applaud the authors for this inclusive work on pain management.

Joyce M. Knestrick, PhD, FNP-BC, FAAN, FAANP
Visiting Professor, George Washington University
Immediate Past President of the American Association of Nurse Practitioners

PREFACE

This book has been a work of love. We wrote it hoping to provide the information we wished we had when we started treating pain.

We discussed writing this book for several years, but never felt it was the right time to pursue it. However, we finally realized the book needed to be written because primary care practitioners were asking for it. Clinicians continue to walk the tightrope, balancing safety and efficacy.

We could tell from listening to nurse practitioners who worked in primary care that they needed evidence-based references for treating their patients with pain. While talking to them, we could see their frustration with the pressures surrounding opioid use; pain was becoming the subject of debate with patients, colleagues, and insurance companies, rather than something to treat. We also noted a lack of information about the therapies used in integrative medicine, which this book covers extensively.

We hope that this book will be a resource for primary care clinicians to use when making decisions to treat pain in their patients and that it will make the hard choices that occur every day in the clinic less stressful and more effective.

Please use this book to improve the pain care you give to your patients. You and they deserve the best care possible.

Yvonne D'Arcy
Deborah Kiley

ACKNOWLEDGMENTS

I would like to thank Dr. Bill McCarberg for his help and support over these many long years and for sharing his extensive pain-management knowledge. He was so very kind as to help me with the naloxone requirements for this book.

I also would like to thank Dr. Kathleen Broglio for the information on medication-assisted therapy (MAT) for treating patients with opioid use disorder. She was kind enough to share her publications and her perspective on the topic.

Yvonne D'Arcy

I am very grateful to the following people in my life who provide support for me and my work, including this book:

Yvonne D'Arcy, who said we need to write this book and mentored me through the process

The staff and patients at the Casa Colina Hospital Pain Program, especially Hal Gottlieb and Don Weir, who taught me about the many dimensions of pain and the importance of self-efficacy in managing pain and life

My nurse practitioner colleagues, who inspire, motivate, mentor, and support me: Barbara Phillips, "Nurse Barb" Dehn, Judy Berg, and LeeAnne Hellesto

Mary Johnson and Lynne Braun at Rush, who helped me find my writing voice

Connie Judd and Cath Barrett, psychiatric-mental health nurse practitioners who proved that you can combine care that is evidence-based, holistic, technically excellent, and compassionate

Dennis Katz and Michael Macione from Hopkinton Drug Pharmacy, who clarified the complexities of using compounding

Kathy, Mary Kate, Deirdre, Jacque, Kelly, Shoshana, Megan, and Ellen, friends who provided encouragement and unconditional support as the pages evolved

The patients who inspire with their resilience and teach me every day

And finally, Steve Floerchinger, MD, and Torrey Smith, ND, who continuously share information and wisdom; your friendship makes me a better person and clinician

Deborah Kiley

PART I

The Foundation of Pain Management

CHAPTER 1

PAIN MANAGEMENT AND THE PRIMARY CARE PRACTITIONER

INTRODUCTION

Nurse practitioners and physician assistants are the backbone of primary care. They see a wide variety of patients who experience different types of pain. Knowing how to deal with a multitude of patients with different pain complaints can help move these patients through the healthcare system efficiently with positive outcomes.

This book provides useful information on treating both simple and complex pain conditions. Clinically pertinent information on assessment, opioid risk assessment, and treatment options help the clinician treat patients most effectively. Case studies provide the clinician with an opportunity to consider realistic pain presentations. Clinical pearls focus on the important aspects of each chapter, and trending points highlight new and upcoming treatments as well as information on specific topics.

THE PROBLEM OF PAIN, THE OPIOID CRISIS, AND THE PRIMARY CARE PRACTITIONER

Pain management has changed drastically over the past 10 years. For many years, the patient with chronic pain was commonly treated with opioids and the doses were titrated upward as needed to control pain. There was a focus on patient report of pain intensity and the use of pain rating scales with numeric values that remained high despite continued dose escalations. In an effort to reduce the pain, opioids were continued long term. Many patients took high-dose opioids for conditions such as low-back pain, abdominal pain, and headaches. At the time, this long-term opioid use, though not ideal, was perceived to be an accepted option for treating the pain so as to make patients more functional. It was not perceived as highly contributory to opioid misuse or the development of a substance abuse disorder. See Box 1.1 for the differences between opioid misuse and opioid abuse.

BOX 1.1

DIFFERENCES BETWEEN OPIOID MISUSE AND OPIOID ABUSE

Opioid misuse: Use of a prescribed medication other than intended, that is, using a pain medication for sleep rather than pain relief

Opioid abuse: Use of a prescribed medication for a purpose other than pain, that is, using a pain medication for its euphoric effect (U.S. Food and Drug Administration [FDA], 2018)

Unfortunately, the amount of opioids being prescribed allowed a large pool of unused drugs to collect in the community, which increased misuse and the potential for abuse. Misuse occurred not only with patients, but also thier family and friends, who knew the patient was using opioid therapy and either stole or asked for medications. Surveys indicate that family and friends were the biggest source of opioids that were being abused (FDA, 2018). Opioid overdose became common and highly publicized. The high rate of opioid misuse contributed to the development of the term *opioid epidemic* to describe the high numbers of opioid misuse and overdose deaths related to opioids or illicit drugs such as heroin.

Today, the climate of opioid use for pain management is quite different. Pain clinics and pain-management practitioners are no longer as prevalent as they had been in the past; nor are they as willing to prescribe opioids for chronic pain patients, often referring them back to their primary care provider after a consult. Today's primary care providers are seeing more and more patients with both acute and chronic pain. At the same time, opioid prescriptions limit the number of pills prescribed and the length of time the opioids can be provided to the patient (Centers for Disease Control and Prevention [CDC], 2017).

Patients who take prescription opioids to control pain face difficulties when trying to move their treatment to a new primary care practice. One hundred and ninety-four primary care clinics were contacted by researchers, who stated they were seeking healthcare for another family member with chronic pain who was opioid dependent. Of the clinics that were contacted, 79 indicated that their practitioners would not provide care to the patient, 81 were willing to schedule an initial consultation, and 33 required more information before they would schedule an appointment for an evaluation (Lagisetty, Healy, Garpestad, Jannausch, & Bohnert, 2019). After receiving additional information about the patient, of the 33 clinics requiring more information, one clinic accepted the patient, four denied the patient, 20 stated they would make a decision after the initial visit, seven referred the patient to a pain clinic, and one asked for medical records to be faxed (Lagisetty et al., 2019). For a patient with chronic pain, the fear of the need for an opioid prescription can severely limit options for care.

Prescribers are being urged to limit the amount of opioids they prescribe to 50 morphine milliequivalents (MME) or less per day for treating chronic pain and to limit the time frame for opioid use postoperatively to 7 days or less (CDC, 2017). The hope was that those limitations would decrease the amount of available prescription opioids for misuse and abuse. Although opioid prescriptions have decreased in number, statistics show that in primary care, a patient who reports pain leaves the office with an opioid prescription 20% of the time (FDA, 2018).

Current evidence shows that long-term opioid use for conditions such as low-back pain does not improve the patients' pain levels, function, or quality of life (CDC, 2017). In addition, long-term use of opioids for chronic pain can lead to abuse and overdose, especially if the patient is taking higher doses (CDC, 2017). This is supported by data from the American Society of Addiction Medicine (ASAM; 2016), which found that of the 20.5 million Americans 12 years of age or older with a substance abuse disorder in 2015, two million had a disorder involving the abuse of prescription pain relievers and 591,000 had a substance use disorder involving heroin.

GUIDELINES AND RECOMMENDATIONS FOR OPIOID PRESCRIBING

Concurrently, the U.S. Food and Drug Administration (FDA) and the CDC issued recommendations and guidelines for prescribing opioids. The overall aim of the new recommendations is to limit the amount of available opioids for abuse in the community and create safe opioid-prescribing practices. Unfortunately, findings indicate that opioids are still commonly obtained from friends and family, allowing for little control over who ultimately abuses the drugs (CDC, 2017; FDA, 2018).

In this age of policy and procedures, what seems to be getting lost in the discussion is the patient who has pain. In opinion articles in the *Wall Street Journal,* patients recount how the use of opioids for trauma pain was being discouraged (Rieder, 2019). After a severe motorcycle accident, Mr. Reider, a bioethicist, was given opioids, but struggled to recover because opioid use was being discouraged (Rieder, 2019).

Patients with chronic pain are finding that they are being asked to taper their opioid dose, and their prescription medications are limited by duration and amount prescribed. In a recent commentary in the *New England Journal of Medicine,* the authors of the CDC guidelines state that it was not their intention to limit opioids for patients who are using them for pain relief. They also stated that when crafting the guidelines their intention was for the guidelines to be used as recommendations rather than strict regulations (Dowell, Haegerich, & Chou, 2019). When using opioids for pain relief, the risk and benefit for the patient should always be the primary concern. If, indeed, opioids are seen to be a benefit, safe prescribing practices can help ensure the safety of the patient and provide pain relief.

CLINICAL PEARL

Surveys have shown that the biggest source of the opioids that are misused or abused come from family and friends. Using urine screens to detect medications that are not prescribed for the patient is one way to see whether friends or family have been sharing medications.

The FDA Blueprint (FDA, 2018) centers around the safe prescribing of long-acting opioids. Long-acting or extended-release opioids are more potent and contain more MME than shorter acting formulas of the same drugs. In patients taking multiple doses of short-acting opioids on a daily basis, use of a long-acting medication can provide improved pain relief with fewer fluctuations in blood levels. Taking extended-release opioids can put these patients at more of a risk of overdose if the medication is abused. Extended-release medications with higher medication amounts can make the patients taking them targets for drug abusers.

Recognizing the heightened risk factors for use of extended-release opioids prompted the FDA to focus on the aspects of safe prescribing. In the FDA Blueprint, the FDA recommends the use of patient–provider agreements, screening tools such as the Opioid Risk Tool (ORT) and urine drug screens, safe disposal, the regular use of state prescription monitoring programs, and educating patients about the increased risks inherent with extended-release medications (FDA, 2018). In addition, pharmaceutical companies that manufacture these drugs have been mandated to fund education programs for opioid prescribers called *Risk Evaluation and Mitigation Strategies* (REMS). Efforts to develop tamper-resistant packaging were also encouraged.

It is important to note that there is risk with use of short-acting opioids as well. Most patients who develop a substance use disorder begin by using short-acting opioids and progress to overdose, substance use disorder, or abuse disorder. The use of short-acting opioids in the postoperative setting has created a group of patients who continue opioid use long after their surgical pain resolves, but continue to take the medication because they fear the pain might return if they discontinued the medication.

THE CDC GUIDELINES FOR PRESCRIBING OPIOIDS

The CDC Guidelines for Prescribing Opioids for Chronic Pain (CDC, 2017) center around decreasing opioid use and dose reduction in patients with chronic pain. The recommendations first state that prescribers should begin pain management with nonopioid and nonpharmacological treatments. If these fail, a trial of the lowest effective dose of short-acting can be used for the shortest possible time period. If opioids are started, the patient needs to be screened for opioid risk using a tool such as the ORT, and if the patient scores as high risk, the guidelines recommend sending the patient for methadone or buprenorphine therapy for pain relief instead. In addition, the CDC encourages limiting opioid prescriptions for postoperative patients to 3 days with a maximum of 7 days.

CLINICAL PEARL

National guidelines recommend the use of urine drug screens to determine whether the prescribed opioid is present or if there are other substances, such as anxiolytics or marijuana, in the urine sample.

RESULTS OF THE CDC PRESCRIPTION GUIDELINE CHANGES

These changes have had a positive effect on opioid use, decreasing the number of opioid prescriptions written. Many insurance providers and state insurance programs have adopted the CDC recommendations for limiting opioid prescriptions. From 2006 to 2016, the number of prescriptions for high-dose opioids with a potency greater than 90 MME per day decreased from 11.5 per 100 persons to 6.1. This was an overall reduction of 46.8% and an average percentage change of 6.6% (CDC, 2017). There are still a significant number of opioid prescriptions being written by prescribers. The CDC is reporting that in 2016, prescribers wrote 66.5 opioid and 25.2 sedative prescriptions for every 100 Americans (CDC, 2017).

Unfortunately, the majority of providers are not following the guidelines, and overdose deaths attributed to opioids are increasing, with 46 people a day dying from overdose (CDC, 2017). The most common drugs implicated in overdose are methadone, oxycodone, and hydrocodone (CDC, 2017); all are commonly prescribed for treating pain. Prescription opioids accounted for 40% of opioid overdose deaths. The introduction of illicitly produced fentanyl for use as a cutting agent for heroin has caught users unaware; the onset of fentanyl is very rapid and the opioid effect is heightened as fentanyl is considered to be 100 times more potent than morphine. The CDC (2017) reports that overdose deaths from synthetic opioids other than methadone increased by 100%, resulting in 19,000 fatalities in 2015 and 2016.

What happens to patients when their healthcare professionals no longer feel that opioid use is appropriate or safe for patients? When the door closes on legal opioids, some patients resort to heroin as a cheaper and easier-to-obtain drug that can relieve pain and provide the euphoric effect many patients with substance abuse disorder crave. Four out of five new heroin users report misusing prescription opioids before using heroine (Jones, 2013). As a result, admissions to drug treatment programs for patients with opioid substance abuse disorders have dramatically increased.

WHAT DO THE CHANGES IN THE PRESCRIBING CLIMATE MEAN TO YOUR PRACTICE?

As frontline healthcare providers, nurse practitioners are being asked to comply with the new recommendations and practices. How have these changes affected your practice? Are you able to comply with the guidelines when prescribing an opioid? What happens when a patient on high-dose opioids is transferred into your practice?

Very recently, the authors of the CDC guidelines were queried by several professional organizations about the impact of the guidelines on patients. The CDC indicated that the guidelines were intended to be recommendations and not inflexible guidelines (Dowell et al., 2019). Patients with cancer and palliative care patients, as well as those with sickle cell disease or postsurgical pain have had the CDC guidelines inappropriately applied to them.

The CDC guidelines and the FDA Blueprint were developed to help prescribers use opioids safely and effectively, while offering information on nonopioid pain-management techniques and medications. It is inevitable that appropriate application of the recent recommendations in pain-management patients will continue to be a discussion among providers, insurance providers, and organizations.

SUMMARY

It is our hope that this book provides information and support for primary care practitioners who are faced with treating patients with pain. This is the type of book I wish I had in my reference library when I first started practicing pain management. I hope you find the information in this book helpful to your practice.

TRENDING IN PAIN MANAGEMENT

- The World Health Organization's *International Classification of Diseases (ICD-11)* has classified chronic pain as a separate disease, not relying on pain as a comorbid condition, as with osteoarthritis (Johnson, 2019; WHO, 2018). Look for more information on this new classification.
- In a *New England Journal of Medicine* article in 2019, the authors of the CDC guidelines indicated that their guidelines were meant to be recommendations, and that restrictions on opioid use were being over-emphasized.
- Look for changes in application of the national guidelines for pain management that take more of a patient-focused approach and use integrative options for pain management.
- Look for development in medications, such as new molecules and integrative therapies, that will lessen the need for opioids.

CASE STUDY

Bill is a construction worker who hurt his back in a traffic accident on his way to work. He comes into his primary care practitioner's office looking for some way to return to work. He states his pain is okay when he is sitting down, but he cannot stand for long and the pain becomes severe in a very short time. He needs to go back to work, but the pain is severely limiting his activity and he knows that he could not work on construction with his current pain level. He asks you for pain medication to help lessen his pain and help him sleep. What are your options?

- The CDC guidelines indicate using nonopioid options for pain relief as the first step in treating the pain. Discuss what type of therapy Bill would consider. Physical therapy and stretching exercises would be helpful to move muscles that are contracting and exacerbating the pain. Other options are massage, acupuncture, and cognitive behavioral therapy. Prescribe a nonopioid medication, such as a nonsteroidal anti-inflammatory drug (NSAID), for pain relief if Bill is a good candidate.
- Assess whether there is a neuropathic component to Bill's pain. If the pain is radiating down one or both legs or Bill describes the pain as electric or shooting, he may have a neuropathic or mixed-pain presentation (musculoskeletal with neuropathic). A neuropathic pain medication, such as a gabapentenoid or a spinal injection, can provide relief for his neuropathic pain.
- Opioids are not indicated for long-term use with back pain. A short course would be okay for the acute pain, but Bill is looking for a way to return to a job in which opioids would be contraindicated for safety reasons. Consider using a nonopioid medication or spinal injection if the pain is neuropathic.

REFERENCES

American Society of Addiction Medicine. (2016). *Opioid addiction 2016: Facts & figures.* Retrieved from www.asam.org

Centers for Disease Control and Prevention. (2017). The current drug overdose epidemic in the United States: Executive summary. *Annual Surveillance Report of Drug Related Risks and Outcomes.* Retrieved from https://www.cdc.gov/drugoverdose/pdf/pubs/2017-cdc-drug-surveillance-report.pdf

Dowell, D., Haegerich, T., & Chou, R. (2019). No shortcuts to safer opioid prescribing. *New England Journal of Medicine, 380*(24), 2285–2287. doi:10.1056/NEJMp1904190

Johnson, M. I. (2019). The landscape of chronic pain: Broader perspectives. *Medicine (Kaunas), 55*(5), 182. doi:10.3390/medicina55050182

Jones, C. M. (2013). Heroin use and heroin risk behaviors among nonmedical users of prescription opioid pain relievers. *Drug and Alcohol Dependence, 132*(1–2), 95–100. doi:10.1016/j.drugalcdep.2013.01.007

Lagisetty, P. A., Healy, N., Garpestad, C., Jannausch, M., & Bohnert, A. (2019). Access to primary care clinics for patients with chronic pain receiving opioids. *JAMA Network Open, 2*, e196928. doi:10.1001/jamanetworkopen.2019.6928

Rieder, T. (2019, June 14). The perilous blessing of opioids. *The Wall Street Journal.* Retrieved from https://www.wsj.com/articles/the-perilous-blessing-of-opioids-11560504600

U. S. Food and Drug Administration. (2018). *The FDA opioid analgesic REMS education blueprint for healthcare providers involved in the treatment and monitoring of patients with pain.* Retrieved from www.FDA.gov

World Health Organization. (2018). *International Classification of Diseases, 11th edition.* Retrieved from who.int/classification/icd/en

ADDITIONAL RESOURCES

Jones, C. M., Paulozzi L. J., & Mack, K. A. (2014). Sources of prescription opioid pain relievers by frequency of past year nonmedical use. *JAMA Internal Medicine, 174*(5), 802–803. doi:10.1001/jamainternmed.2013.12809

Stanos, S., Brodsky, M., Argoff, C., Clauw, D. J., D'Arcy, Y., Donevan, S., . . . Watt, S. (2016) Rethinking chronic pain in a primary care setting. *Postgraduate Medicine, 128*(5), 1–33. doi:10.1080/00325481.2016.1188319

CHAPTER 2

PROBLEMS, SOURCES, AND PATHOPHYSIOLOGY OF PAIN

INTRODUCTION

Pain is the most common reason that patients seek help from healthcare providers (Stanos et al., 2016). It may be acute or chronic, and it may be the result of injury or a chronic condition such as osteoarthritis or cancer. To each patient, pain is a limiting factor in his or her daily life and a financial drain.

Although chronic pain affects patients individually, it has a group effect that is felt in the general population. The number of patients with chronic pain grows annually. Pain is considered to be chronic when it lasts for 6 months or more beyond the normal healing period (American Pain Society [APS], 2008). In 2016, approximately 20% of adults in the United States had chronic pain with about 8% of those patients experiencing high-impact chronic pain (Centers for Disease Control and Prevention [CDC], 2018; National Institutes of Health [NIH], 2018).

> **DEFINITION OF *HIGH-IMPACT CHRONIC PAIN***
>
> *High-impact chronic pain* is defined as pain that limits at least one major life activity. The limitations can be either physical or psychological, such as debilitating anxiety or depression (CDC, 2018; NIH, 2018).

There are some interesting demographics on the chronic pain population, including a prevalence statistic for high-impact chronic pain (CDC, 2018; NIH, 2018):

- Both chronic pain and high-impact chronic pain are more prevalent in patients in poverty.
- Pain is more prevalent in patients with less than a high school education.
- It is more common in adults who have public health insurance (Medicare and Medicaid).

- It is more prevalent in women and older adults.
- It is more common in currently employed adults who have worked in the past.
- Chronic pain is more prevalent in rural populations.

These statistics indicate that primary care providers caring for patients with limited means, caring for older patients, or who practice in rural areas will have more patients with chronic pain in their practices and the effect will be more profound. It also means that there will be less insurance coverage for these patients and more time will need to be spent educating patients who have limited education about their pain.

THE COST OF CHRONIC PAIN

Chronic pain does not respect gender, financial status, race, or age. It can be found in all areas of the U.S. population. The annual cost of chronic pain to the U.S. economy is staggering. The combined estimate of direct medical costs, lost productivity, and disability programs is $560 billion (CDC, 2018). This high financial cost can be tracked effectively, but the personal, more damaging aspects of chronic pain to individual patients are much more difficult to ascertain.

Many patients with chronic pain suffer depression. This may be the result of pain, losing function, or losing important aspects of their personal lives, such as the ability to garden, cook, or perform self-care. Because these losses affect the patients so profoundly, their quality of life decreases and they begin to feel isolated and alone. Healthcare practitioners need to be aware of these changes, assess for depression, and help to set goals that address the patients' need for an improved quality of life.

UNDERSTANDING PAIN

Any number of chronic conditions seen by primary care providers cause pain. Osteoarthritis, diabetic neuropathy, chronic abdominal pain, headache, and low-back pain are all common complaints. Some of these conditions are complex and require long-term treatment plans. Abdominal pain can be caused by adhesions from previous surgeries, Crohn's disease, colitis, or gastroparesis. Pelvic pain in women can be caused by ovarian cysts, endometriosis, uterine fibroids, cystitis, or irritable bowel disease.

In an effort to further define chronic pain, the World Health Organization's *International Classification of Diseases*, 11th Revision, highlights the importance of using biopsychological approaches to manage pain (WHO, 2018). It also provides information about the identification of pain as an independent chronic disease and does not rely on a chronic illness to identify the source of pain (Johnson, 2019). It is interesting to note that the report also identifies a shift to primary care as the site for treating pain (Johnson, 2019).

Given the wide range of pain generators now recognized, the primary care clinician needs to be able to treat both the causative condition and the pain. Considering the many different ways patients experience and describe pain, to treat these patients in primary care requires a long-term plan of care and a great deal of patience and understanding. Using motivational interviewing techniques, such as goal setting, can give these patients more control over their pain and generate more patient satisfaction.

CLINICAL PEARL

All patients with resistant chronic pain should be assessed for a history of sexual or physical abuse. If a factor, unless this is addressed, it will be difficult to make progress with treating the pain.

DEFINITION OF *PAIN*

Pain is defined by the International Association for the Study of Pain (IASP) as "an unpleasant sensory and emotional experience associated with actual or potential tissue damage or described in terms of such damage" (American Pain Society [APS], 2008, p. 1). The IASP is developing a new definition of *pain*. The goal of this revision is to make it clear that pain should not be tied to its stimulus. Also, the new definition describes sensations, such as dysesthesia, or pricking, as unpleasant, but are not considered to be pain (IASP Pain Task Force, 2019). The new definition is: "Pain is an aversive sensory and emotional experience typically caused by, or resembling that caused by, actual or potential tissue injury" (IASP Pain Task Force, 2019). The IASP also reinforces that it is important that the patient's report of pain should be accepted and respected. Nonverbal persons are also considered; the new definition states that any indicators of pain in these patients should be considered a sign of pain.

The Experience of Pain

Everyone alive has experienced pain of some type. Acute pain serves a protective function, allowing the body to identify that there is an injury causing pain. Patients with acute pain expect the pain to resolve, and medication may only be needed for a short time period. Eventually, the patient can expect to return to his or her former lifestyle.

On the other hand, chronic pain has no real purpose and may be caused by any number of past injuries, nerve injuries, or undertreated acute pain. Because chronic pain exists over a period of months, it will have some residual effect and the patient's lifestyle will be affected to some degree. Depending on the level of impact, the patient will try to compensate and look for ways to reduce the pain, so that he or she can be more functional.

PAIN PATHOPHYSIOLOGY

The transmission of pain is a very complex action. There are multiple areas of the body that are involved, from the peripheral nerves to the central nervous system and brain.

The cerebral cortex in the brain serves as a memory bank for past pain experiences; so when new pain occurs, the brain recalls past pain experiences and sends a message to the brain that the sensation being experienced is pain. This allows the descending nervous system to send a response to the pain. Transmission of the pain sensation involves a complex mechanism. Neurons from the peripheral and central nervous system serve as its pathways. A multitude of chemical substances serve as pain inhibitors and facilitators and they travel along the neuronal path.

Adverse childhood events can also influence the way pain is experienced. These events are stored in the brain and their negative effect can be recalled as an influencer of current pain. So that this possibility can be addressed, healthcare providers should ask patients whether they were ever assaulted or abused, or whether they have observed traumatic events.

Pain Transmission

At one time, clinicians believed that pain could be explained using a simple gate-control theory in which the pain impulse caused a gate in the nervous system to open, allowing the sensation of pain to pass from the peripheral nervous system to the central nervous system. The sensation was thought to travel up to the brain, where it was interpreted as pain and processed down the descending neuronal pathway to the periphery of the body (i.e., arms and legs) via the peripheral nervous system, causing a reaction (Figure 2.1). For example, if a woman cooking on a stove put her hand on the hot burner, the immediate response to the pain was to remove her hand from the heat.

Pain Types and Mechanisms

Pain can be categorized in many different ways, but the two most common are ***nociceptive*** pain and ***neuropathic*** pain, with a third new category called ***nociplastic*** pain added recently. There are differences among the three types of pain (Table 2.1).

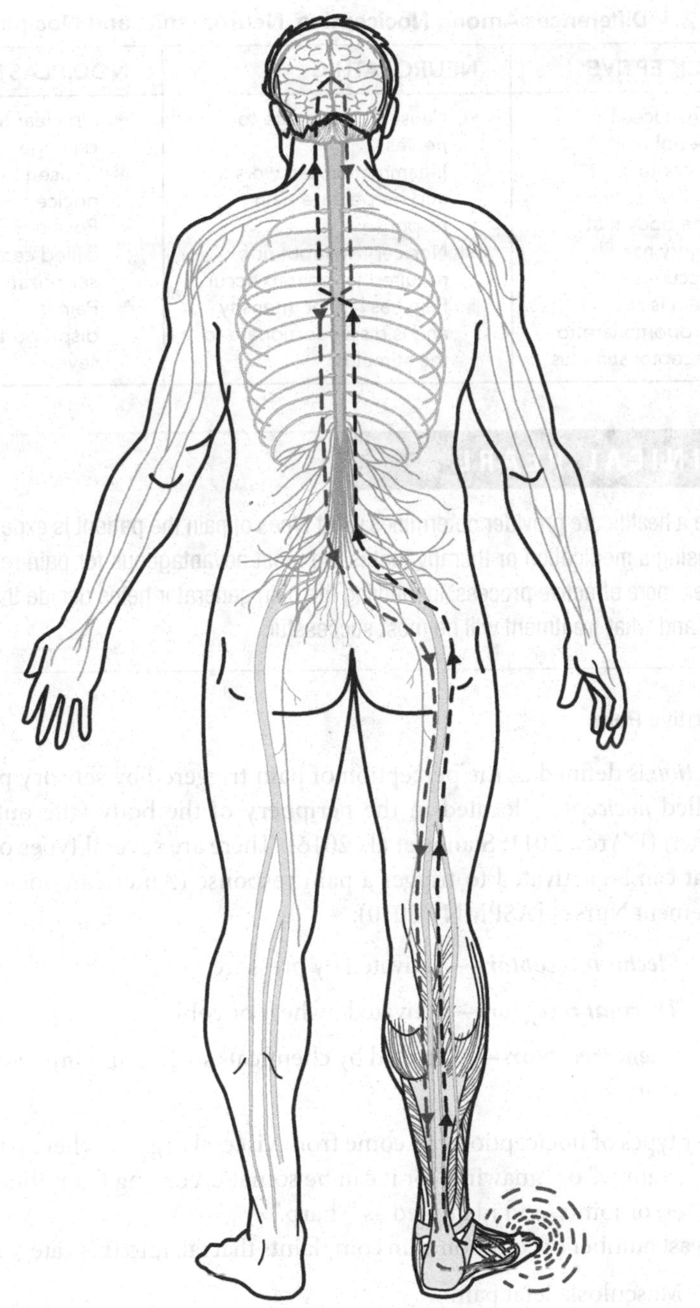

FIGURE 2.1 Diagram illustrating pain transmission: When injury occurs, the sensation travels up to the brain (black arrows) and is interpreted as pain. Then it is processed down the descending neuronal pathway (gray arrows) to the point of injury and causes a reaction.

TABLE 2.1 **Differences Among Nociceptive, Neuropathic, and Nociplastic Pain**

NOCICEPTIVE	NEUROPATHIC	NOCIPLASTIC
■ Produced by peripheral receptors ■ Serves to warn the body that injury has occurred ■ Pain is proportionate to receptor stimulus	■ Caused by damage to nerves ■ Inflammation can worsen and perpetuate pain response ■ Nociceptive input not required for pain to occur ■ Pain has higher intensity and is disproportionate to the stimulus	■ No clear tissue damage ■ Caused by altered nociception ■ Formerly called *central sensitization* ■ Pain is disproportionately severe

CLINICAL PEARL

Once a healthcare provider determines what types of pain the patient is experiencing, choosing a medication or therapy that is the most advantageous for pain relief is an easier, more effective process. Identifying the pain generator helps decide the plan of care and what treatment will be most successful.

Nociceptive Pain

Nociception is defined as the perception of pain triggered by sensory pain receptors called *nociceptors* located in the periphery of the body (the outside, legs, arms, etc.) (D'Arcy, 2011; Stanos et al., 2016). There are several types of nociceptors that can be activated to trigger a pain response (American Society of Pain Management Nurses [ASPMN], 2010):

- ***Mechanoreceptors***—Activated by pressure
- ***Thermal receptors***—Activated by heat or cold
- ***Chemoreceptors***—Activated by chemicals such as inflammatory substances

Other types of nociception can come from visceral organs, where pain is identified as "crampy" or "gnawing," or it can be somatic, coming from the skin, muscles, bones, or joints, and identified as "sharp."

The vast number of common pain complaints that fall into this category include:

- Musculoskeletal pain
- Neck and back pain without neuropathy
- Osteoarthritis and gout
- Rheumatoid arthritis

Neuropathic Pain

Neuropathic pain is one of the most difficult pain conditions to assess and treat. The newest definition of *neuropathic pain* states that it is caused by a lesion or disease of the somatosensory nervous system (Andrews, 2018). A patient with neuropathic pain may have no detectable damage on physical examination or in radiograph scans, and blood tests will be normal.

Sustained inflammation is thought to play a role in the development of neuropathic pain and the continued neuropathic pain response. Inflammation activates a variety of chemicals that are pain producing, such as bradykinin, substance P, hydrogen ions, prostaglandins, histamine, and tumor necrosis factor (TNF). These substances are all known to worsen pain and create changes in the function and structure of surrounding neurons (D'Arcy, 2011). As a result of continued inflammation and the influx of pain-producing substances, the neurons become more permeable to calcium and sodium channels, creating a state of hyperexcitabililty (Benarroch, 2007)

Because the source of the pain resides in the nervous system, it can present as any number of sensations. For example, a patient who is having neuropathic postmastectomy pain may tell the healthcare provider that the pain is severe, a nine out of 10 on a pain scale, and that it shoots across the surgical area. The surgery was performed months ago. No pain medications, such as over-the-counter medications, topical medications, or opioids, have worked. The key here is the pain descriptor.

Patients with neuropathic pain describe their pain as burning, tingling, a strange itching or other sensations, shooting pain, as cold or numbness, or other sensory feelings. In order to treat neuropathic pain, a medication, such as antidepressant, antiepileptic, or serotonin reuptake inhibitor, may need to be used and doses adjusted depending on which medication is selected. Using integrative therapies, such as magnesium or alpha lipoic acid supplements or meditation, can also be tried to see whether they have an effect on the pain.

Pain complaints that fall into this category include:

- Postherpetic neuralgia
- Diabetic peripheral neuropathy
- Spinal stenosis
- Spinal cord injury
- Chemotherapy-induced neuropathies (Stanos et al., 2016)

Nociplastic Pain

Nociplastic pain is the newest term introduced to describe the mechanisms of pain. It is intended to categorize pain that occurs when there is no clear tissue damage. The IASP defines *nociplastic pain* as "pain that arises from altered nociception despite no clear evidence of actual or threatened tissue damage causing the activation of peripheral nociceptors or evidence for disease or lesion of the somatosensory system causing pain" (Aydede & Shriver, 2018, p. 1).

In the past, this term might have been called *central sensitization* or *central hypersensitivity*. It is also important to note that nociplastic pain can occur in conjunction with other types of pain, such as nociceptive and neuropathic pain. Identifying pain as nociplastic can also help healthcare providers choose medication, as patients with nociplastic pain may initially have a response to opioids that decreases dramatically over time (Andrews, 2018). So, if a clinician diagnoses a patient with a nociplastic pain condition, opioids would not be beneficial for treatment.

The pain conditions that fall into this new category include:

- Fibromyalgia
- Complex regional pain syndrome (CRPS)
- Chronic low-back pain
- Irritable bowel syndrome
- Bladder pain syndrome (Andrews, 2018)
- Headaches
- Restless leg syndrome
- Temporomandibular joint disorder (Stanos et al., 2016)

There are advantages to this new term. Patients who may have been misdiagnosed or who have little information on what their pin actually is called may benefit from being told they do have a specific type of pain that has a name. As mentioned, it also allows healthcare providers to choose medications more directly related to the patient's pain and provides pharmaceutical researchers a target to aim for in new-drug development.

Mixed-Pain Presentation

Some patients have the misfortune of developing a pain that has two mechanisms. Often, low-back pain will have a radicular component as well as a musculoskeletal source. Another example is a surgical patient who is not only having acute pain from the surgical injury, but also complains of a neuropathic pain that burns, tingles, or feels painfully cold.

These patients are very complex to treat and require careful assessment allowing the patient to tell the healthcare professional all of the indicators of pain, not just a number on a pain scale. In order to treat these patients, medications for both types of pain may need to be combined to get the best pain relief possible.

The Pain Pathway

The basic route for pain transmission involves the activation of unmyelinated C fibers and myelinated A delta fibers that transmit the pain from the peripheral nervous system to the central nervous system. Myelin acts as an insulating substance that can increase the propagation speed of the nerve impulse and can prevent the impulse from leaving the axon during pain transmission. Unmyelinated C nerve fibers produce pain continuously at a much slower rate (Argoff, 2011).

There are three separate actions in pain transmission along the pain pathway. The neurons serve as a platform for an electrical impulse that can travel along the afferent neuronal pathway, moving the pain stimulus up to the central nervous system for processing.

There are several stages to the transmission of pain:

- *Transduction:* This is the initial stage of pain transmission. As the substances that facilitate pain are produced, for example, bradykinin and TNF, the pain stimulus is created and passed to the neuronal synaptic cleft. As the stimulus progresses, the neurons are depolarized, allowing for the release of chemicals that facilitate the pain stimulus of the afferent nerve. The basis for transduction is the creation of a chemical event that progresses to an electrical event.
- *Transmission:* This occurs when the electrical pain stimulus depolarizes the neurons, while neurotransmitters in the postsynaptic cleft provide information to the presynaptic cleft of the central nervous system neuron. This set of events moves the pain stimulus from the peripheral nervous system to the central nervous system at the dorsal root ganglia.
- *Modulation:* At this stage of the process, neurotransmitters can help increase or decrease the potential for a pain stimulus. As the pain signal proceeds up the afferent pain pathway, it ends in the cerebral cortex, where the stimulus being produced is recognized as pain.

Once the pain signal has been recognized and processed, in the cerebral cortex the descending neuronal pathway, or the efferent pathway, sends the pain signal down from the cerebral cortex, resulting in a response to the pain, such as guarding of the affected area or attempts to move an affected extremity away from the pain.

More simply, the steps in pain transmission include the following:

- A pain stimulus is generated at the peripheral nervous system and moves on the C fibers and A delta fibers up to the dorsal horn of the spinal column.
- The substantia gelatinosa in the dorsal horn can facilitate or inhibit, promote, or stop the progression of the stimulus further up the central nervous system.

- If the stimulus is strong enough or lasts long enough, it is transmitted up through the limbic system to the cerebral cortex.
- Once the stimulus reaches the cerebral cortex, it is identified as pain and a response is generated (ASPMN, 2010).

Today, we know much more about the complexities of how pain is generated, felt, interpreted, and the responses that it creates. We understand it is not as simple as was once thought. Over the years, the finer points of how pain is produced have been studied and refined. We can also look at ways to stop pain transmission by use of medications or techniques such as neural blockade. To a finer point, we can identify where in the cascade of pain transmission a medication can be used to stop or reduce pain.

There are some interesting modifications that the nervous system can undergo in relation to pain:

- Once the pain stimulus enters the nervous system and reaches critical levels of intensity, the T-cell system is activated. This creates a link between the brain and body that connects the subjective and objective experiences of pain.
- If pain sensation increases and continues at higher levels, peripheral sensitization can occur, producing a state of ***neuronal hyperexcitability***. One way this can occur is through a sustained inflammatory response.
- A phenomenon called ***wind-up*** occurs when continued moderate to severe pain causes the N-methyl-D-aspartate (NMDA) receptors to be activated. Once the NMDA receptors are activated, the pain is processed quicker and with more intensity.
- When pain lasts for more than 24 hours, ***neuroplasticity*** can occur in the spinal area of the nervous system. Neuroplasticity accelerates the pain fiber growth and damages the pain inhibition system, with the result being a widespread, more intense pain.
- One result of neuroplasticity is ***peripheral sensitization***. This results in a heightened sensitivity to pain, wherein sensations, such as touch or pressure, become painful (ASPMN, 2010).

The Role of Cytokines, Nerve Growth Factor, and Other Pain Inhibitors and Facilitators

The role of pain facilitation and pain inhibition by chemical substances is an area of growing interest and research. Cytokines are recognized as a group of chemicals that can have proinflammatory or anti-inflammatory action (Zhang & Jianxiong, 2007). They are small secreted proteins released by cells that can have a specific effect on the interactions and communication between cells (Zhang & Jianxiong, 2007).

Cytokines are identified by the cells that produce them or their cellular activity:

- Lymphokine—Produced by lymphocytes
- Monokine—Produced by monocytes
- Chemokine—Cytokines with chemotactic activity
- Interleukin—Cytokines made by leukocytes that act on other leukocytes (Zhang & Jianxiong, 2007)

Cytokines can be produced in one area of the body and move to other distant locations to act. Some of the effects that the cytokines can have are initiation and persistence of pain by activating nociceptive sensory neurons, nerve injury-induced central sensitization, and the development of contralateral hyperalgesia and allodynia (Zhang & Jianxiong, 2007).

There are other pain-facilitating and pain-inhibiting substances acting in the peripheral nervous system that include the following (D'Arcy, 2011):

- Substance P—A neurotransmitter secreted by the free nerve ending of C fibers, whose mechanism is to speed up the nerve transmission
- Bradykinin—Participates in the inflammatory response and hyperalgesia
- Histamine—Released by the mast cells produced in response to tissue trauma
- Serotonin—Can be released by platelets and is produced in response to tissue trauma
- Cyclooxygenase (COX) products (prostaglandin E2 and thromboxane E2)—Act to sensitize and excite fibers, causing hyperexcitability
- Cytokines (interleukin and TNF)—Can sensitize C fiber terminals and participate in the inflammatory and infection process involving mast cells
- Calcitonin gene-related peptide (CGRP)—Located at C fiber nerve endings they produce localized cutaneous vasodilatation, plasma extravasation, and skin sensitization in collaboration with substance P production (ASPMN, 2010)

There is also a group of pain-facilitating and pain-inhibiting substances that can help stop or diminish the body's response to pain with a site of action in the central nervous system:

Pain-facilitating substances are:

- Substance P
- Glutamate—Responsible for the communication between peripheral and central nervous systems and helps to activate the NMDA receptors

- Aspartate
- Cholecystokinin
- CGRP
- Nitric oxide (D'Arcy, 2011)

Pain-inhibiting substances are:

- Dynorphin—An endogenous opioid
- Encephalin
- Norepinephrine
- Serotonin
- Beta-endorphin—An endogenous opioid
- Gamma-aminobutyric acid (GABA) (D'Arcy, 2011)

So, although pain transmission occurs very quickly, within milliseconds, the actual process is very complicated and can be difficult to understand. It does explain why each patient experiences pain in a unique and personal way, depending on the chemical and neuronal status within his or her body.

ACUTE PAIN VERSUS CHRONIC PAIN

Acute pain is something that occurs frequently. It is defined as "a pain that has a short duration and an identifiable cause, such as trauma, injury, or surgery" (APS, 2008, p. 1). Most patients say that they can identify the injury or source of their acute pain and it resolves within a short period of time. The pain resolves over the course of several days and the patient returns to his or her baseline. In many cases, the patient will try to self-treat this type of pain before seeking care for the pain.

The pain pathways for acute and chronic pain are the same, but the transmission process can be altered by neuronal changes and the length of time the pain stimulus occurs. Because patients with chronic pain have extended neuronal pain stimulation, neuroplasticity and wind-up can occur. With acute pain, the pain stimulus lessens over time, so neuronal changes may not occur. Any new pain stimulus for a patient with chronic pain may be intensified since the neuronal system has been altered.

As healthcare providers, it is important to recognize this difference in chronic pain patients. For example, if a patient with chronic pain has surgery, the patient requires more pain medication in the postoperative period since the sensation is heightened and the pain is being transmitted through a neuronal system that has been adversely altered. Recognizing that the patient has hypersensitivity, peripheral sensitization, or wind-up can help provide better pain relief to a patient who already has baseline pain.

SUMMARY

Learning about pain and how it is produced can provide information about the way the patient is experiencing pain and what can be expected. For acute pain, the patient should return to normal functioning without residual pain.

For patients with chronic pain, the pain transmission process has been greatly influenced by substances that facilitate pain and change the way the pain is processed. The extended inflammation that chronic pain causes will make any new pain more painful.

Patients' individual experiences and the differences in pain sensation that they report can make assessment and treatment decisions more difficult for the practitioner who is treating the patient.

TRENDING IN PAIN MANAGEMENT

- Look for new medications and molecules that will act in the nervous system to inhibit pain substances.
- Watch for new medications that will use newly understood pathways, such as the cannabinoid pathway, to relieve pain.
- Look for new molecules that will target specific pain-producing substances, such as TNF, that are longer acting and nonopioid.
- Check for more changes to pain definitions from the IASP.

CASE STUDY

Sarah is a 75-year-old retired music teacher who lives with her husband in their own home. She has diabetes and high blood pressure that are controlled with oral medications. She wears glasses and has hearing aids. She fell recently while getting up to go to the bathroom at night. As a result of her fall, she has broken ribs, a fractured wrist, and a knee injury. She also stubbed her toe quite badly on a bedroom table. When she tells you about her pain, she says, "The pain is better now that I have pain medication but I still have trouble sleeping." She rates her pain at six out of 10 before pain medication. She also tells you she has had numbness in her feet for the past few months that tends to be worse at night. She reports that the pain medication she is using tends to make her feel lightheaded. Six months later, she is still complaining about her toe pain, which seems to have moved up to her ankle. She complains about having difficulty walking and putting pressure on the foot with the toe injury.

(continued)

CASE STUDY (*continued*)

- When you assess the pain that Sarah is experiencing, you realize she has a mixed presentation: nociceptive pain from her ribs, original toe injury, and wrist and neuropathic pain from her feet and toe. Each of these pain types will need to be treated with different types of medications. She can also be categorized as having high-impact chronic pain.
- Because Sarah is an older patient, she should be using reduced doses of any opioid used to treat her pain. Reducing medication dosages may help with her lightheadedness. She may also need to use nonopioids as adjuvant pain relief and lessen the need for any opioids.
- In addition to the neuropathic pain in her feet, Sarah has developed a difficult-to-treat neuropathic condition called *CRPS*. This difficult-to-treat condition will never resolve. It occurs as a result of a crush injury to the toe. The pain is intense and will need medication management with a neuropathic pain medication and a consult to an interventional pain practice for consideration of an injection of implanted spinal cord stimulator.
- Sarah was not wearing her glasses when she fell. She also did not turn on the light in the bathroom. An evaluation by physical therapy for assistive devices to ensure that both she and her living area are safe would be helpful.

REFERENCES

American Pain Society. (2008). *Principles of analgesic use in the treatment of acute pain and cancer pain*. Glenview, IL: Author.

American Society of Pain Management Nurses. (2010). *Core curriculum for pain management nursing*. Dubuque, IA: Kendall Hunt Publications.

Andrews, N. (2018). What's in a name for chronic pain? *Pain Research Forum*. Retrieved from https://www.painresearchforum.org/news/92059

Argoff, C. (2011). Mechanisms of pain transmission and pharmacologic management. *Current Medical Research and Opinion*, *27*(10), 2019–2031. doi:10.1185/03007995.2011.614934

Aydede, M., & Shriver, A. (2018). Recently introduced definition of "nociplastic pain" by the International Association for the Study of Pain needs better formulation. *Pain*, 159(6), 1176–1177. doi:10.1097/j.pain.0000000000001184

Benarroch, E. E. (2007). Sodium channels and pain. *Neurology*, *68*(3), 233–236. doi:10.1212/01.wnl.0000252951.48745.a1

Centers for Disease Control and Prevention. (2018). *Guidelines for prescribing opioids for chronic pain.* Retrieved from https://www.cdc.gov

D'Arcy, Y. (2011). *A compact clinical guide to chronic pain management.* New York, NY: Springer Publishing Company.

IASP Pain Task Force. (2019). *IASP's Proposed new definition of pain released for comment from IASP.* Retrieved from https://www.iasp-pain.org/PublicationsNews/NewsDetail.aspx?ItemNumber=9218

Johnson, M. (2019). The landscape of chronic pain: Broader perspectives. *Medicina, 55*(5), 182. doi:10.3390/medicina55050182

National Institutes of Health. (2018). *Defining the prevalence of chronic pain in the United States.* Retrieved from https://www.nccih.nih.gov/research/research-results/defining-the-prevalence-of-chronic-pain-in-the-united-states

Stanos, S., Brodsky, M., Argoff, C., Clauw, D., D'Arcy, Y., Donevan, S., . . . Watt, S. (2016). Rethinking chronic pain in a primary care setting. *Postgraduate Medicine*, 128(5), 502–515. doi:10.1080/00325481.2016.1188319

World Health Organization. (2018). *International Classification of Diseases, 11th edition.* Retrieved from who.int/classification/icd/en

Zhang, J. M., & Jianxiong, A. (2007). Cytokines, inflammation, and pain. *International Anesthesiology Clinics, 45*(2), 27–37. doi:10.1097/aia.0b013e318034194e

ADDITIONAL RESOURCES

Dahlhamer, J., Lucas, J., Zelaya, C., Nahin, R., Mackey, S., DeBar, L., . . . Helmick, C. (2018). Prevalence of chronic pain and high impact chronic pain among adults—United States, 2016. *Morbidity and Mortality Weekly Report, 67*(36), 1001–1006. doi:10.15585/mmwr.mm6736a2

McCarberg, B., D'Arcy, Y., Parsons, B., Sadosky, A., Thorpe, A., & Behar, R. (2017). Neuropathic pain: A review of etiology, assessment, diagnosis, and treatment for primary care providers. *Current Medical Research and Opinion, 33*(8), 1361–1369. doi:10.1080/03007995.2017.1321532

Yam, M. F., Loh, Y. C., Chu, S. T., Siti, K. A., Nizar, A. M., & Ruliza, B. (2018). General pain pathways of pain sensation and the major neurotransmitters involved in pain regulation. *International Journal of Molecular Science*, 19(8), 2164. doi:10.3390/ijms19082164

CHAPTER 3

PAIN ASSESSMENT: A MULTIDIMENSIONAL APPROACH

INTRODUCTION

Pain assessment is often considered the most difficult part of a clinical pain evaluation. The problem is that the assessment is subjective and some practitioners have difficulty believing the patient's report of pain. The International Association for the Study of Pain (Treede, 2018) states that the patient's report of pain should be believed and valued. However, for primary care practitioners who have extremely busy schedules, the need to make a quick judgment about the patient's pain report and then decide on a treatment may be all that can be done during a visit. Taking the time to go beyond the numeric pain rating and researching the subjective factors that influence the patient's report of pain may be more than can be accomplished in a single visit.

For many years, researchers have been studying the differences between the patients' report of pain and the healthcare providers' assessment of patient pain. In a review of 80 studies that addressed differences in pain assessment, Seers, Derry, Seers, and Moore (2018) found that 61 studies reported underestimation of pain by healthcare professionals compared to patient report. In only one study was overestimation by healthcare professionals reported. The underestimation was more pronounced when pain levels were reported to be severe (Seers et al., 2018).

In a survey of 400 nurse practitioners from various practice areas, there were clear indications that pain assessment presented a continuing problem (D'Arcy, 2009). The respondents did not feel that their basic nurse practitioner (NP) education prepared them to treat patients with chronic pain. Of the respondents, 62% felt they had adequate preparation to assess patients with chronic pain, whereas 38% indicated they did not feel prepared. When the survey respondents were asked whether they felt prepared to treat patients with chronic pain, 44% said they felt prepared, but 56% felt they were not prepared to treat these patients (D'Arcy, 2009). In contrast, 86% of the survey respondents felt they were adequately prepared to assess acute pain. These results may be a response to the need for a more complex assessment for chronic pain than for a simpler assessment of acute pain.

CLINICAL PEARL

Believe the patient's report of pain. Studies have shown that healthcare providers cannot determine pain levels and distrust leads to poor pain management.

Overall, accurate pain assessment continues to be a problem for all healthcare providers. Some practitioners feel unprepared to assess and treat patients with pain and there is strong evidence that healthcare providers tend to underestimate pain in patients.

This chapter offers information on simple one-dimensional pain tools, multidimensional tools more suited for chronic pain, and a new tool developed specifically for primary care providers that is efficient and offers solid information. There is also information on a tool that can be used for patients who are nonverbal or who have Alzheimer's dementia. Some of the tools are easily adapted into electronic medical record systems, which can speed up the assessment process and retain assessments for reference at future appointments.

THE ART OF PAIN ASSESSMENT

Pain is most often reported on an objective scale, such as the 0-to-10 pain intensity scale. This may suffice for acute pain, but for patients with chronic pain, the 0-to-10 scale does not capture what the pain means to the patient. To do a better job of capturing the pain report for a patient with chronic pain, a more comprehensive pain assessment tool, such as the Brief Pain Inventory (BPI), may be necessary.

Assessing a patient for pain is more than just determining a number on a 0-to-10 pain intensity scale. Especially for chronic pain patients, pain is a complex multidimensional condition that requires a more in-depth assessment process. The 0-to-10 scale is best used to determine how much improvement in pain results from a dose of pain medication. A 2-point improvement in the pain score indicates a clinically significant improvement (Farrar, 2001). Using a single-function scale to assess chronic pain will not give the healthcare provider a good picture of what the patient is trying to convey about his or her pain. Using an objective scale to convey a subjective experience will not provide a usable measure of pain for these patients.

The best indicators for acute pain are single-item pain intensity scales, such as the Numeric Pain Rating Scale, which is a numeric pain intensity (NPI) scale, or the Visual Analog Scale (VAS). Even for acute pain, there are aspects of pain assessment that make it important to get a complete picture of the pain. Functionality is key. Determining what the patient could do before experiencing pain, but now cannot do because of the pain, will let you know just how much the pain is impacting the patient's life.

Pain assessment has always been problematic because it relies on patient's self-report of pain. Every person, patient, and provider comes to healthcare with a personal bias. Each of us is a product of our home life, parents, friends, and life experiences. We have a personal sense of what is true or false, right or wrong. This is often called a *gut feeling*. If we come from a background of distrust, we may tend to treat our patients the same way. It is important that healthcare providers trust the patient's report of pain and build a relationship in which the patient can share how the pain is really affecting him or her personally. This is called the *art of pain assessment*.

THE SCIENCE OF PAIN ASSESSMENT

The science of pain assessment centers around the use of valid and reliable measures of pain that can provide a more complete picture of the patient's pain. Using a valid tool will give a reliable measure of pain intensity, the level of interference pain causes with daily activities, and the patient's mood. Because depression is commonly comorbid with pain, a part of the pain assessment should include a depression screening so the healthcare provider can determine whether depression is present and offer to treat it or refer for treatment.

The PEG Scale (pain, enjoyment, general activity) is a new tool developed specifically for use in primary care. It is a three-item pain assessment measure that offers more information than a simple 0-to-10 pain intensity rating. This tool can provide a rating not only of pain intensity, but also indicates pain's interference with enjoyment of life and general activity. It is a simple, easy-to-score tool that is not time-consuming and can be easily converted to an electronic medical record format.

The Process of Assessing Pain

For primary care providers, the pain assessment process may not be something that can be completed in the first visit, especially if the patient has chronic pain. It may require several months of repeat visits to fully determine what kind of pain the patient is having and which treatment works best. Seeing the patient over time also allows the provider to determine just how engaged the patient is in the treatment process as well as the patient's level of compliance with the selected therapies.

When a patient provides a numerical value for pain intensity, such as eight out of 10, this number is an individual perception of the patient's pain. One patient with a pain score of 8 out of 10 may be bedbound, whereas another patient may not be as affected by the pain, having only moderate functional impairment. It is important to determine just what the patients can do at the level of the pain rating.

CLINICAL PEARL

Functionality is a better measure of assessing pain than NPI ratings. Asking the patient what he or she cannot do now because of the pain also gives the healthcare provider an idea of what goals the patient is interested in achieving; for example, increased ability for self-care, able to shop independently, or to perform a particular activity such as attending church.

After determining the numeric rating, a series of standard questions can be used to better pinpoint the pain. Ask the patient about the ***location*** of the pain and any areas that the pain moves or radiates to at any time during the day or night. Some practices use a body diagram that the patient can mark to locate the pain. Because there may be several locations for the pain, it can be helpful to ask the patient to indicate where pain is the worst and where it is less intense.

The next question to ask the patient is what is the ***duration*** of the pain? When did the pain first begin and how long have you had it? You can also ask the patient whether the pain intensity varies during the day and how long these differences last.

Pain intensity questions can provide additional information about the pain. The patient will have already answered the pain question about current pain intensity. If the patient has difficulty using the NPI scale, you can ask the patient to describe the pain as mild, moderate, or severe. The patient should also indicate any time during the day that the pain intensity lessens or increases. If the patient is taking pain medication, ask the patient how long after taking the medication the pain returns. The patient may be experiencing breakthrough pain or end-of-dose failure, and the addition of another type of medication or therapy may extend the pain relief.

Asking the patient to describe the ***quality of the pain*** may give the healthcare provider important information about the type of pain the patient is experiencing. If the patient tells you the pain feels sore, dull, aching, throbbing, or gnawing, the pain is most likely nociceptive pain and it will respond to standard pain medications such as nonsteroidal anti-inflammatory medications. If the patient says the pain feels cold, tingling, burning, painful itching, electric, or shooting, the pain is most likely neuropathic and will require a neuropathic pain medication.

CLINICAL PEARL

Listening carefully to the patient talk about his or her pain can provide some of the best assessment information available. For example, a patient who says his or her pain feels like a blow torch going back and forth across his or her chest is describing a neuropathic pain. Or a patient who says his or her wrist feels like cold ice picks are being inserted into it is also experiencing a neuropathic pain condition, even though the descriptors are very different.

Ask the patient what makes the pain better or what makes it worse. Asking about **alleviating or aggravating factors** can help determine what the patient has already found useful to decrease the pain and what types of activities increase the pain. Most patients have some form of home remedy that they use to treat minor pain. Ask what types of things the patient has already tried and how long the patient used the medication or therapy. If position changes make the pain better, ask how long the pain is better after a position change.

One of the most important aspects of pain assessment is **setting a pain goal** with the patient. Some patients want their pain to be 0 out of 10. For acute pain patients with pain that will resolve, this may be a reasonable goal. For chronic pain patients who have been in pain for 6 months, a 0 out of 10 pain is not a reasonable expectation.

Asking the patient what his or her best and worst pain ratings are during the day can give the healthcare practitioner an idea of the range of the pain. Setting a pain goal that is achievable within those parameters may give the patient comfort in knowing there is something concrete to work toward. Above all, the goal should be achievable and reflect what the patient feels is important.

The pain goal may not be best represented by a number, but may be an activity that the patient has not been able to do but would like to do again. This type of pain goal is centered in increasing **functionality.** Some patients would like to be able to walk around the block; others may want to go to church or shop for groceries independently. Whatever the function goal is, the patient should track his or her ability to perform the activity and whether he or she is better able to do it. Using a diary or patient log in which the patient tracks the distance walked, for example, can indicate how well the pain treatments are working. Using a Fitbit or digital distance tracker is also an acceptable way to help track activity. Overall, the function goal has to be something the patient truly wants and cannot be something that only the practitioner feels is best.

Engaging the patient in the pain assessment process provides the best success. If the patient feels heard and their goals are validated, the practitioner and the patient can form a partnership to work toward maximum pain relief and function for the patient.

Pain-Focused Physical Assessment

After the patient has answered the basic assessment questions, doing a pain-focused physical exam is crucial. Looking distal and proximal to the painful area and asking about referred pain is a start. If the patient is having joint pain, the joint should be put through a full range of motion to see what actions cause the pain. For low-back pain patients, the area of pain should be palpated thoroughly to determine whether there is muscle tightness, spasms, or deformity. Observing the patient while he or she walks to the examination room can provide information about physical status. Noting any limping, guarding, or balance issues can help add to the physical assessment.

A sensory exam is particularly important for patients who may have neuropathic pain. Using a cotton swab, cotton ball, or a pinprick can determine whether there is any loss of sensation or highly sensitive areas. Look for any sign of the following:

- ***Allodynia***—Pain from a sensation that is not normally painful, for example, a handshake or hug
- ***Dysesthesias***—Strange, but clearly uncomfortable sensations, for example, painful itching
- ***Hyperalgesia***—An exaggerated pain response to a sensation that is normally only mildly painful, for example, severe pain from an intravenous needle insertion (McCarberg, D'Arcy, Parsons, Sadosky, & Behar, 2016)

After the assessment questions are answered and the physical exam and inspection are completed, it is very important that all the information be documented. Healthcare practitioners can use the information from the first pain assessment as a guide for developing a plan of care and tracking future outcomes.

PAIN TOOLS

Pain tools come in a variety of formats. Some are designed to be completed by the patient and others are designed to be completed by the healthcare provider. There are tools that work for assessing acute pain, such as a 0-to-10 NPI scale, and others that are more complex and designed to assess chronic pain, such as the Brief Pain Inventory (BPI). These tools include not only the pain intensity rating, but also have questions about satisfaction with pain medications, mood, and ability to participate in physical activity.

Most of the current pain tools have been studied in various populations and tested for reliability and validity. Using a reliable and valid pain assessment tool provides the healthcare practitioner with a way to track pain levels over time and to look at outcomes. A reliable and valid tool ensures that the measurement of pain is done with the highest level of accuracy.

One-Dimensional Pain Assessment Tools

One-dimensional pain tools are designed to measure one aspect of the patient's pain, pain intensity (Breivik et al., 2008). Although the one-dimensional tools are simple to use, they can provide information that is useful for pain assessment. Ackley, Ladwig, Swan, and Tucker (2008) reviewed 164 journal articles on pain assessment and found that single-item pain ratings of pain intensity were reported as valid and reliable indicators of pain intensity. Farrar, Young, Lamoreaux, Werth, and Poole (2001) established that a 2-point or 30% reduction on the numeric pain rating scale was a clinically significant decrease in pain.

The VAS is a very simple scale (Figure 3.1). It consists of a 100-mm line with "no pain" at one end and "pain as bad as it could possibly be" at the other. It was designed originally for research, but can be used clinically as well. To use the VAS, the patient marks a point on the line to indicate pain intensity.

The simplicity of the tool is a plus, but there are some drawbacks as well. Some older patients have difficulty understanding how to mark the pain on the line and there is no real method for comparing pain intensity over time.

For patients who have difficulty using a number to describe their pain, the Verbal Descriptor Scale (VDS) offers a broad option to determine pain severity (Figure 3.2). To use this pain scale, the patient is asked to select the word that best represents the severity of the pain. Asking the patient to point to the word that best describes the pain is also an alternative.

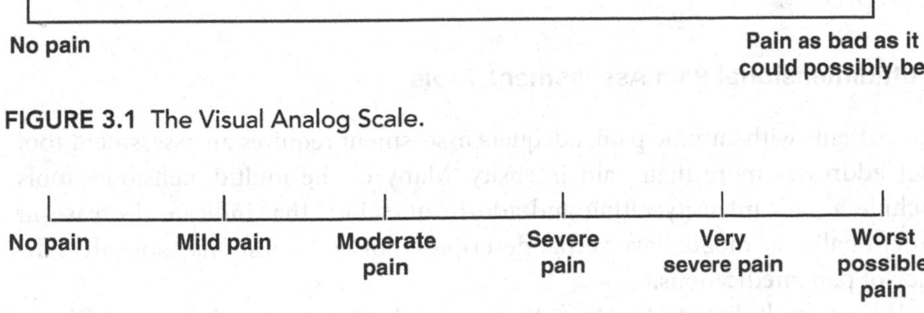

FIGURE 3.1 The Visual Analog Scale.

FIGURE 3.2 The Verbal Descriptor Scale.

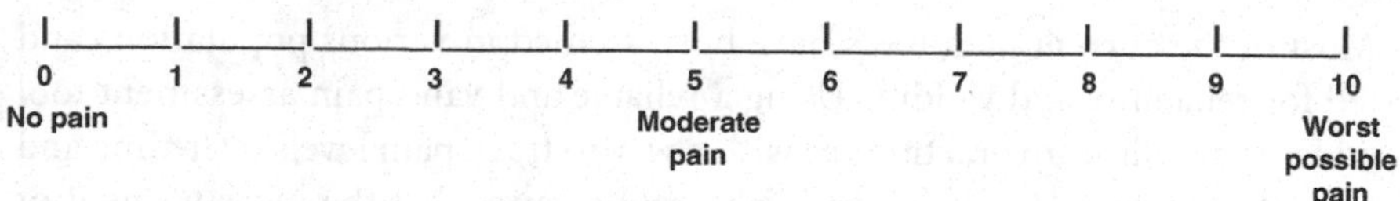

FIGURE 3.3 The Numeric Pain Rating Scale.

As with any scale, there are pluses and minuses. This is a very simple scale and it is easy to use. However, it does not allow for tracking pain over time as descriptors limit comparison.

The NPRS is the most commonly used pain scale today (Figure 3.3). It is best used for acute pain to determine whether a dose of pain medication decreases the pain. The scale itself is an 11-point Likert scale in which 0 represents no pain and 10 represents the worse possible pain. Higher numbers represent more intense pain, whereas lower numbers represent milder pain with lower intensity.

Numeric pain ratings can be categorized as mild, moderate, or severe.

- Mild pain is considered to be in the 1 to 3 range.
- Moderate pain is considered to be in the 4 to 6 range.
- Severe pain is considered to be pain in the 7 to 10 range.

For acute pain, the NPRS can be used effectively. However, to assess chronic pain, the NPRS is used as part of the assessment, but it does not represent the full experience of the pain. Chronic pain is complex. For chronic pain, a multidimensional pain tool, such as the BPI, can provide additional information on mood, pain medications, and activities.

When using tools that are simple and require a word or a number as the response, patients should be told that there is no right or wrong answer. Allowing the patient to choose the number or word representing his or her pain freely is crucial to getting a representative pain rating. It is then up to the healthcare provider to believe the patient's report of pain and act on it appropriately.

Multidimensional Pain Assessment Tools

For patients with chronic pain, adequate assessment requires an assessment tool that addresses more than pain intensity. Many of the multidimensional tools include a pain intensity rating and add-in questions that indicate decrease in functionality or mood, have verbal descriptors, or add questions about the efficacy of pain medications.

The two multidimensional tools that are used most commonly are the BPI and the McGill Pain Questionnaire (MPQ).

Although these pain assessment tools give a wider picture of the patient's pain, they are longer than the one-dimensional tools, and so can be difficult to use in clinical practices. These tools are most often found in specialty pain practices, but have not been widely adapted in primary care practices (Krebs et al., 2009).

Brief Pain Inventory

The BPI is one of the most widely used and best researched multidimensional tools for assessing pain (available at www.mdanderson.org/BPI). It was originally developed to treat long-term pain in cancer patients. It has been validated for use in patients with chronic pain and has been tested in many different countries (Daut, Cleeland, & Flannery, 1983). In all cases, it has been found to be valid and representative of chronic pain across many nationalities and has been translated into a number of languages (Cleeland & Ryan, 1994; Cleeland et al., 1996).

One of the drawbacks of using the BPI is that the patients need to be able to understand the questions and provide information to the clinician.

McGill Pain Questionnaire

The McGill Pain Questionnaire (MPQ) was designed for patients who require a multidimensional assessment of pain (available at www.sralab.org/rehabilitation-measures/mcgill-pain-questionnaire). In addition to chronic pain, it has been tested in a wide variety of conditions, including:

- Experimentally induced pain
- Postprocedural pain
- A number of medical surgical conditions

The tool has been used in a variety of conditions and many different countries. It has been translated into several different languages (McDonald & Weiskopf, 2001; Melzack, 1975, 1987). The only drawback to this tool is its use of a list of verbal descriptors. This makes the tool difficult to score and track.

The PEG Tool

The PEG tool (Exhibit 3.1) is designed to provide a multidimensional pain assessment for primary care patients; it provides some of the same information as the BPI. The questions on activity and enjoyment are based on the BPI and provide some of the same information. The Centers for Disease Control and Prevention (CDC) recommends this tool for use in primary care patients. The tool is designed as a three-item assessment that can be converted into an electronic medical record for tracking over time.

EXHIBIT 3.1

THE PEG TOOL

1. What number best describes you *pain on average* in the past week:

0	1	2	3	4	5	6	7	8	9	10
No pain										Pain as bad as you can imagine

2. What number best describes how, during the past week, pain has interfered with your *enjoyment of life?*

0	1	2	3	4	5	6	7	8	9	10
Does not interfere										Completely interferes

3. What number best describes how, during the past week, pain has interfered with your *general activity?*

0	1	2	3	4	5	6	7	8	9	10
Does not interfere										Completely interferes

Interview version:

1. What number best describes your pain on *average* in the past week, on a scale from 0 to 10, where 0 is "no pain" and 10 is "pain as bad as you can imagine"? (0–10)

   The following two questions ask you to describe how, during the past week, pain has interfered with your life on a "0 to 10" scale, where 0 is "does not interfere at all" and 10 is "completely interferes."

2. What number best describes how, during the past week, pain has interfered with your *enjoyment of life*? (0–10)

3. What number best describes how, during the past week, pain has interfered with your *general activity*? (0–10)

Scoring: The PEG score is the average of the three individual item scores. For clinical use, round to the nearest whole number.

PEG, Pain, Enjoyment, General activity.

Source: Reproduced with permission from Krebs, E., Lorenz, K., Bair, M., Damush, T., Jingwei, W., Sutherland, J., . . . Kroenke, K. (2009). Development and initial validation of the PEG, a three item scale assessing pain intensity and interference. *Journal of General Internal Medicine, 24*(6), 733–738. doi:10.1007/s11606-009-0981-1

In a validation study, the PEG was found to have good reliability, validity, and responsiveness when used in primary care and ambulatory care clinics (Krebs et al., 2009). The PEG was also found to be sensitive to change and was able to differentiate between patients with and without pain improvement at 6 months.

The tool was tested in ambulatory clinics in the Veterans Affairs (VA) system with patients who had chronic pain using a second group of patients who did not have chronic pain as a comparison group.

The PEG is one of the newest pain assessment tools. Its validation study looks very good for the populations that were tested, but more research is needed to give it wider applicability. Two important points:

- It provides information similar to that from the BPI in a shortened, easy-to-use format.
- It was tested on patients with lower back and musculoskeletal pain who are commonly seen in primary care.

Pain Assessment Tools for Specialty Populations

There are groups of patients who have special needs for pain assessment. The young and the elderly are particularly vulnerable patient populations. Nonverbal and demented patients also have special needs for pain assessment since they cannot tell you about their pain.

Pain Assessment in Advanced Dementia Scale

The Pain Assessment in Advanced Dementia (PAINAD) Scale is a pain assessment tool (Table 3.1) developed for use in patients who have Alzheimer's dementia. Because these patients cannot report their pain, it is important to identify the behaviors that indicate pain. Six prime pain behaviors were identified using the Checklist of Nonverbal Pain Indicators (CNPI), developed by Feldt (2000). The behaviors that were felt to best indicate pain in nonverbal patients included:

- Vocalizations
- Facial grimacing
- Bracing
- Rubbing
- Restlessness
- Vocal complaints (Feldt, 2000; Feldt, Ryden, & Miles, 1998)

TABLE 3.1 The PAINAD Scale

	0	1	2
Breathing	Normal	Occasional labored breathing Short period of hyperventilation	Noisy labored breathing Long period of hyperventilation Cheyne–Stokes respiration
Negative vocalization	None	Occasional moan/groan Low-level speech/negative or disapproving quality	Repeated troubled calling out Loud moaning or groaning Crying
Facial expression	Smiling/sad	Frightened; frown	Facial grimacing inexpressive
Body language	Relaxed	Tense; distressed pacing, fidgeting	Rigid, fists clenched, knees pulled up Pulling or pushing away Striking out
Consolability	No need to console	Distracted or reassured by voice or touch	Unable to console, distract, or reassure

Total score __________

Note: Developed at the New England Geriatric Research Education and Clinical Center, EN Rogers Memorial Veterans Hospital, Bedford, MA.

PAINAD, Pain Assessment in Advanced Dementia.

Source: From Warden, V., Hurley, A. C., & Volicer, L. (2003). Development and psychometric evaluation of the Pain Assessment in Advanced Dementia (PAINAD) Scale. *Journal of the American Medical Directors Association, 4*, 9–15.

When you attempt to assess pain in a nonverbal patient, key concepts to consider are:

- Attempt a self-report.
- Search for the potential cause of pain.
- Observe patient behaviors.
- Use surrogate reporting by family or caregivers indicating pain or behaviors/activity changes.
- Attempt an analgesic trial (Herr et al., 2006).

The PAINAD tool uses five different pain behaviors that are rated as either 0, 1, or 2. The zero rating is given for no behaviors noted, and 2 is rated for apparent behaviors. The behaviors that are included in the PAINAD are breathing, negative vocalization, facial expression, body language, and consolability. The behaviors are ranked by severity using the 0-to-2 scale and a score can be obtained. The higher the score, the more pain the patient is having. The difficulty with the PAINAD scale is that it relies on observer ratings that may not be interpreting the patient's behaviors correctly. As stated previously, if pain behaviors are noted, an analgesic trial is indicated.

FACES

The Wong–Baker FACES® Pain Rating Scale (Figure 3.4) was originally developed to assess pain in children too young to use an NPI tool. The original tool has six faces that range from happy and smiling to a sad-looking face with tears. To use the tool, the patient is asked to point to the face that best represents how the pain makes them feel. The Wong–Baker FACES scale has been found to be reliable and valid (Wong & Devito-Thomas, 2006). The scale has also been used in non-Caucasian children and cognitively impaired adults (Wong & DeVito Thomas, 2006). It has also been adapted for use in older adults.

> **CLINICAL PEARL**
>
> When using the Wong–Baker FACES tool, the patient should be asked to pick the face that best describes how the pain makes the patient feel. The patient should not pick a face to depict how he or she looks.

Tools to Measure Functionality

One of the newest areas being developed for assessing pain is the functionality tools. The tool that seems to have the best support is the Clinically Aligned Pain Assessment Tool (CAPA). The originators of the tool feel that it should be able to

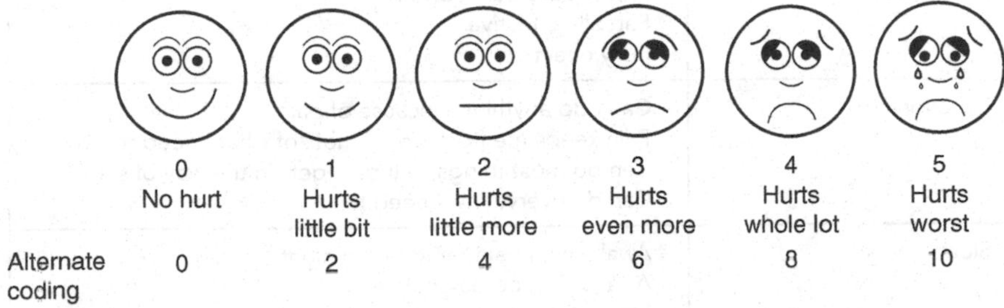

FIGURE 3.4 Wong–Baker FACES Pain Rating Scale.

Source: From Wong, D. L., Hockenberry-Eaton, M., Wilson, D., Winkelstein, M. L., & Schwartz, P. (2001). *Wong's essentials of pediatric nursing* (6th ed.). St. Louis, MO: Mosby Elsevier.

replace the 0 to 10 pain intensity scale. Although the research on the tool is not scant, it does offer some hope that pain assessment can move away from pain intensity toward a functional approach.

Clinically Aligned Pain Assessment Tool

The Clinically Aligned Pain Assessment Tool (CAPA) tool has five elements (Table 3.2):

- Comfort
- Change in pain
- Pain control
- Functioning
- Sleep

Research-wise, the CAPA is a very new tool with minimal research support. Outcomes are difficult to ascertain. However, in a quality-improvement project at the University of Minnesota Medical Center, the use of the CAPA tool was found to improve patient satisfaction scores regarding the item "staff did everything to

TABLE 3.2 The CAPA Tool

QUESTION	RESPONSE
Comfort	Intolerable Tolerable with discomfort Comfortably manageable Negligible pain
Change in pain	Getting worse About the same Getting better
Pain control	Inadequate pain control Partially effective Fully effective
Functioning	Can't do anything because of pain Pain keeps me from doing most of what I need to do Can do most things, but pain gets in the way of some Can do everything I need to
Sleep	Awake with pain most of the night Awake with occasional pain Normal sleep

CAPA, Clinically Aligned Pain Assessment Tool.

Source: From Twining, J., & Padula, C. (2019). Pilot testing the clinically aligned pain assessment (CAPA) measure. *Pain Management Nursing, 20*(5), 462–467. doi:10.1016/j.pmn.2019.02.005

manage pain showing the biggest improvement" (Topham & Drew, 2017). The CAPA tool also meets the regulatory requirement for pain assessment (Topham & Drew, 2017).

SUMMARY

Pain assessment is really a social interaction and a commitment to the process of determining the severity of the patient's pain. Key to the success of the process is the fact that the person to whom the patient entrusts this information believes and values the patient's report of pain. Functional interference caused by pain is also very important and is being included more and more in the assessment process.

There are a wide variety of pain assessment tools available and each has positives and negatives. Choosing a tool that fits the needs of the patient can help hone the process and provide accurate information.

Pain assessment tools are not as refined as they will be in the future. Considering the tools offered in this chapter can provide some direction to help improve clinical pain assessment.

TRENDING IN PAIN MANAGEMENT

- Look for the development of more tools that address the impact on functionality with pain and improvements in the CAPA tool.
- Look for more simple tools like the PEG that provide more than just a simple pain-intensity rating.

CASE STUDY

John is a 55-year-old insurance salesman who hurt his back while pulling his boat out of the lake one Saturday afternoon. He was seen originally in the emergency department for the pain, but was sent back to his primary care provider that Monday for follow-up. At baseline he was deconditioned since his job was is mainly in an office and he does not exercise regularly. He was given nonopioid pain medications and sent to physical therapy, which he could not participate in due to increased pain. A trial of opioid medications did little to relieve the pain, so he was sent to an orthopedist, who recommended surgery. After surgery, John continued to have pain and was not able to return to work full time. His orthopedist does not want to continue prescribing opioids, so he has sent John back to his primary care provider for follow-up.

(*continued*)

CASE STUDY (*continued*)

When you see John, he rates his pain at 8 out of 10. On further assessment with the PEG tool, he says he sleeps very little, has poor pain relief from his pain medications, his function is very impaired, and he has little enjoyment of life. His score is 22 out of 30 on the PEG tool, 22 divided by 3 = 7.3, indicating a severe level impairment from pain. When you listen to John talk about his pain, he relates that the surgical pain is really not as much of an issue as the burning pain that runs down his leg to his foot, which worsens at night.

- After a more complete assessment of John's pain, it becomes apparent that John has neuropathic pain that does not respond to the opioids. After educating John about his pain, gabapentin is started, and John is told the doses will need to be titrated up over time.
- Relaxation and meditation can be helpful to John to help reduce stress and anxiety. John wants to return to work full time, so he is anxious about his continuing pain.
- John will need to set a pain goal that is achievable, He will never be totally pain free, but he can reduce his pain using a variety of pain techniques such as yoga for flexibility, pool therapy, or walking.
- The primary care provider can benefit John the most by reassuring him that he will continue to have support for his recovery and that treatments can be changed as needed to further his needs.

REFERENCES

Ackley, B., Ladwig, G., Swan, B., & Tucker, S. (2008). *Evidence-based nursing care guidelines*. St. Louis, MO: Mosby Elsevier.

Breivik, H., Borchgrevvink, P., Allen, S., Rosseland, L., Romundstad, E., Kvarstein, G., & Stubhaug, A. (2008). Assessment of pain. *British Journal of Anaesthesia, 101*(1), 17–24. doi:10.1093/bja/aen103

Cleeland, C., Nakamura, Y., Mendosa, T., Edwards, K., Douglas, J., & Serlin, R. (1996). Dimensions of the impact of cancer pain in a four country sample: New information from multidimensional scaling. *Pain, 67*, 267–273. doi:10.1016/0304-3959(96)03131-4

Cleeland, C., & Ryan, K. (1994). Pain assessment: Global use of the Brief Pain Inventory. *Annals Academy of Medicine Singapore, 23*, 129–138.

D'Arcy, Y. (2009). Be in the know about pain management. *Nurse Practitioner, 34*(4), 43–47. doi:10.1097/01.NPR.0000348322.40151.2f

Daut, R., Cleeland, C., & Flannery, R. (1983). Development of the Wisconsin Breif Pain Questionnaire to assess pain in cancer or other diseases. *Pain, 17*, 197–210. doi:10.1016/0304-3959(83)90143-4

Farrar, J., Young, J., Lamoreaux, L., Werth, J., & Poole, R. (2001). Clinical importance of changes in chronic pain intensity measured on an 11 point numerical pain rating scale. *Pain, 94*, 149–158. doi:10.1016/S0304-3959(01)00349-9

Feldt, K., Ryden, M., & Miles, S. (1998). Treatment of pain in cognitively impaired compared with cognitively intact older patients with hip fractures. *Journal of the American Geriatrics Society, 46*, 1079–1085. doi:10.1111/j.1532-5415.1998.tb06644.x

Feldt, K. (2000). The Checklist of Non-verbal Pain Indicators (CNPI). *Pain Management Nursing, 1*(1), 13–21. doi:10.1053/jpmn.2000.5031

Herr, K., Coyne, P., Key, T., Manworren, R., McCaffery, M., Merkel, S., . . . American Society for Pain Management Nursing. (2006). Pain assessment in the non verbal patient: Position statement with clinical practice recommendations. *Pain Management Nursing, 7*(2), 44–52. doi:10.1016/j.pmn.2006.02.003

Krebs, E., Lorenz, K., Bair, M., Damush, T., Jingwei, W., Sutherland, J., . . . Kroenke, K. (2009). Development and initial validation of the PEG, a three item scale assessing pain intensity and interference. *Journal of General Internal Medicine, 24*(6), 733–738. doi:10.1007/s11606-009-0981-1

McCarberg, B., D'Arcy, Y., Parsons, B., Sadosky, A., & Behar, R. (2016). Neuropathic pain: A review of etiology, assessment, diagnosis, and treatment

McDonald, D., & Weiskopf, C. (2001). Adult patients' postoperative pain descriptions and responses to the Short Form McGill Pain Questionnaire. *Clinical Nursing Research, 10*(4), 442–452. doi:10.1177/C10N4R8

Melzack, R. (1975). The McGill pain questionnaire: major properties and scoring methods. *Pain, 1*, 277–299. doi:10.1016/0304-3959(75)90044-5

Melzack, R. (1987). The short form McGill pain questionnaire. *Pain*, 30, 191–197. doi:10.1016/0304-3959(87)91074-8

Seers, T., Derry, S., Seers, K., & Moore, A. (2018). Professionals underestimate patients' pain: A comprehensive review. *Pain, 159*(5), 811–818. doi:10.1097/j.pain.0000000000001165

Topham, D., & Drew, D. (2017). Quality improvement project: Replacing the Numeric Rating Scale with a Clinically Aligned Pain Assessment (CAPA) tool. *Pain Management Nursing, 18*(6), 363–371.

Treede, R.-D. (2018). The International Association for the Study of Pain definition of pain: As valid in 2018 as in 1979, but in need of regularly updated footnotes. *Pain Reports, 3*(2), e643. doi:10.1097/PR9.0000000000000643

Twining, J., & Padula, C. (2019). Pilot testing the clinically aligned pain assessment (CAPA) measure. *Pain Management Nursing, 20*(5), 462–467. doi:10.1016/j.pmn.2019.02.005

Warden, V., Hurley, A. C., & Volicer, L. (2003). Development and psychometric evaluation of the Pain Assessment in Advanced Dementia (PAINAD) Scale. *Journal of the American Medical Directors Association, 4*, 9–15. doi:10.1097/01.JAM.0000043422.31640.F7

Wong, D., & DeVito-Thomas. (2006). *The validity, reliability, and preference of the Wong–Baker FACES pain rating scale among Chinese, Japanese, and Thai children*. Retrieved from http://www.mosbysdrugconsult.com/WOW//op08o.html

Wong, D. L., Hockenberry-Eaton, M., Wilson, D., Winkelstein, M. L., & Schwartz, P. (2001). *Wong's essentials of pediatric nursing* (6th ed.). St. Louis, MO: Mosby Elsevier.

ADDITIONAL RESOURCES

D'Arcy, Y. (2011). *A compact clinical guide to chronic pain management*. New York: NY: Springer Publishing Company.

Stanos, S., Brodsky, M., Argoff, C., Clauw, D., D'Arcy, Y., Donevan, S., . . . McCarberg, B. (2016). Rethinking chronic pain in a primary care setting. *Postgraduate Medicine, 128*, 502–515. doi: 10.1080/00325481.2016.1188319

CHAPTER 4

MOTIVATIONAL INTERVIEWING AND OTHER TOOLS FOR EFFECTIVE COMMUNICATION IN PAIN MANAGEMENT

INTRODUCTION

Improving communication positively impacts most clinical interactions. This is especially true when people are in pain. This chapter provides tools to help the patient with pain, the clinician, and everyone in the clinic interact better. Pain can induce fear, anxiety, frustration, distraction, or inaccurate perception of information. Having multiple communication tools available to quickly and effectively identify issues/barriers/ strengths/weaknesses and sort through red flags is especially helpful as more and more patients receive pain management in primary care.

In this chapter, motivational interviewing (MI), the Transtheoretical Model of Behavior Change (TTM), and mindfulness will be highlighted as useful tools in primary care, especially with regard to pain management. They all enhance patient engagement, and over time, create an environment of partnership between patients and staff. This relationship improves encounters and the clinical environment and can also support the change that is frequently needed by patients with chronic and acute pain.

USING THE MI MIND-SET IN PRIMARY CARE

MI, introduced in 1983, has been widely known and discussed, and frequently misinterpreted (Box 4.1). Drs Miller and Rollnick have provided free access to their model, and it has enjoyed extensive acceptance. In 2008, they wrote a paper titled "Ten Things that Motivational Interviewing is Not," describing the positive and negative impacts of the popularity of MI.

Keeley, Engel, Reed, Brody, and Burke (2018) reviewed research on MI training in primary care. The ideal model for training has not been identified; these reseachers found that training in the first year required about 20 hours, with 4 to

BOX 4.1

DEFINITION OF *MI*

MI is a collaborative, person-centered form of questioning intended to elicit and strengthen motivation for change.

MI, motivational interviewing.

Source: From Miller, W. R., & Rollnick, S. (2009). Setting the record straight: What motivational interviewing is not. *PsycEXTRA Dataset.* doi:10.1037/e603162009-007

8 hours annually needed thereafter. As a clinical skill, MI requires formal training that includes didactic and practical components. This training is needed to achieve the change documented in MI programs; however, there are several strategies that primary care clinicians can use to immediately share the benefits of the spirit of MI with their patients.

MI is a very powerful tool to use to help patients change lifestyle behaviors that are impeding pain management; examples include opioid use, smoking, and participation in physical therapy (PT). Individual communication approaches that are included in the model enhance communication, making it an important part of a communication skillset. Use MI when helping a patient with a specific change and incorporate the guiding principles as individual components for routine communication. This strategy supports a positive therapeutic relationship that benefits both patient and clinician. Mastering this approach can add joy to clinical practice while improving the outcomes for patients.

TTM is often confused with MI. Both of them were introduced in the late 1970s, are patient centered, and assist with change. They complement each other, but are different. MI involves the spirit of the clinician, how he or she presents him- or herself and how he or she manages the space where the encounter occurs. TTM helps the clinician to determine a patient's readiness to change a given situation or behavior.

CLINICAL PEARL

Incorporate the spirit of MI into your usual communication by asking questions such as "What would you like to discuss today?"

The Spirit of MI

MI involves a patient-centered approach, acknowledging and incorporating the patient's perspective in setting parameters for dialog as well as setting the stage for change. Miller and Rollnick are clear that MI is not a technique used to manipulate patients, but rather a "spirit" that creates the tone for productive discussion. The four elements of the spirit of MI are partnership, acceptance, compassion, and evocation (Miller & Rollnick, 2013). Miller and Rollnick describe the spirit of MI as "mind-set and heart-set," "these are not prerequisites for the practice of MI ... it is our experience that the practice of MI itself teaches these four habits of the heart" (Miller & Rollnick, 2013, p. 15).

The fundamental principles of MI are expressed in the mnemonics OARS and RULE (Boxes 4.2 and 4.3). OARS describes the communication tools used to practice MI. ***Open questions*** set the stage for true engagement between clinician and patient; used skillfully, they keep dialog moving productively and can save time. ***Affirming*** is a style that acknowledges the positive aspects of another's behavior or presence. This promotes a personal relationship, demonstrating interest in his or her well-being. ***Reflecting*** refers to restating what you believe you heard the patient say. In the beginning of your practice, for example, if he or she says, "It was a miserable week—my pain was unbearable." You could say, "It was a hard week because of your pain." This is a simple reflection; the ability to use complex reflection can be developed with education and practice. ***Summarizing*** combines various facets of the discussion, providing an opportunity for clarification and demonstrating that you were actively listening to the patient. *Reflecting* and *summarizing* require active listening and focus so you will be able to restate what the patient has told you.

Role of MI in Pain Management

MI is a powerful tool to use when discussing discontinuing or tapering opioids, benzodiazepines, alcohol, or tobacco. It was initially used in addiction services

BOX 4.2

OARS: MNEMONIC FOR CORE COMMUNICATION SKILLS

- Open questions
- Affirming
- Reflecting
- Summarizing

Source: From Miller, W. R., & Rollnick, S. (2013). *Motivational interviewing: Helping people change* (3rd ed.). New York, NY: The Guilford Press.

BOX 4.3

RULE: MNEMONIC FOR GUIDING PRINCIPLES OF MI

- Resist the righting reflex.
- Understand and explore the patient's own motivations.
- Listen with empathy.
- Empower the patient, encouraging hope and optimism.

MI, motivational interviewing.

Source: From Rollnick, S., Miller, W. R., & Butler, C. C. (2008). *Motivational interviewing in health care: Helping patients change behavior.* New York, NY: The Guilford Press.

and has spread throughout healthcare settings. Use of MI diffuses adversarial conversations and provides a framework for calm productive exploration of options. The compassionate tone set by this process supports a clinician–patient relationship that supports movement toward change.

- MI is useful for any primary care situation when patients struggle to make lifestyle changes or are stuck in psychosocial or lifestyle behaviors that impair their health. It is an important tool in your communication repertoire.
- The spirit is useful as a fundamental practice in all healthcare interactions and has demonstrated effectiveness with the most challenging situations.

TRANSTHEORETICAL MODEL OF BEHAVIOR CHANGE

To use the concepts included in MI, it is also useful to know the principles of TTM. This model is used in many settings, including primary care, and can be especially helpful when helping patients make lifestyle changes that are critical parts of improving function and reducing pain. TTM accesses and supports the patient's self-efficacy.

TTM was developed by Prochaska and DiClemente in 1982, partially supported as part of a National Cancer Institute grant to investigate smoking cessation (Prochaska & DiClemente, 1982). Since that time, this model has been studied in diverse disease states and populations, with consistent positive outcomes. When you determine where the patient is with regard to his or her readiness for change, and you work within that framework, you can use the spirit of MI to assist the patient through discrepancies and resistance. Incorporating the patient's perspective of his or her pain and what he or she is ready to change to impact this pain is very useful in primary care. It is also useful when discussing all lifestyle decisions encountered in primary care. By actively engaging the patient's perspective, we support the self-efficacy that can improve the patient's pain experience (Jackson, Wang, Wang, & Fan, 2014).

COMPONENTS OF TTM

Prochaska describes the stages of change as a spiral, so it is not a linear process (Box 4.4). In this fluid process, people move forward, backward, and circle around. The TTM presents a model of hope and empowerment; movement from one stage back to another is not failure, but a step in the process. The final stage, termination, occurs when the patient is 100% confident that he or she will not return to the previous behavior (Prochaska & Prochaska, 2016). When TTM is used, the process of change can enhance the patient–clinician relationship and avoid the consequences of adversarial interactions.

CLINICAL PEARL

You can change the tone of a discussion from implying guilt/judgment to one of nonthreatening inquiry by asking *how* or *what* instead of *why*. Example: Instead of asking, "Why did you take extra medication?" Ask, "What did you think would happen when you took the extra medication?"

BOX 4.4

TRANSTHEORETICAL MODEL STAGES OF CHANGE

- Precontemplation
- Contemplation
- Preparation
- Action
- Maintenance
- Termination

Source: From Prochaska, J. O., & Prochaska, J. M. (2016). *Changing to thrive: Using the stages of change to overcome the top threats to your health and happiness.* Center City, MN: Hazelden Publishing.

In TTM, Prochaska discusses the pros and cons of change. When the pros of the status quo outweigh the cons, there will be no behavior change. The role of the physician assistant or nurse practitioner (PA/NP) is to help the patient move toward healthier behaviors using the right tool, either TTM or MI or both, at the right time.

Incorporating the components of MI with the attitudes of mindfulness and using TTM will not only improve care for your patients with pain, but will also support communication among staff and improve your comfort and satisfaction in all encounters. When individual clinicians and staff adhere to these fundamentals, over time, the atmosphere in the clinic becomes calmer, patient engagement increases, and boundaries are more readily set.

Using TTM

To know where the patient is regarding readiness for change, we need to ask the patient. This dialog provides the clinician with information on the patient's perspective of his or her current behavior and sets the stage for engaging the patient in decision-making. For example, during the precontemplation stage, the person is unaware of the need or has no intention of changing. During the contemplation stage, the pros and cons of change are imbalanced, with the cons outweighing the pros. Using "change talk" here can help the patient identify the impact of continuing with the current strategy or the possibility of changing: "What will your life be like in a year if you continue to sit on the couch all day?" "What could your life look like in a year if you start walking every day?"

When we tell someone "you must do this," the programmed response of the brain is "no." When we ask, "What would you like to do?" the internal response is "I can/will do this." This sets the stage to create a plan that will help the patient move toward health.

Assessing Readiness for Change

To determine the patient's stage of readiness for change, ask, "On a scale of 1 to 10, how motivated are you to (change your diet)?" If the patient answers, "5," the next question is, "What makes it 5 and not 4?" This is empowering and allows exploration of what the person is feeling about the behavior.

It is important to use silence/listening and pauses to give the patient time to explore and think. Waiting for 30 seconds for an answer can seem like eternity, but is a very effective use of time. Listen for the patient's answer rather than focusing on what you are going to say next. This changes the dynamic of the conversation and allows for engagement. When you use this approach, notice the difference in patient response from the more common, "Why aren't you better?"

MINDFULNESS

The heading for the first section of his landmark book, *Full Catastrophe Living*, Jon Kabat-Zinn (1990) succinctly describes the practice of Mindfulness as "Paying Attention" (p. 15). It is that simple and profound. To pay attention requires being in the moment, focusing your mind on the patient in the room; this is accomplished by having an intention and assuming an attitude of presence. Being present means focusing only on the moment at hand; this is a powerful clinical tool. To visualize the impact of presence, think about a conversation you have had with a friend and how it felt when you knew the friend was checking his or her email or looking at social media while you were talking, especially if you were discussing something important. Contrast this with what it is like when someone is giving you his or her complete attention. Patients with chronic pain often feel unheard; when they encounter a clinician who gives them nonjudgmental attention, for even a few moments, it can instill calm or hope. The attitudes of a mindfulness practice include nonjudgment, patience, a "beginner's mind," trust, nonstriving, acceptance, and letting go (Kabat-Zinn, 1990, pp. 33–39). Each of these qualities contributes to the quality of presence, being fully in the moment with the person in front of you. Mindfulness is also a very useful pain-management tool that is most easily shared with patients if the clinician has a personal mindfulness practice.

It has been demonstrated that when clinicians practice mindfulness it has a positive impact on both the clinician's well-being and the patient–clinician relationship. Patient rapport and engagement are improved when clinicians practiced mindfulness (Beach et al., 2013). This engagement enhances the use of both TTM and MI.

CLINICAL PEARL

If an appointment is not going well, check how present you are. Being fully present with the patient improves efficiency and can calm challenging situations.

Cultivating a Mindfulness-based approach into your communication pattern improves your comfort and efficiency in interactions. It has been demonstrated to be effective in pain management (Zeidan, Grant, Brown, Mchaffie, & Coghill, 2012). A full schedule can make it a challenge to maintain presence. In today's multitasking culture, the rarity of having anyone's full attention makes it even more powerful. It is also an effective tool to improve an appointment that is escalating in tension. This may seem a paradox; but when you have a truly calm presence, you eliminate one-half of the tension. Frequently, when agitated people feel heard, a situation is diffused.

USING MI AND TTM TO SUPPORT THE CLINICIAN–PATIENT RELATIONSHIP

Incorporate the principles of MI, TTM, and Mindfulness into your standard communication pattern. These approaches are effective individually and are more powerful when practiced together. Some components may already be part of your professional or personal communication style. Exploring the use of them with new patients and established patients, as well as colleagues will decrease the stress, save time, and improve the outcomes.

CLINICAL PEARL

Begin practicing new skills with friends/family, start with practicing presence

Implementing New Communication Approaches in the Clinic

Effective interventions do not need to be complicated; keep them simple. Simple strategies combined with kindness can be life-changing interventions. Begin by practicing being present and nonjudging. If this is a change for you, notice how the staff and patients respond. Spend more time listening and less time talking. Consider taking the first 20% of select encounters to engage with the patient and notice what happens (Rollnick, video, May 2019). Have dialog with the patient, practicing RULE and OARS until they are second nature. Incorporating them into the encounter creates a supportive environment that supports change.

Resisting the righting reflex can be a challenge. Patients come to us to be told what they need to do to fix problems, and we have learned to be directive. Both MI and TTM have demonstrated that a guiding approach using dialog is more effective than trying to "right" their behavior. There are ways to self-manage and consider how you address patients' opinions and desires. If a patient says "I won't go to PT," there are several ways to answer as follows:

- "But you need to" is not a therapeutic answer.
- If you kindly ask, "What it is it about PT that doesn't work for you?", wait and listen for the answer and explore it using OARS; this will help you establish where the patient is in the stages of change and discuss a little longer or wait until another visit.

Another approach is to begin the appointment with, "What can I help you with today?" If someone is not interested in what is on your list of priorities, he or she is not going to hear your sincere discussion. When the person learns that you will address his or her concerns first, he or she is more engaged in the appointment. Of course, not all patients are interested in all aspects of their health, and there are situations where you must be directive; however, you can maintain a consistent nonjudging attitude (this does not mean gullible or enabling) and be firm without being antagonistic. Studies have shown that practices that use MI have more efficient appointments.

- Establish a safe environment where the patient feels heard. Being present helps with this.
- Using questions that open the realm of possibility rather then reinforcing the negative is empowering for patients. When you use this approach, patients will frequently say, "No one has ever asked that before."
- Explore Mindfulness. Practice being present and look at judging. How much do you judge during the day? You may find that you are hardest on yourself. Letting go of this as you can, can be good for you and everyone else.
- When you have comfort with Mindfulness, explore the TTM. Identify the stages of change and note where you and the patients are.

SUMMARY

The techniques in this chapter are effective individually, using the right tool at the right time, and can be synergistic when practiced together. Some components may already be part of your professional or personal communication style. Like any art, communication skills evolve; adding nuance over time can be helpful to patients and gratifying for clinicians. Exploring the use of new components with new patients and established patients, as well as colleagues, will decrease stress and save time.

TRENDING IN PAIN MANAGEMENT

- Watch for increasing emphasis on patient engagement by regulators and payers
- Mindfulness as a tool for mitigating clinician stress
- Innovative trials for teaching MI

CASE STUDY

Mike is a new patient to your practice. He complains of low back pain that has not resolved with medication and a spinal surgery. He comes in today to see you after being referred by another practice for "pain control", and the pain levels remain high. He tells you his pain is very severe, and he needs it to be gone, so that he can go back to his work as a carpenter. He also tells you that he has seen three other healthcare providers who did not help him, and that he has had a surgery that did not work. He is frustrated and angry and tells you that nothing seems to be working for his pain. He is also concerned that he had to fill out forms about his pain, alcohol use, depression, and family history of substance abuse. He cannot see any value in filling out the forms.

You first take a history of all the medications and treatments that Mike has tried to help his pain. He says he did not take some of the pills as they were prescribed needing more to control his pain and refused to use nonsteroidal medications since they were too weak for his pain. He also stopped physical therapy because it hurt him too much and had high co-pay. You use open-ended questions and empathy to establish a relationship and acknowledge how difficult his situation is.

After a thorough physical exam, you sit down to discuss the options for treatment. You tell Mike you can see he has pain. He moves very carefully and tends to guard his back, and has trouble sitting. If he is willing to work with you to set goals and participate in his treatment, you think his pain can be improved. It will take time and it will take different types of therapies for better management of his pain. You ask him what pain level would equal success for him, and discuss that being pain free is not a likely outcome, but working together, the two of you can improve his pain and function using a combination of medications and other therapies such as walking, counseling, and pacing activities. Mike agrees to try your plan of care for 6 weeks to see if there is any improvement.

Mike's plan of care:

- Goal setting. You ask him to express his priorities, and what does he need to accomplish to move his life forward? Establish reasonable/appropriate expectations of pain relief. If a patient expects zero pain, gently and firmly discuss how this goal will interfere with the patient's progress.
- You explore his priorities and include the importance of activity, especially PT, in managing pain and discuss your recommendations and barriers he identifies and identify his internal and external support systems.
- Reconditioning activities. Physical therapy did not work for Mike, so simple walking would be a start at reconditioning. Have Mike keep track of how much he walks daily and see how far he can go in the first few weeks. Massage, acupuncture, and meditation are all options that you can discuss with Mike.

(*continued*)

CASE STUDY (*continued*)

- Non-opioid medications. There is little to no research support for long-term opioids for low back pain. You discuss what he has tried and how he has used them, and recommend a plan going forward.
- You discuss the impact of activity and sleep on mood and function. Screening for depression and anxiety may indicate how actively these need to be addressed.
- Psychology referral to help with frustration and anger could be useful, but may not be available. As indicated, you review Mindfulness exercises and over-the-counter supplements that can be calming.

REFERENCES

Beach, M. C., Roter, D., Korthuis, P. T., Epstein, R. M., Sharp, V., Ratanawongsa, N., . . . Saha, S. (2013). A multicenter study of physician mindfulness and health care quality. *The Annals of Family Medicine, 11*(5), 421–428. doi:10.1370/afm.1507

Jackson, T., Wang, Y., Wang, Y., & Fan, H. (2014). Self-efficacy and chronic pain outcomes: A meta-analytic review. *The Journal of Pain, 15*(8), 800–814. doi:10.1016/j.jpain.2014.05.002

Kabat-Zinn, J. (1990). *Full catastrophe living: Using the wisdom of your body and mind*. DELTA. New York, NY: Bantam Dell.

Keeley, R., Engel, M., Reed, A., Brody, D., & Burke, B. L. (2018). Toward an emerging role for motivational interviewing in primary care. *Current Psychiatry Reports, 20*(6), 41. doi:10.1007/s11920-018-0901-3

Miller, W. R., & Rollnick, S. (2009). Setting the record straight: What motivational interviewing is NOT. *PsycEXTRA Dataset*. doi:10.1037/e603162009-007

Miller, W. R., & Rollnick, S. (2013). *Motivational interviewing: Helping people change* (3rd ed.). New York, NY: The Guilford Press.

Prochaska, J. O., & DiClemente, C. C. (1982). Transtheoretical therapy: Toward a more integrative model of change. *Psychotherapy: Theory, Research & Practice, 19*(3), 276–288. doi:10.1037/h0088437

Prochaska, J. O., & Prochaska, J. M. (2016). *Changing to thrive: Using the stages of change to overcome the top threats to your health and happiness*. Center City, MN: Hazelden Publishing.

Rollnick, S. (May 2019). *SA HIV ATTC: Stephen Rollnick, MI Ready for Translation?*. Valkenberg Hospital. https://www.youtube.com/watch?v=SAntO8nLDMQ

Rollnick, S., Miller, W. R., & Butler, C. C. (2008). *Motivational interviewing in health care: Helping patients change behavior*. New York, NY: The Guilford Press.

Zeidan, F., Grant, J., Brown, C., Mchaffie, J., & Coghill, R. (2012). Mindfulness meditation-related pain relief: Evidence for unique brain mechanisms in the regulation of pain. *Neuroscience Letters, 520*(2), 165–173. doi:10.1016/j.neulet.2012.03.082

ADDITIONAL RESOURCES

Butler, C. C., Simpson, S. A., Hood, K., Cohen, D., Pickles, T., Spanou, C., . . . Rollnick, S. (2013). Training practitioners to deliver opportunistic multiple behavior change counselling in primary care: A cluster randomized trial. *BMJ, 346*, f1191. doi:10.1136/bmj.f1191

Schneiderhan, J., Clauw, D., & Schwenk, T. L. (2017). Primary care of patients with chronic pain. *JAMA, 317*(23), 2367. doi:10.1001/jama.2017.5787

Guides

Encouraging Motivation to Change Reminder Card: https://www.centerforebp.case.edu/client-files/pdf/miremindercard.pdf

Quick Guide for Clinicians on Motivational Interviewing: https://store.samhsa.gov/sites/default/files/d7/priv/sma12-4097.pdf

Videos

Stephen Rollnick

Stephen speaks about Motivational Interviewing: https://www.stephenrollnick.com/about-motivational-interviewing-health

Why learn MI and insights from 25 years of experience: https://www.youtube.com/watch?v=lF1i32ucPvE published in 2013

William Miller

Motivational Interviewing: A Dialogue with the Practice's Co-founder William R. Miller: https://www.youtube.com/watch?v=DSHh6V9yNzg Sept 2017

CHAPTER 5

DEVELOPING A PLAN OF CARE FOR PAIN MANAGEMENT

INTRODUCTION

After assessing the patient for his or her pain complaint, developing a plan of care with achievable outcomes allows the patient to understand how the pain will be managed and what to expect. For patients with pain, having a firm understanding of their pain-management plan can provide a measure of comfort and confidence.

This chapter provides information on how to develop a workable plan for a patient with pain and how to use a patient–provider agreement (PPA) when opioids are being used. It also offers information about software applications and ways to track outcomes digitally.

DETERMINING WHAT IS ACHIEVABLE FOR THE PATIENT

After the initial assessment, setting up a comprehensive plan of care for the patient is essential. For patients with acute pain, the plan can be simplified, but should include information on medications, how long they will be provided, and the intent to taper the patient off of opioid medications once they are no longer needed. The patient may be concerned about this; but if the patient is reassured and helped through the process, it can be achieved with minimal discomfort.

Having a discussion upfront regarding how other medications or opioids will be used and discontinued allows the patient to express concerns and the provider to educate the patient about appropriate use of opioids for relieving pain. If for some reason the patient cannot taper from opioids or is reluctant to continue trying, a referral to a pain clinic, psychologist, or addiction treatment may be needed.

For a patient with chronic pain, the plan of care needs to be more complex and include more aspects of the patient's care. For these patients, multiple disciplines may need to be involved in care, and therefore having a good communication network is crucial to ensuring all practitioners understand the goals of care. Elements of a plan of care for a patient with chronic pain can include:

- Physical and occupational therapy
- Sleep
- Acupuncture or injections
- Counseling for coping and depression
- Medication management
- Behavioral techniques such as biofeedback or mindfulness
- Hypnosis or meditation
- Nutritional management

How do you determine which of these therapies will work for the patient? Depending on the type of pain that the patient is experiencing, some will work better than others. Most patients with chronic pain stop moving because the pain decreases with rest. However, this results in deconditioning, which physical therapy can help remedy. So, for most patients with chronic pain, a physical therapy referral helps to increase function.

For some of the other therapies like meditation, biofeedback, or self-hypnosis, the patient must want to participate for there to be any success. Using motivational interviewing techniques can help identify the therapies that will be successful. For patients who prefer other options, therapies such as acupuncture, transcutaneous electrical stimulation (TENS) units, or chiropractic treatment may be a better fit.

Medication management and nutritional supplements, over the counter or by prescription, can be helpful for some patients. However, patients should be educated about each medication, the side effects, and the risks and benefits. For patients on opioids, boundary setting is key so that there is a clear understanding of what the medication is, the dose, when refills will be available, and where the medication prescription is being filled. The prescriber needs to maintain control of prescribing and set boundaries, and the patient needs to be informed of the consequences of noncompliance with the plan of care.

Because depression and/or anxiety can be comorbid with chronic pain, all patients should be screened for depression. This can be done in the primary care practice or the patient can be referred to a psychologist for screening. If depression is diagnosed, the patient should be treated for the depression along with the pain.

CLINICAL PEARL

Communicating with the patient and determining preferences are key to the success of the plan. Listening to the patient speak about the pain and what the patient feels will help in treating the pain provide insight into what will work in a plan of care.

INCLUDING OTHER DISCIPLINES AND ALTERNATE MEDICATION CHOICES

For a patient with chronic pain, the more disciplines that are included in the process, the more complete the care will be and the more intense the therapy will be. Because these patients have complex needs, using a variety of medications and therapies will provide the best outcomes.

For patients who want to be pain free or hope to get their old lives back, counselors and psychologists can provide the patient with coping skills and help them understand that after developing chronic pain, their lives are changed forever and the new life needs to be embraced. The identified goal is not to remain pain free, but rather to have improved function. Social workers can help patients look for ways to find support groups and programs to help defray costs.

Providers who can offer additional support for patients with chronic pain include:

- Social workers
- Psychologists
- Addiction counselors
- Physical and occupational therapists
- Pharmacists
- Nurses

To find patient-led support groups, the patient can contact the American Chronic Pain Association to see whether a local group is available. Check their website at www.ACPA.com for further information.

Chronic pain needs a combination of medications to help reach the maximum level of relief. Patients with chronic pain may need an antidepressant for neuropathic pain or to enhance sleep. Topical creams and lidocaine patches can be added to oral medications to increase the pain relief. Over-the-counter medications, such as acetaminophen or nonsteroidal anti-inflammatory drugs (NSAIDs), are helpful if the patient is a good candidate.

Educating the patient about using these medications is a key part of getting them to use the medicines both appropriately and as prescribed. Patients often say that acetaminophen is not strong enough for their pain. Using the medications for a 2-week time period at the dosing indicated on the Prescriber Information sheet will allow the patient to see the value of adding it to his or her regimen.

NUTRITIONAL SUPPLEMENTS

Integrative therapies can be very useful in mitigating chronic and acute pain. There are multiple integrative approaches available to decrease inflammation and reduce pain; for example, in addition to eating an anti-inflammatory diet, like the Mediterranean diet, one can add ginger and/or turmeric to food. Some integrative therapies, such as meditation, Qi Gong, and mindfulness, provide potential benefit with minimal risk. Others require analysis of risks and benefits. Use supplements as carefully as prescription medications. Check for interactions and give specific instructions regarding dosing, frequency, and side effects.

Magnesium is an example of a supplement that can be very useful. It plays a role in over 300 cellular reactions, and most people are magnesium deficient. Check drug interactions with magnesium; patients should avoid combining drugs or supplements that could interfere with magnesium absorption.

Magnesium provides multiple benefits, including impacting muscle and nerve pain, and it is calming. Magnesium citrate loosens stools and is helpful for patients who are chronically constipated or if constipation develops with the use of opioids. For patients who have loose stools, magnesium glycinate or taurate does not impact the bowel function as much as magnesium citrate does. Epsom salts provide magnesium. Soaking in a hot tub containing Epsom salts for 20 minutes relaxes the muscles and the magnesium is absorbed through the skin. If the tub is not an option, a foot bath provides similar relief.

Using nutritional supplements and integrative techniques can enhance the patient's plan of care. They can also provide the patient with a sense of control over their treatment options.

USING A PPA TO SET UP THE PLAN FOR OPIOIDS

A PPA offers a way to engage the patient in the plan of care and provides education on their condition and the medications prescribed. The form lists important elements in the treatment plan. The U.S. Food and Drug Administration (FDA; 2018) indicates that a PPA (Exhibit 5.1) should be used for any patient beginning treatment withopioid medications. Once the decision is made to use opioids for treating the patient's pain, the PPA should be explained and signed prior to starting the medications. It is really a "rules of the road" document that explains what is expected of the patient and what the healthcare provider will do.

The PPA

- Explains the respective patient and provider roles,
- Includes responsibilities of the opioid treatment, and
- Improves outcomes, reduces risks, and provides patient education (Pergolizzi et al., 2017).

EXHIBIT 5.1

EXAMPLE OF A PATIENT–PROVIDER AGREEMENT

Patient Agreement Form

Patient Name:

Medical Record Number: **Addressograph Stamp:**

AGREEMENT FOR LONG-TERM CONTROLLED SUBSTANCE PRESCRIPTIONS

The use of ______________________________ (print names of medication(s)) may cause addiction and is only one part of the treatment for: ____________________ (print name of condition, e.g., pain, anxiety, etc.).

The goals of this medicine are:

☐ to improve my ability to work and function at home

☐ to help my ____________________ (print name of condition – e.g., pain, anxiety, etc.) as much as possible without causing dangerous side effects

I have been told that:

1. If I drink alcohol or use street drugs, I may not be able to think clearly and I could become sleepy and risk personal injury.
2. I may get addicted to this medicine.
3. If I or anyone in my family has a history of drug or alcohol problems, there is a greater chance of addiction.
4. If I need to stop this medicine, I must do it slowly or I may get very sick.

I agree to the following:

- I am responsible for my medicines. I will not share, sell, or trade my medicine. I will not take anyone else's medicine.
- I will not increase my medicine until I speak with my doctor or nurse.

(*continued*)

EXHIBIT 5.1 (*continued*)

- My medicine may not be replaced if it is lost, stolen, or used up sooner than prescribed.
- I will keep all appointments set up by my doctor (e.g., primary care, physical therapy, mental health, substance abuse treatment, pain management).
- I will bring the pill bottles with any of the remaining pills to each clinic visit.
- I agree to give a blood or urine sample, if asked, to test for drug use.

Refills

Refills will be made only during regular office hours: Monday through Friday, 8:00 AM–4:30 PM. No refills are available at night or on holidays or weekends. I must call at least three (3) working days ahead (M–F) to ask for a refill of my medicine. **No exceptions will be made**. I will not come to primary care for my refill until I am called by the nurse.

I must keep track of my medications. No early or emergency refills may be made.

Pharmacy

I will only use one pharmacy to get my medicine. My doctor may talk with the pharmacist about my medicines.
The name of my pharmacy is ________________________.

Prescriptions From Other Doctors

If I see another doctor who gives me a controlled-substance medication (for example, a dentist, a doctor from the ED or another hospital, etc.) I must bring this medicine to primary care in the original bottle, even if there are no pills left.

Privacy

While I am taking this medicine, my doctor may need to contact other doctors or family members to get information about my care and/or use of this medicine. I will be asked to sign a release at that time.

Termination of Agreement

If I break any of the rules, or if my doctor decides that this medicine is hurting me more than helping me, this medicine may be stopped by my doctor in a safe way.

I have talked about this agreement with my doctor and I understand the preceding rules.

(*continued*)

EXHIBIT 5.1 (*continued*)

Provider Responsibilities

As your doctor, I agree to perform regular checks to see how well the medicine is working.

I agree to provide primary care for you even if you are no longer getting controlled medicines from me.

Patient's signature Date

Resident physician's signature

Attending physician's signature

☐ This document has been discussed with and signed by the physician and patient. (A signed copy stamped with the patient's insurance card should be sent to the medical records department and a copy given to the patient.)

PPA, patient–provider agreement.

Source: From National Institute on Drug Abuse. (n.d.). *Opioid crisis and pain management: Sample patient agreement forms.* Retrieved from https://www.drugabuse.gov/sites/default/files/SamplePatientAgreementForms.pdf

How well do PPAs work and what do patients and providers think about them? In a multicenter evaluation of a standard PPA document querying 117 patients and 14 providers, Pergolizzi et al. (2017) found that 96% of the patients indicated the PPA was either very helpful or somewhat helpful in deciding the course of treatment. Also, 97% of the same patient group indicated that the document was easy to understand.

In the prescriber group, the healthcare providers felt that the PPA could be administered in 10 minutes or less (Pergolizzi et al., 2017). Also, 72% of the providers felt the PPA could be easily incorporated into their daily practice (Pergolizzi et al., 2017).

In another study on patient and provider perceptions of the PPA, Albrecht et al. (2015) found that general practitioners used the document least, but reported that their liability providers were pressuring them to use it. Both the patient group (40 respondents) and the provider group (40 respondents) indicated that they had a lack of understanding about the purpose and content of the PPA. Many patients indicated that they had been asked to sign a PPA in an emergency department (ED).

In the Albrecht study, prescribers were concerned about the legal status of the document, whereas patients believed the PPA was designed to protect prescribers. It is interesting to note that both groups in the study felt that the PPA would not prevent opioid misuse.

So, although the use of PPAs for patients on opioids has been included in the blueprint for the prescriber continuing-education programs (Center for Drug Evaluation and Research, U.S. FDA, 2012), it has not been widely adopted. More education regarding both the intent and the content of the document is needed so that it is not misunderstood or misused. It is interesting that the liability providers find the document worthwhile and are encouraging its use.

The PPA provides an opportunity to engage with the patient and discuss expectations and consequences of opioid use. It can be framed as a mutual agreement that indicates what the clinician and the patient each agree to. It can be especially useful to establish boundaries when discussing the consequences, for example, when a patient takes more medication than prescribed, with or without requesting an early refill.

MONITORING COMPLIANCE WITH THE IDENTIFIED PLAN OF CARE

In order to achieve the best outcomes, the patient needs to comply with the plan of care. Setting goals and communicating with patients is key to the success of the process. However, tracking compliance can offer a chance for reevaluating the plan of care and revising it to better fit the patient's needs.

There are indications that using paper-and-pencil tracking in a diary or log can help the patient track progress. Today, there are a number of digital applications available that can help a patient track sleep and activity. A device, such as a Fitbit, can be used to track daily activity and sleep. To use such a device, the patient needs to be somewhat savvy about using the technology.

There are also considerations about data safety when using an app that could be accessed by someone who is not meant to have it, or when patients may not realize who can see their information if they choose to share it with friends on the Internet via the app. Before using an app and putting data into it, investigate how the data will be collected and shared with outside vendors.

Other helpful apps include:

- **AHRQ Question Builder:** Designed for patients with chronic disease, this free app can track questions they have, questions they may ask, and pictures. The patient can also record appointments in a phone calendar.

The patient controls all the information unless he or she chooses to share it with family or clinicians.

Available at www.ahrq.gov/news/newsroom/press-releases/new-questionbuilder.html

- **Mindfulness, meditation, or sleep apps, for example, Headspace, Calm, Insight Timer:** Many of these apps offer free content with an option to upgrade for a fee. Programs can be used for meditation or to promote sleep. The healthcare provider should be familiar with these apps to be able to determine which app he or she wants to recommend and what options are useful within the app.
- **Cardiac Coherence:** This app is free for Android users and has a low fee if using iOS systems. The app uses a 5-minute breathing timer that facilitates cardiac coherence, which can be calming. This activates the parasympathetic nervous system, decreasing the dominance of sympathetic nervous system. This app gives the patient a point of focus and does not require any mental effort other than focusing on breathing while following a moving ball. It is not a meditation app, but is calming and can be useful for someone who is not willing to use meditation.

CLINICAL PEARL

Nothing is free. Your data is valuable to someone; decide what you are willing to share.

EDUCATE PATIENTS USING OPIOIDS ON MEDICATION SAFETY AND DISPOSAL

Educating patients about medications and their side effects goes a long way toward achieving success of the pain-management plan. Even if the medications prescribed are not opioids, the patient should be educated on the medication, dose, rationale for using it, and its side effects.

If the patient is taking opioids, there are several key concepts that the patient needs to know to maintain medication safety. The patient on opioids should be told the following:

- Never share the medications. There is risk of overdose if the patient's family members or friends share the medication.
- Keep the medication safe. The FDA Blueprint recommends use of a locked box rather than a medicine chest, where the public has access to the medication.

- Take the medication as prescribed. Report any sedation or side effects to the prescriber.
- Do not combine sedating medications, such as sleeping medications or benzodiazepines, or use alcohol when on opioids. The increased sedative effect can be lethal.
- If the patient becomes oversedated, 911 should be called immediately. If naloxone is available, a dose should be administered and respiratory support started immediately.

When patients need to dispose of opioid medications, they should be flushed down the toilet or contaminated in some way with dirty kitty litter, old coffee grounds, or another distasteful substance. There are also gel bags available for disposal. Visit www.mallinckrodt.com/corporate-responsibility/responsible-use/medication-disposal for more information.

In some areas, there are take-back days during which police departments and pharmacies offer containers in which old, unused medication can be disposed. The one thing the patient should not do is just throw them out in the regular trash, where anyone searching the trash could retrieve them for use.

SUMMARY

Developing an effective pain-management plan for patients with chronic pain requires the clinician to foster a relationship with patients while using a multidisciplinary approach in which communication regularly takes place. The patient and provider are responsible for compliance with the plan of care and for tracking outcomes. Using a PPA for a patient on opioids can provide a structure for the process and offers education to the patient about his or her medication use. If the plan of care is successful, the patient will be a partner in the process and enjoy the benefits of positive outcomes.

TRENDING IN PAIN MANAGEMENT

- Look for new and better ways to track patient compliance and to progress toward the identified goals such as sleep and activity.
- Look for new ways to dispose of medication.
- Keep abreast of new state and federal regulations regarding medication use and disposal.

CASE STUDY

Sara is a 35-year-old patient with chronic migraine headaches. She has at least six headaches per month. Each time she is significantly disabled by severe pain, nausea, and visual impairment. Sara was a nurse on a medical–surgical unit in a local hospital, so she understands her headaches and has tried multiple medications for pain relief with mixed results. Sara is currently unemployed because her headaches make it impossible for her to maintain a consistent presence at work.

When you examine Sara, she is not having a headache. She does have a rather extensive file of neurological studies and MRI results. She is hoping you can help her get some pain relief for these headaches because she needs to go back to work. Her medication choices are limited since she works with patients. Sara admits to feeling depressed and anxious because she had to leave her nursing position as a result of her headaches.

- Setting up a plan of care for Sara will be challenging because she will need medications, coping skills, behavioral interventions, and depression treatment.
- Sara's exam is benign at this visit. She appears anxious and emotional. Her former neurological exams indicate chronic migraine headaches triggered by light and sound.
- Sara's goal is to return to work.
- Using one of the newer migraine medications intended to abort headaches and another to treat a headache is helpful. Using an antidepressant at night for migraine maintenance and depression is the way to help both conditions. Sara is also a candidate for BOTOX injections.
- Sara will need ongoing support. She will also need a referral to psychology for anxiety and depression treatment and monitoring.
- In order to track Sara's progress, you suggest she use a diary to note her headaches and a digital tracker to monitor her sleep patterns and activity.
- Using integrative and lifestyle changes to prevent headaches can also help Sara cope with her recurrent headaches.

REFERENCES

Albrecht, J., Khokhar, B., Pradel, F., Campbell, M., Palmer, J., Harris, I., & Palumbo, F. (2015). Perceptions of patient provider agreements. *Journal of Pharmaceutical Health Services Research, 6*(3), 139–144. doi:10.1111/jphs.12099

Center for Drug Evaluation and Research. U. S. Food and Drug Administration. (2012). Blueprint for prescriber continuing education program. *Journal of Pain and Palliative Care Pharmacotherapy, 26*(2), 127–130. doi:10.3109/15360288.2012.680013

U.S. Food and Drug Administration. (2018). *The FDA opioid analgesic REMS education blueprint for healthcare providers involved in the treatment and monitoring of patients with pain.* Retrieved from https://www.fda.gov/media/99496/download

National Institute on Drug Abuse. (n.d.). *NIDAMED: Clinical resources.* Retrieved from www.drugabuse.gov/nidamed-medical-health-professionals

Pergolizzi, J., Curro, F., Colo, N., Ghods, M., Vena, D., Taylor, R., . . . LeQuang, J. (2017). A multicentre evaluation of an opioid patient-provider agreement. *Postgraduate Medical Journal, 93*(1104), 613–617. doi:10.1136/postgradmedj-2016-134607

PART II

Medication Management

CHAPTER 6

SELECTING A MEDICATION TO FIT PATIENTS' PAIN-MANAGEMENT NEEDS

INTRODUCTION

Because pain is the most common complaint of patients seeing a healthcare provider, after determining where the pain is located, the real issue is which medication the healthcare provider (HCP) should choose to treat the pain. Given the large number of medications and therapies that can be used to treat pain, choosing a medication that fits the patient's needs and that will be successful is crucial.

One of the worse scenarios is to have the patient try the medication and then stop using it without telling the provider. Some of the reasons that patients give for stopping a prescribed medication are side effects, such as confusion, lightheadedness, and nausea, or a seemingly simple side effect, such as constipation. Many patients who are given prescriptions fail to fill them or stop taking the medication without an adequate trial. They often say the medication "just didn't work." This results in continued pain complaints from patients and frustration for both providers and patients. Patient education about medications and their potential side effects with continued review at subsequent visits can help target any problem areas.

CLINICAL PEARL

Failure to ask about use of over-the-counter medications or supplements can result in a medication interaction that can prove dangerous.

Primary care providers have busy schedules and limited time available to see patients. Determining which medication might be the best for the patient can be time-consuming. There are some ways to help with the decision-making process, such as following national guidelines and looking at what type of pain the patient is experiencing to choose a suitable medication for the specific type of pain (Stanos et al., 2016). Using other clinic staff to explain the medications to the patient and how to use them can also cut down on time. Using preprinted handouts with medication information and side effect information can help the patient understand medications that are being prescribed.

HOW TO USE A NATIONAL GUIDELINE TO CHOOSE A MEDICATION FOR LOW-BACK PAIN

Low-back pain (LBP) is a very common complaint encountered by primary care practitioners. It affects most Americans at some time in their lives to some degree, especially between the ages of 30 and 50 years (D'Arcy, 2011). LBP can occur spontaneously or be the result of overuse, wear and tear, osteoarthritis, or an injury, such as a herniated nucleus pulposus (HNP), caused by tissue trauma. It is very common for patients to try self-treatment with heat, over-the-counter medications, or rest. When these options fail, the patient comes to the primary care provider to get help with the pain and loss of function.

Chou and Huffman (2007) and Chout et al. (2007) developed evidence-based guidelines for the American Pain Society that address LBP. Because LBP is a common complaint seen by primary care providers, using the recommendations suggested by the guidelines can be helpful. These guidelines can provide confidence and support for both prescribing medications and the use of radiology and physical therapy. Unfortunately, in a study of 720 family care providers, only 25% provided care consistent with the national guideline recommendations (Cherkin, Wheeler, Barlow, & Deyo, 1998; McCarberg, Stanos, & D'Arcy, 2012).

The national guidelines for acute LBP include:

- Using nonsteroidal anti-inflammatory drugs (NSAIDs), such as ibuprofen and naproxen, at normal daily doses if the patient is a good candidate
- Using skeletal muscle relaxants
- Encouraging the patient to remain active rather than being on bedrest and/or using opioids
- Limiting the use of radiographic studies to patients with severe pain or a neurological complication such as urinary incontinence as a result of the injury (Chou et al., 2007)

For patients with chronic LBP, the choices for treatment are a little different. Using NSAIDs or acetaminophen long term can have negative effects on liver and kidney function. There is also the possibility of a gastrointestinal bleed; so long-term treatment with NSAIDs is not recommended.

For those patients with failed back syndrome or long-term nociceptive or neuropathic pain, a different set of medications and treatments are recommended. For LBP, the recommended treatment options are as follows:

- Nonmedication-based therapy such as chiropractic care, acupuncture, yoga, or exercise therapy
- Antidepressants (tricyclic antidepressant [TCA])
- Benzodiazepines (can cause oversedation and should not be combined with opioids [Centers for Disease Control and Prevention [CDC], 2017])
- Opioids, tramadol (Chou, 2009)
- Duloxetine (Chou et al., 2017)

As with all medications, the prescriber has to weigh the risks and benefits for long-term therapy with any medication. There are pros and cons for use of tricyclics. They are usually considered for LBP with a neuropathic component. The most commonly used is amitriptyline, but the medication has a number of anticholinergic effects, such as drowsiness and dry mouth, which patients should be educated about before initiation of the medication. Amitriptyline is not recommended for patients over the age of 65 related to the risk of hypotension potentially resulting in falls (McCarberg et al., 2012).

Benzodiazepines have been implicated in the increased risk of opioid overdose when the medications are combined, and as such, they have fallen out of favor. As a group, the medications are highly sedating. The CDC guideline indicates that using a benzodiazepine with an opioid is contraindicated (CDC, 2017).

Anticonvulsants have shown to offer some improvement with LBP, especially LBP with a neuropathic component. If gabapentin is used, the prescriber will have to titrate the doses upward to achieve a therapeutic effect, as only 10% is bioavailable to the patient. Although this is an off-label use for these medications, they are commonly being prescribed with positive effects.

The use of opioids for chronic LBP requires much discussion. The decision to start a trial of opioids should be undertaken only after much consideration and conversation with the patient. The discussion should center on the fact that these medications will be used as a trial to see whether there is good benefit to the patient and an increase in functionality. Some studies have indicated that opioids are ineffective for long-term use in chronic pain, whereas others have shown modest benefit (McCarberg et al., 2017). Screening the patient for opioid risk and using a patient–provider agreement (PPA) is recommended for all patients being started on an opioid trial.

Guidelines can provide structure for treating patients with chronic pain conditions, such as osteoarthritis and fibromyalgia, and conditions with high rates of disability such as LBP. They can help the prescriber decide which medication regimen would produce the best outcome for the patient. However, many practitioners still choose to use medications that are not recommended and unfortunately get poorer outcomes for their patients.

USING THE PAIN TO DETERMINE WHAT MEDICATIONS TO CHOOSE

Determining the type of pain is very important when considering the medication to use to treat it. This is especially true when the pain has a neuropathic or nociplastic source. Using opioids to treat neuropathic pain will not produce the relief needed. The pain is being generated by a neuronal source, not a nociceptive injury. In a data review from March 2008 to February 2012, 52% of patients with painful diabetic neuropathy, fibromyalgia, or arthritis were prescribed opioids as part of a first-line treatment after a trial of over-the-counter NSAIDs (Stanos et al., 2016). Such choices have resulted in poor pain relief, patient demands for increased doses, and opioid dependence.

CLINICAL PEARL

Using a neuropathic medication for neuropathic pain will result in better pain relief with no opioid dependence.

For most patients with aches, sprains, strains, or simple musculoskeletal pain, the usual pain medications, such as NSAIDs or acetaminophen, or combination opioids, such as hydrocodone acetaminophen compounds short term if the pain is severe, are sufficient. The addition of a nonpharmacological therapy, such as heat or ice, can improve pain relief. The expectation is that the patient will return to baseline after a short period of time.

For patients who have chronic pain, the scenario is very different. For most long-term conditions, such as arthritis or painful diabetic neuropathy, the realistic goal is not a 0/10 pain level, but rather managing the pain and decreasing it to the lowest possible intensity. For these patients, the plan of care is more complex.

When a patient continues to complain of pain and the prescribed medication is not effective for adequate pain relief, and the dose increases have failed to produce any benefit, consider that the pain may have a neuropathic component. For these patients, a reevaluation of the pain is needed. Ask the patient to describe all areas of pain and listen for descriptors such as painful numbness, tingling, shooting, stabbing, or burning. Conditions that indicate neuropathic pain include:

- Hyperalgesia
- Allodynia
- Hypoalgesia
- Paresthesia
- Dysesthesia
- Hypoesthesia (McCarberg et al., 2016)

These should raise suspicion that the pain has a neuropathic generator and will need a neuropathic pain medication. These medications can be used alone or in combination with other classes of medications such as opioids. NeuPSIG national recommendations on medications to treat neuropathic pain and taken from the meta-analysis by Dworkin et al. (2010) and Finnerup et al. (2015) include:

First-line medications

- TCAs, such as nortriptyline and desipramine, with starting dosages of 25 mg at night, with titration upward as tolerated
- Selective serotonin–norepinephrine reuptake inhibitors (SSNRIs), such as duloxetine and venlafaxine, starting at doses of 30 and 37.5 mg, respectively, once per day
- Calcium channel ligands, also called *membrane stabilizers*, such as gabapentin and pregabalin; starting doses for gabapentin are 100 to 300 mg daily titrating upward to an effective dose; pregabalin doses start at 50 mg three times daily or 75 mg twice per day

Second-line medications

- Topical 5% lidocaine patches are indicated for peripheral neuropathy, no more than three patches every 12 hours.
- Capsaicin cream applied to the affected area is indicated for peripheral neuropathy.

Third-line medications

- Tramadol—Start with a dose of 50 mg once or twice daily
- Opioid agonists, morphine, oxycodone, methadone, levorphanol—Starting dose of morphine is 10 to 15 mg every 4 hours as needed; use equianalgesic dosing used for other medications
- Botulinum toxin A is recommended for peripheral neuropathy only

The medications indicated for neuropathic pain can be used alone or in combination. It is essential to continue to monitor the patient's pain and the patient's response to the medications, and titrate the dosages as needed.

Nociplastic pain is the newest of the pain categories; it waspreviously called *central sensitization* or *central hypersensitivity*. It is important to note that nociplastic pain can occur in conjunction with other types of pain, that is, nociceptive and neuropathic pain. Identifying pain as nociplastic is helpful as patients with nociplastic pain may initially show a response to opioids that decreases dramatically over time (Andrews, 2018). If a clinician diagnoses the patient with a nociplastic pain condition, opioids would not be beneficial for treatment. The conditions that fall into this category are all difficult to treat, for example, fibromylagia, complex regional pain syndrome, and some bladder syndromes. Medications that could prove to be effective include gabapentin, TCAs, and the SSNRIs. Because each patient is unique, it is necessary to try one medication and titrate to the effective dose. If this medication is not sucessful, switch to another class.

CLINICAL PEARL

Knowing what type of pain the patient has is a powerful clue as to what type of medication will be effective for pain control.

USING THE PATIENT ASSESSMENT AND SCREENING TO DETERMINE THE BEST OPTION FOR TREATING PAIN

Using a pain-focused assessment and examination can highlight the areas that the patient describes as painful. For patients with chronic pain, a comprehensive tool, such as the Brief Pain Inventory or even the three-question pain, enjoyment of life, and general activity (PEG) tool, can provide insight into the pain. Looking for the source and type of pain can help determine which medication might be the best for the patient.

Questioning the patient about the medications and treatments that they have used in the past can identify problem areas. Making specific inquiries about over-the-counter medications, supplements, or cannabis or cannabidiol (CBD) oil can elicit a more complete picture of medication use. When the patient tells the healthcare provider that they have taken a particular medication, asking what dose the patient used and for how long can determine whether the patient gave the medication an appropriate trial and any problems that caused the patient to stop the medication. Some patients tell the healthcare provider that a particular medication "doesn't work," when in reality, they only tried a dose or two.

If opioids are going to be used to treat pain, an opioid screening tool, such as the Opioid Risk Tool (ORT), will need to be used to determine the level of risk. For low-risk and medium-risk patients, regular monitoring should be sufficient to maintain safe opioid practice. For patients who fall into high-risk categories, the CDC (2016) recommends sending the patients for methadone or suboxone treatment.

CLINICAL PEARL

Using a valid and reliable tool to assess for pain as well as a screening tool to determine opioid risk can help provide support for medication choices that the healthcare provider is making.

SPECIAL CONSIDERATIONS FOR MEDICATION MANAGEMENT

Some patient groups require special consideration when selecting a medication to treat pain. Some patients have changed physiology, such as those who are on chronic opioids and those with surgical or new pain, or those with many comorbidities, such as older patients. Whatever the condition patients may have, there are some special considerations to remember when choosing a medication.

Geriatric Patients

Patients who are older than 65 are usually considered to be geriatric. Because these patients have a changed physiology, they require dose and medication choices that fit their age and condition. Prescribers may find prescribing for older patients challenging, because there are concerns about disorientation, confusion, and unintentional overdose in this population. Even older adults without renal disease or heart failure can have decreased renal function that allows opioid medications to accumulate and not clear, resulting in oversedation.

Opioids are seen as being a high risk for this population despite the fact that some older patients do well with low-dose opioids and have an increased quality of life, allowing them to be more active. As such, older patients are often undertreated even with nonopioid analgesics, such as NSAIDS, because of risks for those with cardiac disease who are on blood thinners.

Age-related physical changes include:

- Decreased renal clearance
- Decreased hepatic function
- Higher ratio of fat to lean muscle

- Decreased serum protein levels
- Reduced first-pass metabolism (D'Arcy & Bruckenthal, 2011)

The CDC (2016) recommendations for using opioids in older patients include assessing the patient for cognitive functioning, doing a medication review to determine the risk of medication interactions, and educating patients about using only the medications that are prescribed as they are prescribed. Because of the reduced clearance potential and possibility of changed cardiac, renal, or hepatic function in older patients, there is a risk for unintentional overdose that could cause a fall or injury or respiratory depression. When opioids are being used in older patients, the need for education and discussion about side effects, such as constipation, is also an integral part of the care plan.

CLINICAL PEARL

When starting older patients on opioids, use conservative dosing beginning at lower rates, decreasing the initial doses by 25% to 50% (U.S. Food and Drug Administration, 2018).

Patients With New Acute Pain Who Are on Chronic Opioids

As patients with chronic pain continue to experience nociceptive pain, peripheral sensitization can occur. The tissue damage releases bradykinin, leukotrienes, substance P, and prostaglandins, all of which facilitate pain production. As this pain continues, there is increased sensitivity in the peripheral neurons, allowing for more sensitivity to the continued pain production and new pain stimuli. Consequently, the neuronal activation thresholds are lowered and increased neuronal fire rates result. These patients can develop hyperalgesia and allodynia in the damaged tissue, further increasing the sensation of pain (Stanos et al., 2016).

When patients on chronic opioids develop a new pain as the result of surgery or other injury, their highly sensitized systems require more pain medication than their baseline doses to control their pain. The usual process is to continue the usual pain medications and add in either extraoral immediate-release medication or intravenous (IV) opioids. The additional medications can be titrated off once the new pain resolves.

CLINICAL PEARL

When patients on chronic opioids have surgery, they should take their usual dose prior to the procedure and resume the usual dose as soon as possible after the procedure. In this way, there will be no void in the pain relief.

Patients on Medication Management

Patients with opioid use disorder (OUD) who are on medication-assisted treatment (MAT) with methadone, naltrexone, or suboxone will require a thorough assessment and careful medication dosing when they report new pain or have surgery. Of note, the use of these medications for treating OUD has decreased the overall mortality rates in this population. In 2016, there were 350,000 patients being treated with methadone, 60,000 being treated with buprenorphine, and more than 10,000 being treated with naltrexone (Broglio & Matzo, 2018). The chances are good that a primary care provider will see one of these patients for pain.

The term *substance use disorder (SUD)*, of which OUD is one type, replaces the older term *addiction*. In order to be diagnosed with OUD, a patient must meet the diagnostic criteria outlined in the Fifth Edition of the *Diagnostic and Statistical Manual of Mental Disorders* (*DSM-5;* American Psychiatric Association, 2013) published in 2013. These patients demonstrate impaired control, risky use behaviors, social impairment, and tolerance and withdrawal (Broglio & Matzo, 2018).

In order to provide treatment for a number of patients who need care, a physician, nurse practitioner, or physician's assistant can take the recommended coursework and obtain a special waiver to their license that allows the provider to take a specific number of patients into their practice to provide the drugs recognized as treatment options—methadone, buprenorphine, or naltrexone—used specifically to treati OUD. The common doses for these medications are as follows:

- Methadone: 60 to 120 mg per day by mouth
- Buprenorphine: 8 to 24 mg daily after induction via sublingual or transmucosal administration
- Naltrexone: 380 mg monthly via intramuscular (IM) injection

When doing a medication review with a patient, it is essential to clarify what these medications are being used for: Methadone in particular can be used for pain management as well as OUD treatment.

When a patient on methadone has a new pain occurrence, such as surgery, it is important to continue the daily dose of methadone and add additional pain medication for the new pain. In order to ascertain the correct dose of methadone required, the care provider will need to contact the methadone-dispensing facility as the methadone doses being used to treat OUD are not reported to the state monitoring program and will not appear on those records.

Buprenorphine, a mixed mu agonist–antagonist medication, can be used for pain as well; so it is important to know why buprenorphine is being used. To treat a patient with new pain who is on buprenorphine MAT, discontinue buprenorphine and provide opioids. This means that high-dose opioids will be required and the patient will need careful monitoring for respiratory depression and withdrawal.

Once the new pain is resolving, the patient should be in a mild state of withdrawal before the MAT buprenorphine is restarted (Broglio & Matzo, 2018).

For patients who are on naltrexone, an opioid antagonist used for MAT, the medication will need to be stopped 72 hours prior to surgery or IM naltrexone should be discontinued 1 month prior to surgery. Patients on naltrexone MAT who have a trauma or unexpected surgery will need high-dose opioids to overcome the reversal effects of naltrexone. Careful monitoring is also needed to ensure that the patient does not have adverse effects, respiratory depression, or unrelieved pain.

SUMMARY

Deciding which medication to use for patients with pain can be a challenge. Using national guidelines, patient assessment, and taking special care with patients who are older or who have a new pain but are on chronic opioids can help guide medication decisions.

As always, MAT patients are special patients who need careful handling for pain. Using nonopioids and integrative therapies can help the patient relax and achieve better pain control. And finally, make sure that all medication choices and their rationales are documented, so that the outcomes can be tracked.

TRENDING IN PAIN MANAGEMENT

- Look for more information on nociplastic pain and the conditions that fall under this pain category and recommendations for medications to treat them.
- Look for more developing information on treating patients with SUD who have chronic or acute pain.
- National guidelines will continue to evolve and updates available as changes are made.

CASE STUDY

Selena is a 35-year-old woman who has low-back pain (LBP). She first started having the pain about 4 years ago after a fall from a four-wheel vehicle. She has had two surgeries to help relieve her pain, which have been semi-successful. She has a little more function, but no better pain control. She works as a day-care teacher and needs to be able to sit on the floor and stand for long periods of time. She takes 30 mg of extended-release oxycodone twice a day with some short-acting oxycodone

(*continued*)

CASE STUDY (*continued*)

for breakthrough pain. She does not like the opioids and would prefer a different type of treatment plan. She rates her pain as 5/10.

What medications would you try?

- Selena has chronic LBP. She is young and long-term use of opioids can become problematic. The first issue to resolve is how the current plan fits into the recommendations of the LBP guidelines. Because long-term opioids are not indicated, you will need to look at what types of medications will help Selena get through her day and allow her to sleep.
- When you examine Selena, she tells you about the numbness she feels in her lower leg and shows you how the numbness radiates down her leg. You realize that Selena has both musculoskeletal pain and neuropathic pain. This requires the addition of a neuropathic medication such as gabapentin or amitriptyline. As you start the new medication, you monitor Selena for pain relief and note she has decreased pain levels.
- At this point, you can begin to titrate Selena's opioid doses to lower levels every 10 days. You can monitor her for signs of increased pain and withdrawal.
- Selena also needs some techniques to help her that are not medication related. She thinks she can do mindfulness exercises and yoga. Because she is active at her job, she needs techniques that she can use at her discretion.
- Once Selena gets better pain relief, tapering the opioids to the lowest possible level or discontinuing them altogether would be a good outcome. Selena is motivated and should have good success with the plan of care.

Using the recommendations for a national guideline and discovering just what types of pain Selena has can help create a better plan of care for this patient.

REFERENCES

American Psychiatric Association. (2013). *Diagnostic and statistical manual of mental disorders* (5th ed.). Arlington, VA: American Psychiatric Publishing.

Andrews, N. (2018). *What's in a name for chronic pain?* Pain Research Forum. Retrieved from https://www.painresearchforum.org/news/92059-whats-name-chronic-pain

Broglio, K., & Matzo, M. (2018). Acute pain management for people with opioid use disorder. *American Journal of Nursing, 118*(10), 4–10.

Centers for Disease Control and Prevention. (2016). *CDC guidelines for prescribing opioids for chronic pain*. Retrieved from https://www.cdc.gov/mmwr/volumes/65/rr/rr6501e1.htm

Centers for Disease Control and Prevention. (2017). *The current drug overdose epidemic in the United States: Executive Summary*. Annual Surveillance Report of Drug Related Risks and Outcomes. Retrieved from https://www.cdc.gov/drugoverdose/pdf/pubs/2017-cdc-drug-surveillance-report.pdf

Cherkin, D., Wheeler, K., Barlow, W., & Deyo, R. (1998). Medication use for low back pain in primary care. *Spine, 23*, 607–614. doi:10.1097/00007632-199803010-00015

Chou, R., Devo, R., Friedly, J., Skelly, A., Weimer, M., Fu, R., . . . Grusing, S. (2017). Systematic pharmacological therapies for low back pain: A systematic review for and American College of Physicians Clinical Practice Guideline. *Annals of Internal Medicine, 166*(7), 480–492. doi:10.7326/M16-2458

Chou, R., Fanciullo, G. J., Fine, P. G., Adler, J. A., Ballantyne, J. C., Davies, P., . . . Miaskowski, C. (2009). Clinical guidelines for the use of chronic opioid therapy in chronic noncancer pain. *The Journal of Pain, 10*(2), 113–130.e22. doi:10.1016/j.jpain.2008.10.008

Chou, R., Qaseem, A., Snow, V., Casey, D., Cross, J., Shekelle, P., & Owens, D. (2007) Diagnosis and treatment of low back pain: A joint clinical practice guidelines from the American College of Physicians and the American Pain Society. *Annals of Internal Medicine, 147*(7), 478–491. doi:10.7326/0003-4819-147-7-200710020-00006

D'Arcy, Y. (2011). *A compact clinical guide to chronic pain management*. New York, NY: Springer Publishing Company.

D'Arcy, Y., & Bruckenthal, P. (2011). *Safe prescribing for nurse practitioners*. New York, NY: Oxford University Press.

Dworkin, R., O'Connor, A., Audette, J., Baron, R., Gourlay, G., Haanpaa, M., . . . Wells, C. D. (2010). Recommendations for the pharmacological management of neuropathic pain: An overview and literature update. *Mayo Clinic Proceedings, 85*, S3–S14. doi:10.4065/mcp.2009.0649

Finnerup, N., Attai, N., Haroutounian, S., McHicol, E., Baron, R., Dworkin, R., . . . Wallace, M. (2015). Pharmacology for neuropathic pain in adults: a systematic review and meta-analysis. *Lancet, 14*(2), 162–173. doi:10.1016/S1474-4422(14)70251-0

McCarberg, B., D'Arcy, Y., Parsons, B., Sadosky, A., Thorpe, A., & Behar, R. (2016). Neuropathic pain: A review of etiology, assessment, diagnosis, and treatment. *Current Medical Research Opinion, 33*(8), 1361–1369. doi:10.1080/03007995.2017.1321532

McCarberg, B., Stanos, S., & D'Arcy, Y. (2012). *Back and neck pain*. New York, NY: Oxford University Press.

McCarberg, B. H., & Barkin, R. L. (2001). Long-acting opioids for chronic pain: Pharmacotherapeutic opportunities to enhance compliance, quality of life, and analgesia. *American Journal of Therapeutics, 8*(3), 181–186. doi:10.1097/00045391-200105000-00006

Stanos, S., Brodsky, M., Argoff, C., Clauw, D., D'Arcy, Y., Donevan, S., . . . Watt, S. (2016). Rethinking chronic pain in a primary care setting. *Postgraduate Medicine, 128*, 502–515. doi:10.1080/00325481.2016.1188319

U. S. Food and Drug Administration. (2018). *The FDA opioid analgesic REMS education blueprint for healthcare providers involved in the treatment and monitoring of patients with pain*. Retrieved from https://www.fda.gov/media/99496/download

ADDITIONAL RESOURCES

Chou, R., & Huffman, L. (2007). Medications for acute and chronic low back pain: A review of the evidence for an American Pain Society/American College of Physicians clinical practice guideline. *Annals of Internal Medicine, 147*(7), 505–514. doi:10.7326/0003-4819-147-7-200710020-00008

Johnson, M. (2019). The landscape of chronic pain: Broader perspectives. *Medicina (Kaunas), 55*(5), 182. doi:10.3390/medicina55050182

CHAPTER 7

OVER-THE-COUNTER MEDICATIONS, NONOPIOID MEDICATIONS, AND SUPPLEMENTS FOR PAIN MANAGEMENT

INTRODUCTION

When you have determined that a patient would benefit from analgesia and have identified the probable pain generators, the next task is selecting an appropriate agent from the plethora of products available, both over the counter (OTC) and by prescription (legend). There are many medication choices that can be effective for pain once the type of pain is determined. In addition, lifestyle change is one of the most fundamental interventions needed to lessen chronic pain.

Product selection begins by identifying the pain generator, determining its severity, and establishing whether it is acute or chronic. This is followed by consideration of individual patient circumstances, including comorbidities, personal preferences, financial constraints, and personal and formulary restrictions. Concern regarding the risk of addiction, now known as *opioid use disorder*, has increased the use of nonopioid medications.

CLINICAL PEARL

Before deciding on an agent, consider the patient's formulary limitations, discretionary income, and preference for allopathic or integrative approaches.

CLINICAL PEARL

Dosage ranges given are representative of what is found in the literature. It is essential, as with all medications, that the prescriber consider comorbidities, polypharmacy interactions, age, and cardiac, renal, or hepatic disease when selecting any agent and choosing a dose and duration.

Membrane stabilizers and muscle relaxants, higher dose nonsteroidal anti-inflammatory drugs (NSAIDs), and compounded medications are only available by prescription. NSAIDs, acetaminophen, and aspirin (ASA) are available OTC. Supplements are generally available OTC. Most often, patients with pain try to self-treat with something they can purchase at their local drug store. When the OTC medications fail, they seek help from their primary care provider.

OTC medications can play an important role in managing patients' pain; unfortunately, there is a belief that OTCs are safe without regard for personal circumstances or dosage/amount/duration. When asking patients about their use of OTC medications, be sure to ask what the dose is and how long the patient has used the medication.

Educational resources have been created by the U.S. Food and Drug Administration (FDA; Center for Drug Evaluation and Research, 2015), drug manufacturers (Get Relief Responsibly, n.d.), and others; see Additional Resources at the end of the chapter. You can review these websites and select materials for your patients in written or digital form or refer them specifically to the site that will address their situation.

The variety and combinations of OTC medications can be confusing and overwhelming. It is daunting to go to the grocery or drug store and try to select one medication. It is good to know what is available in your community as well as the challenges faced by people trying to navigate the choices on the shelves.

When recommending OTC drugs or supplements, use the same detail you use for legend drugs. Provide the patient with written instructions, including name of the medication, dose, side effects, frequency, and duration. Projecting a manner that reflects confidence in the recommendation will improve effectiveness. If you casually say, "You could try this," the recommendation has much less power than if you say, "Let's try this, it can be very helpful."

Combination preparations can be ordered preformulated, such as acetaminophen with caffeine (Excedrin) or ibuprofen with famotidine (Duexis). They can also be customized using a compounding pharmacy, for example, providing a personalized prescription for patients who need a specific combination or delivery method, such as a topical cream, or require medication without artificial dyes.

Many medications for pain management have black box warnings regarding use in *pregnant and older patients* as well as the drug's adverse *effects, including gastrointestinal (GI), cardiovascular, and mental health/suicide risk. Know these warnings before prescribing any drugs in the class.*

ANALGESICS

Acetaminophen (Tylenol)

Mechanism of action is unclear.

Forms: 325-mg, 500-mg tabs or caplets

Dosing: 1 to 2 caplets q4–5h prn, max 10 tabs/24 hours, do not exceed 1 g every 4 hours, or 4 g/d from all sources. Some clinicians recommend patients limit chronic use of acetaminophen to 3 g/d to protect against additional sources of acetaminophen hidden in pain and cold preparations. Provide patients with examples of these products, such as Dayquil, generic sinus medicine with pain relief, Contac, Robitussin. Be mindful of acetaminophen burden when patients are taking regular doses of prescription medication containing acetaminophen, such as Vicodin or Tylenol with codeine. For patients who use Internet resources, a list of websites with extensive information on safe OTC medications is included in the Additional Resources at the end of this chapter.

ANTI-INFLAMMATORIES

Salicylates

Aspirin

Available forms: 325-mg 500-mg tabs, 60- to 600-mg suppository

81-mg-tab dose for secondary prevention of atherosclerotic cardiovascular disease (ASCVD)

Dosing: For pain/fever 325 to 650 mg q4h prn max 4 g/d

Patients who take ASA need to be educated about side effects such as gastrointestinal bleeding or tinnitus.

Nonsteroidal Anti-Inflammatory Drugs

NSAIDs are available in many different formulations with variations in dosing and tolerability. The class effects are constant. NSAIDs have had a black box warning since 2005 regarding GI bleeding as well as renal and cardiovascular adverse effects.

The two most commonly used are ibuprofen (Advil) and naproxen (Naprosyn). They are each available OTC and in prescription strength. NSAIDs are also available as combination products (see "Combination Products" section). Recommendations for NSAIDs indicate they should be used at the lowest effective dose and for the shortest period of time. It is a good practice to inquire specifically at office visits how patients are using NSAIDs, including all types, dosage, and frequency, and to discuss any indicated changes such as decreasing dosage or stopping unsafe use (such as combining NSAIDs).

Available forms: OTC, legend, oral, topical, compounded, injectable

Mechanisms of action: All NSAIDs inhibit cyclooxygenase mediators of inflammation; Cox-2 selective inhibition (celecoxib) decreases GI side effects.

Ibuprofen (Advil, Motrin) strengths OTC: 200 mg; prescription: 400, 600, 800 mg

Forms: Oral, topical, and compounded

Dosing equivalents: Naproxen 200 mg = naproxen sodium 220 mg
naproxen 500 mg = naproxen sodium 550 mg

Naproxen sodium (OTC Aleve 220 mg)

Naproxen (Naprosyn)

Forms: 250-, 375-, 500-mg tabs

Dosing: 1 cap BID is usual dose; use the lowest effective dose for the shortest time

Diclofenac (Voltaren, Cataflam)

Prescription only

Forms: Oral, topical, compounded

Delayed-release tabs: 25-, 50-, 75-mg tabs, extended-release tabs: 100-mg tab

Dosing: Use the lowest effective dose for the shortest necessary time

For osteoarthritis (OA): 50 mg BID–TID, max 150 mg/d or 75 mg BID; extended release, 100 mg once/day

Topical gel (Voltaren), liquid (Pennsaid), patch (Flector), compounded

Diclofenac is commonly used in topical preparations, See "Topicals" section for dosing.

CLINICAL PEARL

Research continues on the safety profiles and indications for various NSAIDs. Watch for evolving recommendations and concerns.

Celecoxib (Celebrex)

Selective inhibitor of COX-2 enzymes

Dosing: 100- and 200-mg capsules 100 to 200 mg twice/day

In 2018, the FDA approved a change in guidance regarding the cardiovascular risk of celecoxib, finding 100 mg BID noninferior to naproxen and ibuprofen (Center for Drug Evaluation and Research, 2018). A retrospective analysis published in the *Journal of the American College of Cardiology (ACC)* in April 2019 recommends balancing the risks and benefits of prescribing celecoxib for elderly patients with risk factors for aortic stenosis and recommends additional study of risks (Bowler, Raddatz, Johnson, Lindman, & Merryman, 2019).

Ketorolac (Acular), *the only intravenous (IV) NSAID,* is indicated only for moderately severe acute pain. Ketorolac can be useful when a patient needs immediate relief. It is not indicated for minor or chronic pain. Remember that the cardiovascular and renal side effects common to all NSAIDs are the same with intramuscular (IM)/IV dosing. *Administration of ketorolac is contraindicated for patients currently receiving ASA or NSAIDs.*

Dosage: 10-mg tabs; prefilled syringe 60 mg/2 mL (IM/IV), use the lowest effective dose. You will not get any additional pain relief if a dose above 30 mg is used; there is only more risk for side effects above this dose (American Pain Society [APS], 2008).

CLINICAL PEARL

Consult the package insert for specific black box warnings specific to ketorolac before prescribing. Use is limited to 5 days following IM/IV dosing.

Steroids

Methylprednisolone (Medrol Dose Pack)
The ultimate anti-inflammatory, steroids should only be used when benefits clearly outweigh the risks. Although they can provide dramatic relief, it is important to consider the risk of potential adverse effects and to have a plan of use. The Medrol Dose Pack provides methylprednisolone as 4-mg tablets in a packet with a built-in taper. This decreases the problems that occur with prolonged use of a steroid and simplifies instructions for the patient.

Writing on the use of steroids as adjunct for pain in palliative care, Vyvey (2010) describes the use of steroids as adjunct for pain in palliative care as based primarily on expert opinion and empirical evidence. It may be tempting to reach for the dose pack for its temporary impact. Before prescribing though, consider alternative treatments and have a plan for what you will do next. Would the patient benefit from a local steroid injection rather than the dose pack or perhaps a different oral medication?

Precautions: Advise patients about potential sleep disruption or mood changes as well as elevation of blood sugars secondary to steroid use, so that the patient is prepared for these.

CLINICAL PEARL

If a patient requires a steroid, what is the next step in the plan? Take this seriously and use the drug thoughtfully.

Supplements

A wide variety of anti-inflammatory supplements is available in many forms: food, oral capsules, powders, and topicals. The use of supplements of various types is increasing and it is very likely that most of your patients have tried a supplement. Ask each patient what supplements he or she has tried and what he or she currently uses. Supplement-drug interactions can occur and need to be considered when prescribing. Medscape has an online drug–OTC–supplement interaction tool (Drug Interaction Checker, n.d.).

Glucosamine with or without chondroitin and curcumin are two very commonly used supplements, for example.

Glucosamine with or without chondroitin

Glucosamine and chondroitin are components of cartilage that are used as supplements to decrease pain; there is evidence that they also impact progression of joint space narrowing. Glucosamine sulfate with or without chondroitin sulfate has been demonstrated to be safe and to decrease OA pain in the knee and to stop progression of joint space narrowing. There is no evidence of impact on OA of the lumbar spine (Gaby, 2017). Glucosamine sulfate has been found to be more consistently useful than glucosamine hydrochloride; this may account for differences in clinical studies. There is variability in the amount of active ingredient in supplement brands; consider these factors if a patient is not responding. Some people may see improvement in a few weeks, whereas others may require 6 months to show benefit (Rakel, 2018).

Dosage: Glucosamine sulfate 500 mg TID, chondroitin sulfate 400 mg two to three times/day

Precautions: Potential reaction to glucosamine in patients with shellfish allergy

Curcumin (active ingredient in turmeric): This is used worldwide for healing, cooking, and ceremonies. Turmeric has antioxidant and anti-inflammatory properties. As the plant turmeric, it has been used for 4,000 years. It has been extensively studied and declared "Generally Regarded as Safe (GRAS)" by the FDA. You may be surprised how many of your patients have tried it or are using it.

Dose: Available as a supplement in combination or alone (Meriva, CuraPro, Curaphen, Turmeric), the root of turmeric is used in several cultures for cooking. It is available as a supplement (curcumin) and as a spice (turmeric), both powdered and whole root. Curcumin has low bioavailability; this is improved with addition of piperine (black pepper).

Dosage: A dose of 500 mg four times/day or 1,000 mg twice/day is commonly used (Rakel, 2018).

Precautions: It is possible that high doses of curcumin may be antithrombotic; caution patients who take anticoagulants (Kim, Ku, & Bae, 2012).

MUSCLE RELAXANTS

Used for relief of pain associated with muscle spasm, all muscle relaxants can cause sedation; patient response will vary. As with any potentially sedating medication, initiate therapy when patients can be at home and are not responsible for others, like small children, and do not drive or perform potentially hazardous activities until they know how they will respond to the medication. Some people can only tolerate muscle relaxants at night, but find them very helpful in providing the relief needed for sleep.

Forms available: Oral tablets and capsules, topical

Metaxalone (Skelaxin): 400-, 800-mg scored tablets three to four times/day

Generally less sedating than cyclobenzaprine or tizanidine

Tizanidine (Zanaflex): 2-, 4-mg tabs (generic); 2-, 4-, 6-mg capsules (branded)

Dose: 2 to 8 mg one to three times/day. Maximum daily dose is 36 mg. Individualize dosing. Tizanidine can cause drowsiness, with severity varying patient to patient. Some people cannot tolerate daytime dosing; others are able to take a low dose during the day and a higher dose at night.

Precautions: Start low and titrate up as tolerated/needed; have the patient begin the medication at night when there is no need to drive. Some patients prefer to take tizanidine when they are already in bed.

Cyclobenzaprine (Flexeril): 5-, 10-mg tablets; compounded topical

Precautions: Some patients find this drug very sedating; have the patient start at night when there is no need to drive. Sedation or dry mouth may be intolerable for some patients. Structurally related to tricyclic antidepressants (TCAs), it is contraindicated with monoamine oxidase inhibitors (MAOIs), and may cause serotonin syndrome.

Dose: 5 to 10 mg up to TID

CLINICAL PEARL

Do not prescribe carisoprodol (Soma). If a patient who presents is taking it, advise the patient you will not prescribe it and gradually taper them off of it.

See Box 7.1 for information on managing patients taking carisoprodol (Soma).

BOX 7.1

MANAGEMENT OF PATIENTS TAKING CARISOPRODOL

In the past, many patients were given the muscle relaxant carisoprodol (Soma), which is now a Schedule IV Controlled Substance. Patients taking carisoprodol may develop sedation over time due to the primary metabolite, the tranquilizer meprobamate. Do not abruptly discontinue use of carisoprodol; taper gradually and monitor the patient. Seek consultation with a pain-management or addiction specialist if needed.

MEDICATIONS FOR NEUROPATHIC PAIN

Gabapentinoids/Antiepileptic Drugs

Dizziness, drowsiness, and sedation are the class effects of antiepileptic drugs (AEDs). Titrate up when starting and taper down when discontinuing. Mental fogginess frequently impacts dose tolerance.

Gabapentin and pregabalin impact voltage-gated calcium channels in the central nervous system (CNS) and are widely used off label for neuropathic pain

(Dworkin et al., 2007). The Canadian Pain Society's revised consensus statement 2014 on neuropathic pain recommends gabapentinoids, TCAs, and serotonin–norepinephrine reuptake inhibitors (SNRIs) as the first-line treatment with cannabinoids as the third-line treatment for neuropathic pain (Moulin et al., 2014).

Pregabalin and gabapentin are both available as oral capsules; gabapentin is also used in compounded topical preparations. Apart from their wide use in treating neuropathic pain, Tomic et al. suggest that AEDs have an anti-inflammatory effect in addition to the known neuropathic benefit, and that using AEDs in combination with other medications will have synergistic benefits (Tomić, Pecikoza, Micov, Vučković, & Stepanović-Petrović, 2018). Gabapentin or pregabalin can improve quality of life for patients with lumbar stenosis (Bansal et al., 2016; Takahashi et al., 2014).

As indicated, AEDs can be sedating; start low and go slow and go lower and start slower with older patients. Use a written titration schedule. Gabapentin has nonlinear kinetics, with *bioavailability decreasing as the dose increases.* Pregabalin has consistent bioavailability across doses.

Gabapentin is a scheduled drug in some states, whereas pregabalin is a Drug Enforcement Administration (DEA, 2017) Schedule V drug.

Gabapentin (Neurontin)

This drug is indicated for neuropathic pain. Start doses at night. Caution patient about possible dizziness/drowsiness. Dosing must be *individualized for each patient for efficacy and tolerance.*

Forms: 100-, 300-, 400-mg hard-shell capsules; 600-, 800-mg scored tablets; solution 50 mg/mL

Topical compounded preparation: Begin with hs dosing; some patients may only tolerate 100 mg at hs to start. Evaluate cognitive impact and increase dosage as tolerated/needed using the lowest effective dose.

There are two challenges with prescribing gabapentin: side-effect tolerance and determining the effective dose for each patient. It may take time for the patient to tolerate dosage increases, requiring patience in both prescriber and patient.

The nonlinear pharmacokinetics of gabapentin mean that the patient shows less effect as doses increase. At 1,200 mg/d in three divided doses, bioavailability drops to <50% and continues to decrease with higher dosages (Bockbrader et al., 2010).

Dosage for neuropathic pain: 300 to 1,200 mg TID, max 3,600 mg/d; taper when discontinuing

Pregabalin (Lyrica)

Pregabalin in generic form was approved in July 2019.

Forms: 25, 50, 75, 100, 150, 200, 225, and 300 mg

Dosing is individualized. Approved dosing: Begin with 150 mg/d in divided doses; some clinicians begin with 50 mg BID if tolerated. Start with the first dose in the evening in case of drowsiness. Speed of dosage titration will depend on patient's pain and cognitive response. Some patients report distal swelling. Taper when discontinuing.

- Diabetic neuropathy: 50 to 100 mg TID max 600 mg/d; doses over 300 mg/d increase adverse effect risk with unlikely benefit
- Fibromyalgia 150 to 225 mg BID; max 450 mg/d

It is not unusual for payers to require failure of gabapentin before authorizing pregabalin.

Supplements

Magnesium

Magnesium is a macromineral that is essential in over 300 chemical reactions, including transmembrane ion movements and enzymatic reactions. Most people are deficient in magnesium and benefit from supplementation. Magnesium impacts calcium channels and (N-methyl-D-aspartate NMDA) receptors, decreasing hypersensitivity. With good potential for positively impacting chronic pain, expanded use of this safe and useful mineral continues (Kirkland, Sarlo, & Holton, 2018).

Forms: Capsules, tablets, and powder for oral use; Epsom salt (magnesium sulfate) for use in bath solution and topical oil

Magnesium citrate stimulates bowel function and can be useful for patients with constipation; if patients tend toward loose stools, a different salt is indicated. Magnesium glycinate is well absorbed and tolerated. Magnesium taurate is also well tolerated. Magnesium has few adverse effects. Dosage can be limited by bowel tolerance. As with any medication, use caution when prescribing for patients with renal disease. An Epsom-salt bath or foot bath at hs can be relaxing, and also provides magnesium, which is absorbed transdermally.

Local Anesthetic

Lidocaine (Lidoderm): Used topically, lidocaine inhibits nerve impulse conduction. The only FDA-approved use of Lidoderm is for postherpetic neuralgia. Topical *lidocaine* (4%) is used by patients and clinicians for a variety of neuropathic and joint complaints.

Forms: Prescription (5% Lidoderm, lidocaine patch, lidocaine ointment), compounded

OTC (4% lidocaine: Salonpas, Aspercreme): Also available as ointment and roll-on.

ANTIDEPRESSANTS

All medications in this group carry a black box warning for suicidality.

Tricyclic Antidepressants (TCAs)

TCAs impact pain through reuptake of norepinephrine.

Class effect adverse reactions include dry mouth, sedation, blurred vision, angle closure glaucoma, urinary retention, and cardiovascular effects.

CLINICAL PEARL

Avoid all TCAs in older patients due to their high anticholinergic profile as well as risk for sedation and orthostatic hypotension.

Source: From 2019 American Geriatrics Society Beers Criteria® Update Expert Panel. (2019). American Geriatrics Society 2019 updated AGS Beers Criteria® for potentially inappropriate medication use in older adults. *Journal of the American Geriatrics Society, 67*(4), 674–694. doi:10.1111/jgs.15767

All TCAs require dose titration.

Amitriptyline (Elavil): There are adverse cardiovascular effects and drug interactions to amitriptyline. In 2015, a Cochrane review found that amitriptyline provides 25% more relief than placebo and 25% of people will have an adverse effect (Moore, Derry, Aldington, Cole, & Wiffen, 2015). Serious cardiovascular reactions include orthostatic hypotension, hypertension, arrhythmias, QT prolongation, and myocardial infarction (MI).

Nortriptyline (Pamelor): Begin with 10 to 25 mg at hs, titrate to effective dose (50–150 mg) (APS, 2008).

Desipramine (Norpramin): Begin with 25 mg/d, titrate to effective dose (50–150 mg) (APS, 2008).

Dosage: 10-, 25-, 50-, 75-, 100-, and 150-mg tabs

It can take 2 to 6 weeks to see the impact of amitriptyline. Give at hs. Start low and titrate up as needed and tolerated.

CLINICAL PEARL

Duloxetine, Celexa, and venlafaxine decrease neuropathic pain through an increase in serotonin and norepinephrine levels by decreasing reuptake.

Serotonin–Norepinephrine Reuptake Inhibitors

2019 Beers Criteria Update: Avoid SNRIs in patients with history of fall or fracture (AGS, 2019).

Duloxetine (Cymbalta)

Dosage forms: 20, 30, 60 mg caps

Start at 20 to 30 mg/d for a week, may increase up to 60 mg/d as needed/tolerated. Recommended dose for neuropathic pain, fibromyalgia, chronic musculoskeletal pain: 60 mg/d. Cochrane review 2014 found 60 mg of duloxetine to be useful for neuropathy and fibromyalgia (Lunn, Hughes, & Wiffen, 2014).

Venlafaxine (Effexor)

Venlafaxine has a dose-dependent effect. Serotonin dominates at a lower dose and the effect of norepinephrine is seen at higher doses. Norepinephrine is the likely component that impacts neuropathic pain.

Forms: Tabs of 25, 37.5, 50, 75, 100 mg

Begin with 37.5 mg once or twice a day. Titrate up over 4 to 6 weeks; increase by 75 mg/wk; max dose 225 mg (Dworkin et al., 2007). Use with caution in patients with cardiac disease (risk of cardiac conduction abnormality and hypertension). Gradually reduce dose when discontinuing to avoid withdrawal. Dosing over 150 mg provides a greater norepinephrine effect, so a higher dose may be more effective; note that it also carries more side effects.

Side effects: Nausea, diaphoresis, and headache

Selective Serotonin Reuptake Inhibitor

Citalopram (Celexa)

Forms: 10, 20, 40 mg tablets; start with 10 to 20 mg/d; effective dose is 20 to 40 mg/d (APS, 2008).

TOPICALS

Capsaicin

Form: OTC topical cream—0.025%, 0.075%, 0.1% cream (found in many branded products: Zostrix, Therapatch warm, Pain Enz)

Used for 2 weeks, capsaicin restructures C fiber transmission of pain, decreasing the transmission potential.

Apply up to four times/day; avoid broken or irritated skin, *do not contact mucous membranes.* Avoid occlusive dressings.

Diclofenac

Diclofenac gel (Voltaren gel): Available in branded and generic form, 1% gel; 2 g QID, max 8 g/joint/d up to 32 g/d total; do not apply to broken skin. Gel has up to 10% systemic absorption.

Diclofenac patch 1.3% (Flector patch): Apply one patch BID; minimal systemic absorption

Diclofenac with dimethyl sulfoxide (DMSO) (Pennsaid) solution: 1.5%, 2%; apply to knee two sprays 2% solution or 40 drops 1.5% solution per knee QID; avoid occlusive dressings; solution has up to 6% absorption

Also available in various OTC preparations that include 4% lidocaine, with or without menthols, in patches and ointments

Lidocaine

Prescription Lidocaine 5% (Lidoderm); Only approved by the FDA for postherpetic neuralgia; extensive off-label use for neuropathy and joint pain

Dosing is 12 hours on, 12 hours off. Advise patients not to use the patch to participate in an activity that would be limited by pain, but to use it after they have been active; this is a great opportunity to discuss when pain can be useful to limit injury. Some people with sensitivity to adhesives may not tolerate the patch. See "Compounding" section for information on compounded topical preparations.

The proliferation of OTC pain patches reflects manufacturers' response to the market for effective pain relief and also illustrates the challenges faced in choosing OTC products. Many different formulations are marketed with similar names. Advise patients to read labels carefully and provide handouts or access to websites offering information.

A few examples of what patients may find when searching store aisles for pain relief: Aspercreme and Salonpas patches contain 4% lidocaine. Salonpas also makes a pain-relief patch that contains 10% menthol salicylate and 3% menthol. Icy Hot contains 4% lidocaine + 1% menthol.

The prescription Lidoderm patch is FDA approved for postherpetic neuralgia, but has been used widely with varying efficacy for multiple other complaints. When Lidoderm patches are not an option due to high copays or insurance denials, at 4%, the OTC form offers a useful alternative.

CLINICAL PEARL

Always dispose of any patch, OTC medication, or prescription with care. Keep away from children and pets. Any patch can have residual active ingredients that can be harmful.

COMBINATION PRODUCTS: COMPOUNDED AND PRESCRIPTION

OTC Combinations

Remember to consider total acetaminophen and NSAID burden, and to remind patients to monitor this, especially during cold-and-flu season.

NSAIDs, ASA, and acetaminophen are available in countless OTC branded products alone or combined with antihistamines and decongestants (Tylenol Cold Max, Sudafed PE, Excedrin Migraine, Motrin, Tylenol). Remind patients that similar product names can contain different active ingredients, and it is *essential to read labels* on the back of the package.

Prescription Combinations

NSAID–GI protector combinations carry the NSAID black box warning for cardiovascular (CV) and GI side effects.

Two products decrease the risk of gastric ulcer: famotidine (an H2 blocker) and esomeprazole (proton-pump inhibitor [PPI]).

Consider all risks and benefits as well as possible alternatives when prescribing combination drugs. Use only if necessary and for the shortest possible time. For localized joint pain, a topical NSAID could provide more benefit with less risk than an oral NSAID. To decrease gastric risk, consider acetaminophen as an alternative to an NSAID. Engaging in physical therapy (PT) to improve strength and function can also decrease the need for NSAIDs.

Ibuprofen/famotidine (Duexis): Contains 800 mg of ibuprofen and 26.6 mg of famotidine) in coated tablets

Dose: 1 tab TID

Naproxen/esomeprazole (Vimovo): Contains 375 mg of naproxen and 20 mg of esomeprazole or 500 mg of naproxen and 20 mg of esomeprazole in delayed-release tablets

Dose: 1 tab BID at least 30 minutes before a meal

Compounded

All compounded medications require a prescription regardless of content. Compounded medications have not been reviewed or approved by the FDA and use is off label.

The FDA describes *compounding* as a practice in which a licensed pharmacist, a licensed physician, or a person under the supervision of a licensed pharmacist combines, mixes, or alters ingredients of a drug to create a medication tailored to the needs of an individual patient. The FDA states that although compounded drugs can serve an important medical need for certain patients, they also present a risk to patients (Center for Drug Evaluation and Research, 2019). It is important to remember that any prescription or supplement prescribed or recommended presents risks and benefits.

The FDA has regulations addressing compounded medications, but the medications are not FDA approved; however, substances used by compounding pharmacies are of pharmaceutical grade. The FDA website has resources on regulations and guidelines regarding compounding (Center for Drug Evaluation and Research, 2019).

Compounded medications can be very effective and require the same care be taken in dosing frequency and concentration as other legend drugs. These drugs are available through compounding pharmacies, which may be local or accessible online.

CLINICAL PEARL

Compounded medications are generally not covered by insurance.

As indicated, compounding allows the use of individualized formulas to meet specific patient needs. Compounding pharmacists have special training in formulation and utilization of compounded medications and may be able to provide medications in a format tolerated by patients who cannot use standard oral-dosing forms. For pain management, compounded medications can be used topically to combine multiple agents with different mechanisms of action. Diclofenac, ibuprofen, ketamine, gabapentin, lidocaine, and others may be used in different concentrations and combinations. To safely use compounded medications, you must know the mechanism of action of each agent as well as dosing recommendations. If you choose to use compounded medication, establish a relationship with a compounding pharmacist whom you can trust as a resource on options, including medication options and carriers. Ask questions, consult with and discuss patient needs with the pharmacist. Ask the pharmacist for guidance regarding the base of the formula if you have any questions. There are multiple carriers available to make topical preparations; the characteristics of the carrier have an impact on the absorption rate and total available medication.

Understand the effects of the various components in the compounded medication suggested; you are responsible for knowing the characteristics of the base which carries the medication and the active components, including sensitivities and interactions. Understand the indications for various topical components base for carriers. The compounding pharmacist can help with this.

CLINICAL PEARL

Provide an environment in which patients feel safe sharing information about anything they use for pain or other health applications.

MISCELLANEOUS

It is important to know everything that patients use to manage their pain and other health concerns. Some things are benign, others dangerous, and others may be providing significant benefit.

If a patient reports doing or ingesting something you are not familiar with, maintain a nonjudgmental position and explain that you cannot advise the patient on how this may interact with what you prescribe, and that you will need to check it out. Take the time to investigate for your own edification and to determine whether something presents a risk or benefit for the patient.

Some products develop popular use before their adoption by medical science. Patients may decide to use these products without consulting their clinicians, or may request a prescription for a substance you are not familiar with. Kratom and cannabis have been used by patients for pain management without prescription for years. Low-dose naltrexone (LDN) has been used off label for pain management as well. As a compounded medication, it requires a prescription. It is gaining in popularity, and you may have patients who request it.

Treatments based on using plants have different characteristics from chemicals formulated for legend drugs. You will see complex interactions that may or may not be evident until more research is done. This is currently the situation with cannabis. LDN is similarly complex; understanding of mechanisms of action is evolving. Using low doses of naltrexone can have an immune-modulating effect working on the innate immune system. Could the impact be due to targeting an underlying mechanism that we poorly understand? This could be what is going on when it is so helpful for some people with multiple sclerosis (MS), fibromyalgia, and migraine, yet does not help others. LDN is also being researched for cancer treatment; more information will follow.

Kratom

The FDA has not approved kratom for any use; the DEA lists it as a drug and chemical of concern (DEA, 2017).

Kratom is a tropical tree grown in South East Asia; its leaves are purchased by patients over the Internet. The FDA and the DEA continue to investigate kratom and have issued warnings regarding its use. It is considered an opioid by the FDA and is not recognized as a supplement (Veltri & Grundmann, 2019). It is an addictive sedative that can cause hallucinations, delusion, and confusion.

Some patients report that it is very effective for managing their pain or mitigating withdrawal symptoms. There are risks of herb–drug interactions, which will not appear in online interaction checkers.

Cannabinoids

Studies demonstrate positive benefits of cannabinoids in managing pain (Vučković, Srebro, Vujović, Vučetić, & Prostran, 2018), with mixed opinions among researchers regarding methodology and outcomes.

"The endocannabinoid system (ECS) is a widespread neuromodulatory system that plays important roles in CNS development, synaptic plasticity, and the response to endogenous and environmental insults" (Lu & Mackie, 2016). This is a complex system with multiple feedback loops; understanding the effects of various components of the ECS is evolving.

CB1 and CB2 are cannabinoid receptors. CB1 receptors are located primarily in the CNS, whereas CB2 receptors are primarily peripheral and impact the immune system (Alger, 2013). The effect of ingestion of exogenous cannabinoids (THC and CBD) is due to their impact on the endogenous ECS.

As a natural plant-derived product, cannabis contains many active substances with complex molecular and submolecular structures (terpenes). The cannabis plant contains 80 to 100 exogenous cannabinoids, and the most well known are THC and CBD.

Cannabis (Marijuana and Hemp)

Marijuana is classified by the DEA as a Class I Controlled Substance. Confusion about differences between hemp and marijuana continues. The 2018 Farm Bill legalized the growing of hemp, which is defined as *Cannabis sativa* with <0.03% tetrahydrocannabinol (THC).

Marijuana, which can also be called *weed, pot, dope,* or *cannabis*, refers to the dried flowers and leaves of the cannabis plant. It contains mind-altering (psychoactive) compounds like THC, as well as other active compounds like cannabidiol (CBD) that are not mind altering (Centers for Disease Control and Prevention [CDC], 2018).

Patients have used cannabis to address pain for many years. It remains a Schedule I drug federally, but many states now allow medical and/or recreational use of marijuana. Attitudes toward and use of THC and CBD are rapidly evolving as science progresses and regulations change. You may or may not choose to recommend CBD or cannabis in some form. If you do or do not recommend it, you will have patients who use it; therefore, you will need to understand how it works as well as local laws and derive a plan for how you will approach the use of cannabis products.

This agricultural product is being used by a diverse set of people for a wide range of effects. As a plant-based product, it has many interacting compounds that impact each consumer differently; epigenetic metabolic pathways and physiology of types of pain likely result in a high degree of variability in response. Plant pharmacology does not exist in a one-component vacuum; interrelationships among components are part of what makes cannabis effective.

Research is ongoing from multiple perspectives; more data accumulates each month. An open and thoughtful approach using critical analysis is needed to separate fact from myth when interpreting this data. How the plant material is processed, individual epigenetic metabolic pathways, and type of pain are some of the variables to consider. Ultimately, *you are responsible for what you prescribe or recommend to patients.* Support your patients with science-based information and discuss their personal choices.

Popular use, science, and myth about cannabis confuse the situation. There is conflicting information regarding CBD and THC, and conflicting state and local laws make cannabis complicated. Cannabinoids have been reported to impact pain, and many patients are trying CBD products in all forms, with varying effects and success.

Evidence and policy will continue to change; stay up to date on current federal and state laws. The National Council of State Boards of Nursing (NCSBN) and the Federation of State Medical Boards (FSMB) have published guidelines on the use of medical marijuana (FSMB, 2016).

FDA-Approved Products (Epidolex)

Most THC and CBD products are accessed independently by patients OTC. There is only one FDA-approved CBD product, Epidolex. It is CBD that is 99% pure and contains no other cannabinoids; it is approved for treatment of specific childhood seizure disorders. Other preparations are available internationally, and clinical trials are underway in the United States. Dronabinol (Marinol) is a synthetic THC and a Schedule III Controlled Substance. It is FDA approved for nausea and vomiting associated with chemotherapy, and anorexia associated with weight loss in patients with AIDS.

THC and CBD

There is discussion of the impact of various molecules on each other for positive synergy or to mitigate adverse effects (also known as the entourage effect).

The interactions and efficacy of THC and CBD are not fully understood; the science is evolving. Patient response will vary among different products, sources, and routes of administration (Box 7.2). Drug–herb interactions exist, including potential sedation. Check potential interactions when prescribing any medication for patients using cannabis products (Drug Interaction Checker, n.d.). Because of the perceived efficacy and popularity of THC and CBD, many research studies

BOX 7.2

DRUG INTERACTIONS WITH THC AND CBD

As THC and CBD are used more widely, adverse effects and interactions are being reported. In January 2019, Damkier et al. (2019) described a case report of edible cannabis *increasing international normalized ratio (INR) values over 10* in a patient with a mechanical heart valve on warfarin. The *Medscape* drug supplement interaction checker (Drug Interaction Checker, n.d.) is a source of information on known interactions.

CBD, cannabidiol; THC, tetrahydrocannabinol.

are being conducted on them. These studies offer increasing understanding of the individual components of the plants, but this is still in its infancy.

Tetrahydrocannabinol

Analyzing data recorded in the RELEAF app between June 2016 and October 2018, Li et al. reviewed patient reports of the effectiveness of THC. Patients reported an average pain reduction of 3 points on a 10-point scale, with use of whole flowers being the most effective. Higher THC levels were associated with increased pain relief and more side effects. CBD was not associated with pain relief (Li et al., 2019).

Precautions: The study of THC became more complicated when multiple vaping illnesses and deaths occurred in 2019. THC has been associated with 1,604 cases of e-cigarette or vaping-use associated lung injury (EVALI) and 34 confirmed deaths in the United States as of October 22, 2019 (CDC, 2019).

Because of the strong correlation with the use of vaping products that contain THC, the CDC recommends using no vaping products that contain THC, and until specific causes of deaths are determined, not to consider using any vaping products.

Cannabidiol

CBD is available from multiple sources; purity and quality will vary. It can be hard to know whether CBD comes from hemp or marijuana.

CBD forms: Edibles, topicals, cosmetics, tinctures, inhalants, drops, or sprays; OTC CBD mixtures vary and purity of cannabinoids differs.

CLINICAL PEARL

Look at cannabis' activity through the lens of a biologist. Cannabinoid pathways are being studied, and there are likely additional feedback loops and synergies that are not yet understood.

Low-Dose Naltrexone

Use is off label. Low-dose naltrexone (LDN) is not FDA approved. *Information in this chapter is for general information only and should not be used for prescribing purposes. If you wish to prescribe LDN, education or consultation with someone experienced in the use of LDN are needed.*

Action: LDN impacts the immune response via action on toll-like receptors (TLR) and opioid receptors and by other unclear mechanisms.

LDN is used in doses of 1.0 to 4.5 mg/d, profoundly less than the 50 mg of naltrexone dose used to reverse the effect of opioids. People worldwide have reported using it *off label* with success for neuropathic pain, and your patients may ask for it. LDN has been generally found to be a safe medication, *but it will cause withdrawal symptoms if given to a patient taking opioids.* If you choose to prescribe LDN, you will need to study its unique characteristics and dosing fully. Younger, Parkitny, and McLain (2014) postulate that LDN may be a glial cell modulator, with anti-inflammatory effects in the CNS, and that although early studies are promising and many patients report benefit, more research is needed.

In preliminary studies, Younger and colleagues have found LDN to be effective in managing fibromyalgia and reducing inflammation (Younger, Noor, McCue, & Mackey, 2013; Younger et al., 2014). The *LDN Book* provides an overview of the pharmacology and current understanding of the efficacy of LDN.

LDN is a unique substance that has multiple modes of action. It is only available from compounding pharmacies. It can be taken orally or transdermally. If GI upset occurs, this may be corrected by using a liposomal form. The Boston Veterans Affairs (VA) is currently conducting a clinical trial of LDN for osteoarthritis and inflammatory arthritis (VA Office of Research and Development, 2020). Because this medication is gaining popularity with patients, your patients may ask you for LDN to treat for multiple conditions, including for pain management.

Response to this medication is individual and requires careful mindful titration. Prescribing requires an individualized approach. Dosage is 0.5 to 4.5 mg, titrated to individual patient response. It will cause *withdrawal if the patient is taking opioids,* so it cannot be used with opioids. As stated, this dose is not commercially manufactured and must be ordered from a compounding pharmacy.

LIFESTYLE CHANGE: THE MOST COST-EFFECTIVE OTC REMEDY

Lifestyle changes, including better sleep, movement, food, and mind–body practices, can impact pain and quality of life. Sleep research supports emphasizing restorative sleep as an important component of pain management. Supporting positive lifestyle change is a key component of any pain-management plan.

Sleep

Inadequate sleep contributes to many comorbidities; helping patients to get enough good-quality sleep can be a challenge in primary care. Taking the time to improve sleep without use of prescription hypnotics can improve quality of life and potentially decrease the need for OTC or prescription medication.

We frequently encounter patients who cannot sleep because of pain. Researchers are finding that lack of sleep causes increased pain, resulting in patients moving in a cycle that can be challenging to reverse.

A study of healthy young men demonstrated that sleep deprivation enhances pain responsivity and blunts areas that modulate pain (Krause, Prather, Wager, Lindquist, & Walker, 2019). Finan, Goodin, and Smith (2013) found that sleep impairments reliably predict new incidents and exacerbations of chronic pain and suggest that sleep impairments are a stronger, more reliable predictor of pain than pain is of sleep impairments.

Strategies to improve sleep include the following (Walker, 2018):

- Sleep hygiene should be followed, that is, establish a routine that includes a consistent bedtime and stopping use of all screens and monitors 2 hours before going to bed.
- If you must use the phone or computer, use a blue light filter.
- Sleep in a cool room.
- Avoid caffeine during the afternoon and alcohol before bed.
- Taking a warm bath in the evening can also be sleep promoting.

CLINICAL PEARL

Tincture of time and lifestyle changes are important and cost-effective OTC interventions. Provide patients with information on how to use them.

SUMMARY

As the demand for nonopioid approaches to managing chronic pain increases, it is important to stay current on research and determine risks and benefits of all medications. Medications can provide pain relief to support patients as they heal; the impact of medication can be increased by adding exercise and movement.

Individualized therapy is needed for all pain management. Many factors impact optimal therapy, and they range from helpful to harmful. Opioids may be the safest medication choice for one person and contraindicated for another. No medication or supplement is always good or always bad.

Be Sure Patients Know How to Choose and Use Medication Safely

- Be mindful of all possible sources of medication/supplements in anything they take.
- Give precise instruction on how to take medications.
- Give instruction on how long it will take to see effects and possible adverse effects.
- Know drug interactions.
- Know the risks and benefits of OTC medications.
- Know how to read labels, including looking at not only the brand name on the front, but also the ingredients on the back. Read manufacturer dosing instructions. Be alert for duplication of substances in different medications. Note how much medication is in each tablet and how many tablets/dose have to be taken.
- Supplements may have slower onset and longer lasting impact than prescribed medications.
- Titration schedule: Have preformatted handouts ready for medications that require titration, for example, tizanidine, gabapentin, pregabalin.

Key factors that impact selection of agents to manage pain include:

- Cost to the patient
- Patient age
- Comorbidities
- Type of pain

- Addiction risk
- Sedation potential and risk depending on patient occupation and social situation

NSAIDs carry the risk of GI bleed, hypertension, as well as renal and hepatic compromise. They can be effective, and do not impact the mental status, but oral NSAIDs are high risk, and alternatives should be considered.

Be sure patients are aware of how to safely use acetaminophen, especially what the the maximum safe daily dose is for them as well as the risks of hidden sources. Use published tools to educate patients, and advise them to err on the side of caution.

Start low and go slow with membrane stabilizers and some muscle relaxants, which can be sedating. Use caution when prescribing potentially sedating medication for older patients who are at increased risk of falls and other complications.

Human biology and psychosocial factors are complex. Despite scientific advances, there is much we do not understand. Keep this in mindand hear what the patient has to say. Use your best judgment, informed by experience and education with respect to the body's capacity to heal, as you provide care for patients with big and small problems.

In primary care, it is useful to have a menu of medications useful for each type of pain that you see, with a safety profile that can be managed in the primary care environment. Know the potential adverse effects of drug classes and specific medications.

TRENDING IN PAIN MANAGEMENT

- Use of new agents and off-label use of existing agents to manage pain is emerging.
- Research is being done on new targets for pain medication; there is promising research on peptides and monoclonal antibodies.
- Use of liposomal formulations to enhance tolerability and absorption of oral medications will expand.
- Research and therapies based on inflammatory pathways, autoimmune responses, and the innate immune system will increase.
- There will be ongoing research and changes in regulations regarding uses of cannabis/THC/CBD products.
- Very low-dose naltrexone (VLDN) is being studied to replace or decrease the need for opioids.

CASE STUDY

Rafael is a 55-year-old accountant. He played sports in high school and college. He works at a computer 10 hours/day, goes to the gym once or twice a month, and practices judo twice per week. Last week, during his judo practice, he injured his knee; pain was so severe that he went to urgent care. X-rays of the knee demonstrated moderate degenerative joint disease without fracture. He was given tramadol # 10 and advised to follow up with primary care.

He presents for follow-up today and reports that his knee pain is better (5/10). He found the tramadol helpful, but would like to avoid pain medication. He has been taking ibuprofen four capsules three to four times/day with the tramadol. Last dose of tramadol was 2 days ago.

- To avoid the systemic side effects of NSAIDs, you prescribe diclofenac gel (Voltaren) applied to the knee two to three times/day.
- If he does not have coverage for diclofenac, an OTC lidocaine patch could provide relief. You instruct him to use the lidocaine patch hs or during the day at work and not to use the patch during workouts as the knee pain can be protective during a workout. You also advise him to limit his activity to avoid stress on the joint. He can apply the patch at night to provide relief/facilitate rest.
- Recommend glucosamine 500 mg TID, advising him that it may take weeks or months to notice the effect, and that in addition to providing pain relief for OA, it may prevent progression of his degenerative joint disease.
- Rafael uses turmeric in his diet, and you encourage him to continue, reminding him that absorption is increased when turmeric is combined with black pepper.
- You prescribe PT—a regular therapeutic exercise program for core stability and strengthening of the knee—reinforcing the importance of PT.
- You ask Rafael to return in a month for follow-up.

REFERENCES

Alger, B. E. (2013). Getting high on the endocannabinoid system. *Cerebrum: The Dana Forum on Brain Science, 2013*, 14. Retrieved from https://www.ncbi.nlm.nih.gov/pubmed/24765232

American Pain Society. (2008). *Principles of analgesic use in the treatment of acute and cancer pain*. Glenview, IL: Author.

Bansal, S., Lubelski, D., Thompson, N. R., Shah, A. A., Mazanec, D. J., Benzel, E. C., & Khalaf, T. (2016). Membrane-stabilizing agents improve quality-of-life outcomes for patients with lumbar stenosis. *Global Spine Journal, 6*(2), 139–146. doi:10.1055/s-0035-1557144

Bockbrader, H. N., Wesche, D., Miller, R., Chapel, S., Janiczek, N., & Burger, P. (2010). A comparison of the pharmacokinetics and pharmacodynamics of pregabalin and gabapentin. *Clinical Pharmacokinetics, 49*(10), 661–669. doi:10.2165/11536200-000000000-00000

Bowler, M. A., Raddatz, M. A., Johnson, C. L., Lindman, B. R., & Merryman, W. D. (2019). Celecoxib is associated with dystrophic calcification and aortic valve stenosis. *JACC: Basic to Translational Science, 4*(2), 135–143. doi:10.1016/j.jacbts.2018.12.003

Center for Drug Evaluation and Research. *Educational resources: Understanding over-the-counter medicine*. U.S. Food and Drug Administration, FDA. Retrieved from https://www.fda.gov/drugs/understanding-over-counter-medicines/educational-resources-understanding-over-counter-medicine

Center for Drug Evaluation and Research. *FDA approves labeling supplement for Celebrex (Celecoxib)*. U.S. Food and Drug Administration, FDA. Retrieved from https://www.fda.gov/drugs/drug-safety-and-availability/cder-statement-fda-approves-labeling-supplement-celebrex-celecoxib

Center for Drug Evaluation and Research. *Human drug compounding*. U.S. Food and Drug Administration, FDA. Retrieved from https://www.fda.gov/drugs/guidance-compliance-regulatory-information/human-drug-compounding

Centers for Disease Control and Prevention. (2018). *What is marijuana?* Retrieved from https://www.cdc.gov/marijuana/faqs/what-is-marijuana.html

Centers for Disease Control and Prevention. (2019). *Outbreak of lung injury associated with the use of E-cigarette, or vaping, products*. Retrieved from https://www.cdc.gov/tobacco/basic_information/e-cigarettes/severe-lung-disease.html

Damkier, P., Lassen, D., Christensen, M. M. H., Madsen, K. G., Hellfritzsch, M., & Pottegård, A. (2019). Interaction between warfarin and cannabis. *Basic & Clinical Pharmacology & Toxicology, 124*(1), 28–31. doi:10.1111/bcpt.13152

Drug Enforcement Administration. (2017). *Kratom*. Retrieved from https://www.dea.gov/factsheets/kratom

Drug Interaction Checker. (n.d.). Drug interactions checker. *Medscape*. Retrieved from https://reference.medscape.com/drug-interactionchecker

Dworkin, R. H., O'Connor, A. B., Backonja, M., Farrar, J. T., Finnerup, N. B., Jensen, T. S., . . . Wallace, M. S. (2007). Pharmacologic management of neuropathic pain: Evidence-based recommendations. *Pain, 132*(3), 237–251. doi:10.1016/j.pain.2007.08.033

Federation of State Medical Boards. (2016). *Model Guidelines for the Recommendation of Marijuana in patient care*. Retrieved from https://www.fsmb.org/siteassets/advocacy/policies/model-guidelines-for-the-recommendation-of-marijuana-in-patient-care.pdf

Finan, P. H., Goodin, B. R., & Smith, M. T. (2013). The association of sleep and pain: an update and a path forward. *Journal of Pain: Official Journal of the American Pain Society, 14*(12), 1539–1552. doi:10.1016/j.jpain.2013.08.007

Gaby, A. R. (2017). *Nutritional medicine* (2nd ed.). Concord, NH: Fritz Perlberg Publishing.

Get Relief Responsibly. (n.d.). *OTC pain medication info, safety, dosage, & resources*. Retrieved from https://www.getreliefresponsibly.com

Kirkland, A. E., Sarlo, G. L., & Holton, K. F. (2018). The role of magnesium in neurological disorders. *Nutrients, 10*(6), 730. doi:10.3390/nu10060730

Kim, D-C., Ku, S-K., & Bae, J-S. (2012). Anticoagulant activities of curcumin and its derivative. *BMB Reports, 45*(4), 221–226. doi:10.5483/bmbrep.2012.45.4.221

Krause, A. J., Prather, A. A., Wager, T. D., Lindquist, M. A., & Walker, M. P. (2019). The pain of sleep loss: A brain characterization in humans. *Journal of Neuroscience: The Official Journal of the Society for Neuroscience, 39*(12), 2291–2300. doi:10.1523/JNEUROSCI.2408-18.2018

Li, X., Vigil, J. M., Stith, S. S., Brockelman, F., Keeling, K., & Hall, B. (2019). The effectiveness of self-directed medical cannabis treatment for pain. *Complementary Therapies in Medicine, 46*, 123–130. doi:10.1016/j.ctim.2019.07.022

Lu, H., & Mackie, K. (2016). An introduction to the endogenous cannabinoid system. *Biological Psychiatry, 79*(7), 516–525. doi:10.1016/j.biopsych.2015.07.028

Lunn, M. P., Hughes, R. A. C., & Wiffen, P. J. (2014). Duloxetine for treating painful neuropathy, chronic pain or fibromyalgia. *Cochrane Database of Systematic Reviews.* doi:10.1002/14651858.cd007115.pub3

Moore, R. A., Derry, S., Aldington, D., Cole, P., & Wiffen, P. J. (2015). Amitriptyline for neuropathic pain in adults. *Cochrane Database of Systematic Reviews.* doi:10.1002/14651858.cd008242.pub3

Moulin, D., Boulanger, A., Clark, A. J., Clarke, H., Dao, T., Finley, G. A., . . . Williamson, O. D. (2014). Pharmacological management of chronic neuropathic pain: revised consensus statement from the Canadian Pain Society. *Pain Research & Management, 19*(6), 328–335. doi:10.1155/2014/754693

National Council of State Boards of Nursing. (n.d.). *The world leader in nursing regulatory knowledge.* Retrieved from https://www.ncsbn.org

Rakel, D. (2018). *Integrative medicine* (4th ed.). New York, NY: Elsevier.

Takahashi, N., Arai, I., Kayama, S., Ichiji, K., Fukuda, H., Kaga, T., & Konno, S. (2014). Therapeutic efficacy of pregabalin in patients with leg symptoms due to lumbar spinal stenosis. *Fukushima Journal of Medical Science, 60*(1), 35–42. doi:10.5387/fms.2013-22

Tomić, M., Pecikoza, U., Micov, A., Vučković, S., & Stepanović-Petrović, R. (2018). Antiepileptic drugs as analgesics/adjuvants in inflammatory pain: Current preclinical evidence. *Pharmacology & Therapeutics, 192*, 42–64. doi:10.1016/j.pharmthera.2018.06.002

2019 American Geriatrics Society Beers Criteria Update Expert Panel. (2019). American Geriatrics Society 2019 updated AGS Beers Criteria® for potentially inappropriate medication use in older adults. *Journal of the American Geriatrics Society, 67*(4), 674–694. doi:10.1111/jgs.15767

VA Office of Research and Development. (2020, January). *Low dose naltrexone for chronic pain from arthritis.* Retrieved from https://clinicaltrials.gov/ct2/show/NCT03008590

Veltri, C., & Grundmann, O. (2019). Current perspectives on the impact of Kratom use. *Substance Abuse and Rehabilitation, 10*, 23–31. doi:10.2147/SAR.S164261

Vučković, S, Srebro, D., Vujović, K. S., Vučetić, C., & Prostran, M. (2018). Cannabinoids and pain: New insights from old molecules. *Frontiers in Pharmacology, 9*, 1259. doi:10.3389/fphar.2018.01259

Vyvey, M. (2010). Steroids as pain relief adjuvants. *Canadian Family Physician Medecin de Famille Canadien, 56*(12), 1295–1297, e415. Retrieved from https://www.ncbi.nlm.nih.gov/pubmed/21156893

Walker, M. (2018). *Why we sleep: Unlocking the power of sleep and dreams.* New York, NY: Scribner's.

Younger, J., Noor, N., McCue, R., & Mackey, S. (2013). Low-dose naltrexone for the treatment of fibromyalgia: Findings of a small, randomized, double-blind, placebo-controlled, counterbalanced, crossover trial assessing daily pain levels. *Arthritis and Rheumatism, 65*(2), 529–538. doi:10.1002/art.37734

Younger, J., Parkitny, L., & McLain, D. (2014). The use of low-dose naltrexone (LDN) as a novel anti-inflammatory treatment for chronic pain. *Clinical Rheumatology, 33*(4), 451–459. doi:10.1007/s10067-014-2517-2

ADDITIONAL RESOURCES

OTC Information

https://bemedwise.org
https://www.fda.gov/drugs/understanding-over-counter-medicines/educational-resources-understanding-over-counter-medicine
https://www.getreliefresponsibly.com
https://www.knowyourdose.org

Cannabis

FDA Regulation resource links: https://www.fda.gov/news-events/public-health-focus/fda-regulation-cannabis-and-cannabis-derived-products-including-cannabidiol-cbd

FDA Role in Regulation of cannabis products PowerPoint: https://www.fda.gov/media/128156/download

Low-Dose Naltrexone

Elsegood, L. (Ed.). (2016). *The LDN book: How a little-known generic drug—low dose naltrexone—could revolutionize treatment for autoimmune diseases, cancer, autism, depression, and more.* White River Junction, VT: Chelsea Green Publishing.

The LDN Research Trust website has links to current clinical trials as well as testimonials and outcomes reported by prescribers and pharmacists who are using LDN for off-label use: https://www.ldnresearchtrust.org

CHAPTER 8

RISK SCREENING TOOLS FOR PRESCRIBING OPIOIDS FOR PAIN RELIEF

INTRODUCTION

Pain-management guidelines recommend evaluation of risk factors prior to prescribing opioids (Centers for Disease Control and Prevention [CDC], 2018). Use of research-based screening tools can support safe and effective prescribing and pain management. In this chapter, we discuss when, why, and how to use these tools and describe several common tools. The sensitivity and specificity of the tools varies, and research continues; it is important to identify several tools that fit your clinical flow and patient population and use clinical judgment and experience when interpreting the results.

Tool categories include evaluating the risk of opioid use before starting opioids, the risk of abuse or diversion by patients already taking opioids, and screening for anxiety or depression. It is essential that the screening tools be used thoughtfully and appropriately; they are not diagnostic tools, they assist in determining risk. Screening tools provide guidance for prescribers to evaluate patient risk of opioid use disorder (OUD) thoughtfully, yet there is minimal evidence regarding the validity of these tests. In a review of studies of opioid screening tools, Chou et al. (2009) found that additional research is needed.

Dr. Lynne Webster (2019) wrote a compelling description of the double-edged sword of screening- tool use, advocating for patients and reminding prescribers that the Opioid Risk Tool (ORT) should not be used to withhold pain medication from people only because they answer yes to the presence of preadolescent sexual abuse.

USING SCREENING TOOLS

Any skill improves with consistent practice. When you use a tool consistently, interpretation speed and accuracy improve. Documentation of the results of the

BOX 8.1

SCREENING TOOLS COMMONLY USED TO DETERMINE OPIOID RISK

Opioid Risk Tool (ORT)

Diagnosis Intractability Risk Efficacy (DIRE)

Screener and Opioid Assessment for Patients with Pain (SOAPP-R)

Current Opioid Misuse Measure (COMM)

Patient Health Questionnaire-9 (PHQ-9)

The Generalized Anxiety Disorder (GAD-7)

tool and your rationale for subsequent therapy provides support for clinical decisions (Box 8.1).

Most of these tools are available only in English. The Screener and Opioid Assessment for Patients with Pain (SOAPP-R) has a validated Spanish form (Butler et al., 2013). The Patient Health Questionnaire—9 (PHQ-9) and the Generalized Anxiety Disorder (GAD-7), which screen for depression and anxiety, are available in multiple languages (www.phqscreeners.com). Some tools are self-administered. Other tools are administered by the clinician. Some tools are available in digital formats, including apps for tablets. In addition, Urine Drug Screening (UDS) and Prescription Drug Monitoring Program (PDMP) provide information about clinical decision-making.

CLINICAL PEARL

Environmental and genetic factors should influence how closely a patient's opioid use is monitored. However, a history of experiencing preadolescent sexual abuse does not mean a person will necessarily develop an OUD. It is only a risk factor. It does not determine the outcome of using opioids, although it may partially indicate the level of monitoring, support, and education that would be appropriate.—Lynne Webster, MD

OUD, opioid use disorder.

Source: Reproduced with permission from Webster, L. (2019). The Opioid Risk Tool has been weaponized against pain patients. *Pain News Network*. Retrieved from https://www.painnewsnetwork.org/stories/2019/9/21/the-opioid-risk-tool-has-been-weaponized-against-pain-patients

Why Use Screening Tools?

As more patients with pain are being managed in primary care, clinicians are faced with the challenge of evaluating not only a pain complaint, but also the risk of OUD. You cannot determine a patient's risk solely based on his or her appearance or presentation. Screening tools provide additional useful information to determine a patient's risk of OUD. Documentation of screening in clinical notes provides support for your decision-making. It is important to document why opioids are being used and how you are protecting your patient from addiction, abuse, and diverting the drugs. Consistent use of the screening tools increases one's ability to use them efficiently. In 2017, an estimated 18 million people misused prescription medications at least once in the prior year (Substance Abuse and Mental Health Services Administration [SAMHSA] Report, 2017). It is hoped that policy and procedure changes and development of new strategies for managing pain and addiction will decrease these numbers.

CLINICAL PEARL

Maintain a therapeutic relationship; the goal is to provide the best care for the patient, not to label each person according to his or her risk of substance abuse.

Developing clinical interviewing skills to engage the patient in discussion informed by results of evaluation tools increases the probability of an accurate assessment. It is a challenge not to overestimate or underestimate the risk of OUD; using multiple tools informed by experience optimizes the probability of accuracy. If you are not confident or experienced, have a plan to consult with an experienced primary care colleague or relevant specialist for additional support. Treat everyone with respect while remaining vigilant regarding possible manipulation. When using the tools as part of your routine, you can increase your skill in reading clues that caution is indicated or more information required, combining art and science.

CLINICAL PEARL

All skills improve with familiarity and practice. Choose the tools that fit the needs of your practice and use them often.

TOOL SELECTION

Choose a tool or two to use for prescreening and ongoing screening. Practice using the tools, then determine which are most relevant for your patient population and continue to use them. If tools have been selected by your practice, familiarize yourself with them and use them consistently. You may find that incorporating some of the questions from various tools into your menu of clinical questions asked strengthens your clinical interview.

The ORT is easily administered and scored and widely used as an initial assessment. Moore, Jones, Browder, Daffron, and Passik (2009) compared the ORT, SOAPP-R, and Diagnosis Intractability Risk Efficacy (DIRE) and found that the SOAPP-R was the most reliable indicator of need to discontinue opioids due to abuse, and that combining the clinical interview with the SOAPP-R provided the most sensitive test. Taking time to thoughtfully examine the questions in the screening tests will help you to understand the implications of your patient's scores and can also enhance your understanding of the risk factors of addiction, the impact of life and genetic events, and the power of your clinical evaluation. These tools are useful for screening, but require clinical judgment for appropriate use. Document screening-tool results and the clinical decision-making that accompanies them.

CLINICAL PEARL

By fine-tuning and consistently increasing the sensitivity of your subjective and objective assessment of patients, you will increase the quality and safety of your pain-management and opioid prescribing.

PRESCRIPTION DRUG MONITORING PROGRAMS

In 2019, 49 states had PDMPs, which provide online data regarding controlled substance prescriptions. These databases are evolving and becoming more robust. Program components and regulations regarding access vary from state to state and continue to evolve. Some electronic medical records (EMRs) incorporate links to the PDMP in the clinical note, providing smooth access and documentation that the PDMP was opened.

Know your state regulations regarding accessing PDMPs prior to prescribing, the process for updating the database, and how current the information is. The CDC, the Substance Abuse and Mental Health Services Administration, and the Bureau of Justice Assistance are encouraging all states to require PDMP use to avoid prescribing irregularities including opioid prescribing by multiple prescribers, for example (Vestal, 2018). Review of the PDMP is part of the CDC guidelines (2018).

Document that you have checked the PDMP and what you found. Is it consistent with patient report of use? Use of PDMP for each pain-management visit is an important part of safe prescribing.

SCREENING TOOLS

Opioid Risk Tool

The ORT is widely used and referenced on most sites that describe tools used to evaluate opioid risk. It can be administered in 1 minute, providing important screening information in diverse settings. Developed by Lynne Webster (Webster & Webster, 2005), the ORT is used prior to initiating opioid therapy. It consists of five categories with a total of 10 questions, whose scoring is the sum of the weighted responses. The ORT considers family history and personal history of substance abuse, age and gender of the patient, and any sexual abuse prior to adolescence. Scores are weighted and totaled.

The sum of the patient responses determines whether they are at low, medium, or high risk for future opioid abuse.

Scoring is as follows:

- 3 or lower = low risk
- 4 to 7 = moderate risk
- 8 or above = high risk

Described as the ORT-OUD, a revised ORT has been developed. Cheatle, Compton, Dhingra, Wasser, and Obrien (2019) found that eliminating the preadolescent sexual abuse question for females and eliminating weighting of responses produced a simpler screen and consistent or superior results. The revised ORT (ORT-OUD) was published in January 2019 (Cheatle et al., 2019). More information on the utility of the ORT-OUD will emerge as more trials are done and more clinicians use it in practice. Look at both of these opioid-risk tools and decide whether one of them is the best fit for your patient population, knowing that the new tool offers less historical data.

The ORT is available as an app (in MDCalc) and in various online calculators. It can also be printed and given to patients to complete prior to their visit or verbally administered by the prescriber or the support staff.

CLINICAL PEARL

It is essential that screening tests be used for screening, not diagnosis. If a patient screens at low or high risk, it remains the responsibility of the prescriber to remain vigilant and gather more information as indicated.

Diagnosis Intractability Risk Efficacy

The DIRE (Belgrade, Schamber, & Lindgren, 2006) is used to predict the risk of addiction/OUD and the potential risk of prescribing opioids. The DIRE has seven categories: diagnosis, intractability, psychological risk, chemical health risk, reliability risk, social support risk, and efficacy. Each category is scored 1 to 3 based on clinician's rating of patient characteristics. The sum of category scores is totaled to determine the risk.

The DIRE is completed by the clinician, who assesses the patient's status based on his or her evaluation. This requires clinician time each time the tool is used and requires practice for the clinician to become proficient in using the tool. It is included in screening guideline documents and may be useful depending on your patient population.

Scoring the DIRE is as follows:

- A score of 7 to 13 shows the patient is not a suitable candidate for long-term opioid analgesia.
- A score of 14–21 indicates the patient is a good candidate.

The DIRE is available as an app (MDCalc.com) and can be printed for use by the prescriber.

Screener and Opioid Assessment for Patients with Pain

SOAPP-R is available as a 5-, 14-, or 24-item tool that is completed by the patient and scored by the clinician. Items address patient mood, feelings, behavior, and experience with alcohol or drugs; responses are weighted 0 to 4 (never to very often).

The SOAPP-R is designed to assist clinicians in determining how closely to monitor a patient who is prescribed opioids. This tool has been refined multiple times and has multiple forms. The SOAPP-R was validated in 2008 (Butler et al., 2013).

Scoring in SOAPP-R is as follows:

- 22 or greater = high risk
- 10 to 21 = moderate risk
- 9 or less = low risk

SOAPP-R is available in Spanish and English. The Spanish translation was validated by Butler et al. in 2013.

Current Opioid Misuse Measure

COMM is designed to monitor ongoing risk of opioid abuse. The COMM provides an adjunct tool for ongoing monitoring of patients taking opioids. It is a patient self-report tool used to measure aberrant behavior risk in patients using chronic opioid therapy and identifies the patients who are currently misusing opioids (Butler et al., 2010). The patient completes the tool, which is then scored by the clinician. It takes about 10 minutes for the patient to complete the form, which includes 17 items with questions regarding behavior in six areas over the past 30 days. It can be used when establishing care with a new patient who is already taking opioids, and used periodically to monitor patients taking opioids chronically.

Scoring in the tool is as follows:

- 9 or higher = increased risk of misusing medication
- 8 or less = lower risk of misuse

Cutoff scores were chosen to capture patients at risk of misusing medication; therefore, the COMM is more likely to identify a patient as high risk (false positive) incorrectly than to miss a potential abuser.

Patient Health Questionnaire-9 and the Generalized Anxiety Disorder-7

PHQ-9 and GAD-7 are widely used and effective tools to screen patients for depression and anxiety quickly. Mood impacts pain and pain impacts mood. The PHQ-9 is a brief measure of depression severity (Kroenke, Spitzer, & Williams, 2001). The GAD-7 screens for anxiety (Spitzer, Kroenke, Williams, & Löwe, 2006). These tools are easy to score (Exhibit 8.1).

It is useful to screen all patients at their first visit, providing a baseline with insight into mood and areas for follow-up that could be missed in a brief clinical encounter. The tools can also be repeated, giving insight into progress or deterioration. They are very quick to use, easy to include in the electronic health record

EXHIBIT 8.1

PHQ-9 AND GAD-7 SCREENING TOOLS

PHQ-9: Screens for Severity of Depression

Score	
0–4:	to minimal
5–9:	Mild
10–14:	moderate
15–19:	moderately severe
20–27:	severe

GAD-7: Screens for Severity of Anxiety

Score	
5:	mild anxiety
10:	moderate anxiety
15:	severe anxiety

(EHR), and available online and in an app. Using these tools can also open up topics to discuss with patients, as they are willing. Although they are not specific for opioid risk, they provide added insight. Recognizing depression and anxiety is an important part of primary care. The PHQ-9 and GAD-7, when used consistently, are useful adjuncts for assessment in all patients, especially those with pain.

Translated into many languages, forms for these assessments are available online at www.phqscreeners.com/select-screener and can be printed. The design of the form is consistent with the English versions, allowing the patient to complete the form in their native language and the clinician to calculate the results. The forms are only language translations and do not reflect testing for cultural reliability. The Patient Health Questionnaire (PHQ) Screeners website (phqscreeners.com) includes scoring rubrics, instructions, and additional considerations and guidance regarding use of the tools (Patient Health Questionnaire Screeners, n.d.). The PHQ-9 and GAD-7 are not diagnostic tools; they provide screening for anxiety and depression, and the results provide guidance for further evaluation.

URINE DRUG SCREENING

Testing for the presence of prescription and other substances via UDS is an important part of key decision-making. It is essential to have a clear policy regarding when and how UDS is used. Many pain-management clinicians require the results of UDS prior to prescribing opioids in any nonurgent situation. UDS is part of the CDC guidelines (2018; see Exhibits 8.2 and 8.3).

EXHIBIT 8.2

USING OPIOID SCREENING TOOLS IN PRACTICE

Incorporate tools into your workflow, including ORT, UDS, PHQ-9, GAD-7.

- Check the PDMP before you see the patient; this is part of his or her relevant history.
- Include the screening tools when a patient presents seeking treatment for a pain complaint.
- If any new patient taking opioids prescribed by another clinician presents to you, use the COMM to screen for current abuse risk and check the PDMP before prescribing any sedating medications.
- Be aware of all medications and supplements the patient is taking; include monitoring for indications of any substance abuse.

(*continued*)

EXHIBIT 8.2 (*continued*)

- Do not leap to judgments about people who are taking any type of medication. Although opioid abuse is a national problem, there are many people who use their medications responsibly and depend on them to function and have a good quality of life.
- A balanced assessment uses art and science to determine the risk and benefit of opioids.
- Expand the information in your clinical assessment to support initial decision-making and follow-up; incorporate the use of tools into your regular assessment process. Screening tools provide information to use with the other data you collect.
- For all patients who require pain management, evaluate the whole picture and determine probable pain generators and what treatment is indicated. This includes consideration of drug interactions with medications the patient is taking as well as comorbidities such as diabetes or hypertension. Consider the opioid risk as another comorbidity—no more or less. You can use screening tools plus your clinical experience to optimally prescribe all medications.
- Use the *lowest effective* dose of any medication. The goal is to manage pain, not eliminate it.

COMM, Current Opioid Misuse Measure; GAD-7, the Generalized Anxiety Disorder-7; ORT, Opioid Risk Tool; PDMP, Prescription Drug Monitoring Program; PHQ-9, Patient Health Questionnaire-9; UDS, urine drug screening.

EXHIBIT 8.3

OPIOID-PRESCRIBING APPROACHES DETERMINED BY PATIENT'S RISK OF OUD

- *Low risk (ORT = 3 or less, SOAPP-R = less than 9):* Continue to monitor as indicated, including checking the PDMP before prescribing opioids and UDS as indicated per the clinical protocol. Document what you do and why. When starting an opioid trial, set an expectation that the medication is to support other therapies and is not the long-term plan. Use the lowest effective dose for the shortest time.
- *Moderate risk (ORT = 4–7, SOAPP-R = 10–21):* This is the most challenging category and requires careful analysis of risk and benefit. Explore the risk factors with the patient and the current standard of care for using opioids in pain management. When possible, choose a nonopioid intervention as your initial strategy. If you decide to prescribe an opioid, set the expectation that this will be a time-limited treatment

(*continued*)

EXHIBIT 8.3 (continued)

and that you will be working with the patient to prevent problems. You may decide to prescribe a small amount at a low dose and return for early follow-up in 1 to 2 weeks. When in doubt, check with an expert colleague before prescribing.

- *High risk (ORT 8 or above, SOAPP-R = 22 or greater):* If you do not have experience prescribing for patients at high risk, consult with pain management or a colleague experienced in managing high-risk patients *before* prescribing opioids. These patients may require referral or comanagement.

ORT, Opioid Risk Tool; OUD, opioid use disorder; SOAPP-R, Screener and Opioid Assessment for Patients with Pain.

Additional screening tools are available, and many of them are open access. Additional resources available for these tools are listed at the end of the chapter.

CLINICAL PEARL

Document the ways in which you follow guidelines for prescribing and the impact of treatment on patient's pain and function.

SUMMARY

Incorporate the use of relevant screening tools into your clinical workflow. Use the tools for screening, not diagnosis. Use the screening score as part of your ongoing patient management, regardless of the initial assessment of risk. If evaluation raises concerns regarding the risk of addiction or diversion, consider referral or consult with a pain-management or addiction specialist, or appropriate behavioral health professional.

Screen for the following:

- Risk of opioid abuse
- Risk of other substance abuse, including alcohol and OUD
- Risk of problems with ongoing opioid therapy
- Depression and anxiety
- Inappropriate use of prescription medications

Comply with the federal and state regulations regarding prescribing opioids. Jody Lutz (2019) compiled an online resource list of each state's guidelines. There are many tools available, and research is ongoing to refine and shorten the current tools and to develop new tools. A list of additional resources offering more information that can be used for your practice is included at the end of the chapter. Do not give away your power as a clinician. Determine the risks of prescribing opioids and what you are willing to prescribe. Skillful use of screening tools can provide direction when conducting your interview and examination. You cannot give away the liability, it remains yours, but risk can be mitigated by using recognized screening tools in combination with clinical evaluation and thorough documentation. There are many available therapeutic options, including physical therapy, antidepressants, muscle relaxants, membrane stabilizers, and anti-inflammatory and integrative approaches. Think of opioids as the last option, not the first.

TRENDING IN PAIN MANAGEMENT

- Look for more digital screening tools and integration of established tools into the EMR.
- Watch for changes in state and federal PDMP programs.
- Watch for evolution of ORT and ORT-OUD.

CASE STUDY

David is a 40-year-old male who has been in your practice for 5 years. He is healthy, has a sedentary job, takes no prescription medication, has no recreational drug use, and drinks alcohol three to four times per week. He has only come to the office three times in 5 years, once for viral symptoms and twice for musculoskeletal pain resulting from overtraining at the gym. He presents today complaining of severe low -back pain and inability to sleep.

His pain is 6/10 at night; his back feels tight and there is no weakness. He has been getting poor sleep since doing deadlifts this past week. Pain is aching and stabbing, localized to his lower and mid-back. He is in no acute distress, but is clearly uncomfortable, with a guarded posture. On exam, he has significant paraspinal spasm with no weakness or neurological deficit. The PDMP reflects no record of prescriptions for controlled substances in the past 2 years. His PHQ-9 was zero 5 years ago and is 5 today; his GAD-7 remains at 4. His opioid risk is moderate based on his ORT score of 4, based on his age, gender, and family history of alcohol abuse.

Based on physical exam, your treatment plan includes physical therapy with over-the-counter nonsteroidal anti-inflammatory drugs (NSAIDs) and a muscle relaxant to take as needed and tolerated. You counsel him regarding the impact of consistent

(*continued*)

CASE STUDY (*continued*)

alcohol consumption on the liver and advise him not to drink alcohol when taking the muscle relaxant. An Epsom salt bath at bedtime may facilitate sleep.

His exam does not indicate use of opioids. You refer him to a physical therapist, prescribe a muscle relaxant, and advise to return for follow-up as indicated. As you close the visit, he requests pain medication to allow him to sleep.

1. Should he be given opioids?

   Not today. His screening tests do not indicate high risk, but opioids are not indicated for his physical findings. You advise him that the muscle relaxant with the NSAID and the Epsom salt bath will help with sleep.

2. Does his ORT make him ineligible for opioids?

   No. If his symptoms warranted a short course of an opioid, a trial could be discussed, including the fact that his age and family history put him at risk of addiction. In this situation, the screening tool results provide an opportunity for patient education that can help him to be proactive in avoiding problems. This encounter also provides an opportunity to educate him that opioids are for pain management, not for sleep.

REFERENCES

Belgrade, M. J., Schamber, C. D., & Lindgren, B. R. (2006). The DIRE score: Predicting outcomes of opioid prescribing for chronic pain. *Journal of Pain*, *7*(9), 671–681. doi:10.1016/j.jpain.2006.03.001

Butler, S. F., Budman, S. H., Fanciullo, G. J., & Jamison, R. N. (2010). Cross validation of the Current Opioid Misuse Measure (COMM) to monitor chronic pain patients on opioid therapy. *Clinical Journal of Pain*, *26*(9), 770–776. doi:10.1097/AJP.0b013e3181f195ba

Butler, S. F., Fernandez, K., Benoit, C., Budman, S. H., & Jamison, R. N. (2008). Validation of the revised screener and opioid assessment for patients with pain (SOAPP-R). *J Pain*, *9*(4), 360–372. doi: 10.1016/j.jpain.2007.11.014

Butler, S. F., Zacharoff, K. L., Budman, S. H., Jamison, R. N., Black, R., Dawsey, R., & Ondarza, A. (2013). Spanish translation and linguistic validation of the Screener and Opioid Assessment for Patients with Pain-Revised (SOAPP-R). *Pain Medicine*, *14*(7), 1032–1038. doi:10.1111/pme.12098

Centers for Disease Control and Prevention. (2018). *CDC guidelines prescribing opioids for chronic pain*. Retrieved from https://www.cdc.gov/drugoverdose/prescribing/guideline.html

Cheatle, M. D., Compton, P. A., Dhingra, L., Wasser, T. E., & O'Brien, C. P. (2019). Development of the revised opioid risk tool to predict opioid use disorder in patients with chronic nonmalignant pain. *Journal of Pain*, *20*(7), 842–851. doi:10.1016/j.jpain.2019.01.011

Chou, R., Fanciullo, G. J., Fine, P. G., Miaskowski, C., Passik, S. D., & Portenoy, R. K. (2009). Opioids for chronic noncancer pain: Prediction and identification of aberrant drug-related behaviors: A review of the evidence for an American Pain Society and American Academy of Pain Medicine Clinical Practice Guideline. *Journal of Pain*, *10*(2), 131–146. doi:10.1016/j.jpain.2008.10.009

Kroenke, K., Spitzer, R. L., & Williams, J. B. W. (2001). The PHQ-9. *Journal of General Internal Medicine*, *16*(9), 606–613. doi: 10.1046/j.1525-1497.2001.016009606.x

Lutz, J. (2019, October 10). *Opioid prescribing guidelines, a state by state overview*. Retrieved from https://www.affirmhealth.com/blog/opioid-prescribing-guidelines-a-state-by-state-overview

Moore, T. M., Jones, T., Browder, J. H., Daffron, S., & Passik, S. D. (2009). A comparison of common screening methods for predicting aberrant drug-related behavior among patients receiving opioids for chronic pain management. *Pain Medicine*, *10*(8), 1426–1433. doi:10.1111/j.1526-4637.2009.00743.x

Patient Health Questionnaire Screeners. (n.d.). *Screener overview*. Retrieved from https://www.phqscreeners.com/select-screener

Spitzer, R. L., Kroenke, K., Williams, J. B. W., & Löwe, B. (2006). A brief measure for assessing generalized anxiety disorder. *Archives of Internal Medicine*, *166*(10), 1092. doi:10.1001/archinte.166.10.1092

Substance Abuse and Mental Health Services Administration Report. (2017). *NSDUH detailed tables*. Retrieved from https://www.samhsa.gov/data/report/2017-nsduh-detailed-tables

Vestal, C. (2018, January 15). States require doctors to use prescription drug monitoring systems for patients. *The Washington Post*. Retrieved from https://www.washingtonpost.com/national/health-science/states-require-doctors-to-use-prescription-drug-monitoring-systems-for-patients/2018/01/12/c76807b8-f009-11e7-97bf-bba379b809ab_story.html

Webster, L. (2019). The Opioid Risk Tool has been weaponized against pain patients. *Pain News Network*. Retrieved from https://www.painnewsnetwork.org/stories/2019/9/21/the-opioid-risk-tool-has-been-weaponized-against-pain-patients

Webster, L. R., & Webster, R. M. (2005). Predicting aberrant behaviors in opioid-treated patients: preliminary validation of the opioid risk tool. *Pain Medicine*, *6*(6), 432–442. doi:10.1111/j.1526-4637.2005.00072.x

ADDITIONAL RESOURCES

Screening-Tool Links

CO*RE Tools Repository with links to assessment tools and screeners: http://core-rems.org/opioid-education/tools

National Council of State Boards of Nursing (NCSBN) Opioid Toolkit resources: https://www.ncsbn.org/opioid-toolkit.htm

National Institute on Drug Abuse (NIDA) Screening and Assessment Tools Chart with links to tools: https://www.drugabuse.gov/nidamed-medical-health-professionals/screening-tools-resources/chart-screening-tools

State of Washington Association of Medical Directors Group (AMDG): Offers links to various downloadable patient assessment tools: http://www.agencymeddirectors.wa.gov/AssessmentTools.asp

Regulation Links

PDMP Training and Assistance Center: Offers iinformation on national and state legislation and resources: http://www.pdmpassist.org

Digital Tools

CDC opioid guideline app: https://www.cdc.gov/drugoverdose/prescribing/app.html
Apps for select screening tools— iOS and Android: www.MDcalc.com
  DIRE
  GAD-7
  Hamilton Anxiety Rating Scale
  Hamilton Depression Rating Scale
  ORT
  PHQ-9

CHAPTER 9

THE OPIOID DILEMMA: USING OPIOIDS IN PRACTICE

INTRODUCTION

The use of opioids in clinical practice has changed dramatically over the past 10 years. For many years, it was very common for a patient who complained of pain to be given a prescription for an opioid medication with no concern about the unused portion of the prescribed amount. Currently, the Centers for Disease Control and Prevention (CDC; 2016) is attempting to limit the number of days patients are prescribed opioids and the number of tablets given with each prescription. For example, the recommendation from the CDC is to provide 3 days of opioids for acute postoperative pain, with 7 days being the maximum. Unfortunately, postoperative pain may last longer, requiring a longer prescription for pain relief during the rehabilitation period.

Preoperative patient education should include information on other methods of managing pain, such as local anesthetic pumps, as well as how opioids will be used, titrated down, and discontinued once surgical pain is reduced to manageable levels. Without this education, patients may assume that the opioid medications will continue until all pain is resolved or to prevent the return of postoperative pain.

Somehow, patients seem to be getting lost in the discussions about what a reasonable pain-management goal is. Patients should expect to have some pain, but the healthcare providers' efforts should be aimed at providing the best pain management possible using safe prescribing. Measuring the risks and benefits of opioid use is an ongoing process and should continue until opioids are discontinued.

The recent dramatic shift in opioid prescribing is the result of increased opioid abuse, both of prescription medications and illegal street drugs, causing a significant increase in overdose deaths. Data suggest that 27 million Americans use illicit drugs, which includes the nonmedical use of prescription drugs, with 7 million of these users meeting the criteria for a substance use disorder (SUD), formerly termed *addiction* (Bachhuber, Weiner, Mitchell, & Samet, 2016). Of the 7 million Americans who qualify for a diagnosis of SUD, 1.9 million people have disorders related to the nonmedical use of prescription pain relievers (Bachhuber et al., 2016).

CLINICAL PEARL

SUD is the term currently used to describe what was formerly called *addiction*. It is diagnosed using the *Diagnostic and Statistical Manual of Mental Disorders*, Fifth Edition (*DSM-5*; American Psychiatric Association [APA], 2013) criteria. Opioid use disorder (OUD) is a category under SUD, along with other conditions such as alcohol use disorder.

The human toll of opioid abuse is enormous and rising. Fatal overdose deaths related to opioids have tripled and fatal overdose deaths related to sedative use have quintupled since 1999 (Bachhuber et al., 2016). These deaths are a result of both prescription opioid use and illegal drugs. Once a patient is unable to obtain opioids by prescription, the options are illegal sources, where there is no quality assurance and contamination with other substances is common. Currently, there is a large influx of fentanyl from China that is mixed with heroin to create a faster and elevated high, which patients with OUD are seeking.

Unfortunately, treatment options for these individuals have been reduced, and few, if any, opportunities for OUD treatment exist. The use of medication-assisted treatment (MAT) with methadone or buprenorphine fills the gap. Primary care providers who meet the education requirement for MAT practice can treat patients for SUD with a special waiver attached to their license. This is still a developing practice, and there is a great need for treatment to help patients with SUD.

Many experts have tried to determine what caused this opioid epidemic. The practice of overprescribing opioids has been examined and addressed by the CDC by adding pill limits and time limits to prescriptions. Some experts feel the creation of pain as the fifth vital sign in 1996 by the American Pain Society (APS) encouraged practitioners to be generous with pain medications (Brown, 2018). Others feel that The Joint Commission (TJC) issued citations to institutions for lack of pain control, creating a climate that encouraged generous prescriptive practices. However, examination of the prescription data reveals that opioid prescriptions were steadily increasing in the 10 years prior to the institution of TJC standards in 2001 (Brown, 2018).

Past prescriptive practices left patients feeling that the answer to their pain was the use of opioids. Patients may feel their pain is being untreated or dismissed if they do not receive a prescription for a pain medication. Patients may also find false information on the Internet, leaving them confused and dissatisfied. Because pain management is migrating to primary care, this debate will continue for some time, and educating patients on when opioids are appropriate for use and prescribers on how to use opioids safely will be an ongoing process.

CURRENT STATUS OF OPIOID USE IN PRIMARY CARE

Primary care providers see a large number of patients who cite pain as a major complaint. Patients with migraine headaches, osteoarthritis, and low-back pain are seen daily in primary care practices throughout the United States. How these patients are treated can vary from practice to practice and from state to state.

Primary care providers are on the frontline of our healthcare system, and they are in the forefront of what is being termed the *opioid epidemic*. They are the first healthcare practitioners that patients with chronic pain see, and they account for 50% of all prescription opioids dispensed (Bachhuber et al., 2016). Recently, a study of opioid prescribing in primary care used 678,319 electronic health records (EHRs) to determine that physicians were 33% more likely to provide an opioid prescription to patients who had appointments later in the day. They were also 17% more likely to prescribe opioids to patients who had appointments that were running 60 minutes or more behind schedule, compared to patients with appointments that started on time. All patients in the study had not received an opioid prescription within the past year (Naprash & Barnett, 2019). Why this practice was taking place did not surprise pain-management experts reviewing the article, given that the pressures of time, productivity, development of complex care plans for opioid use, and documentation are added to the decision-making process (Bucheit, 2019).

Formal pressure is being placed on primary care practitioners by the U.S. Food and Drug Administration (FDA) and the CDC. The recommendations of their new guidelines highlight the need for assessment, screening for opioid risk, safe opioid prescribing, and patient education. Finding the time in a busy clinic day to comply with these requirements is a monumental job. In addition, state insurance programs and insurance providers are weighing in and putting pressure on providers to make sure they are compliant with opioid risk screening and patient–provider agreements (PPAs).

To be a primary care practitioner in the current climate requires creating a delicate balance of patient expectations, a lack of time, and the need for being complaint with national guidelines and recommendations. Using safe prescribing practices can help refine the process, allow the healthcare provider (HCP) to offer adequate pain relief, and provide security with decision-making. The requirement by many states that license renewal is linked to pain-management education programs provides an opportunity for practitioner education that can make opioid prescribing an easier process.

OPIOID-PATIENT PATHOPHYSIOLOGY

Over the past few years, opioid prescribing for both men and women has increased dramatically. There are differences in both the availability of the medications and the outcomes of prescribing them. Women are a more vulnerable population in that women can become pregnant, have estrogen—a known pain potentiator—and gender differences in prescription opioid use and abuse exist (Back, Lawson, Singleton, & Brady, 2011; Green, Serrano, Licari, Budman, & Nutler, 2009). This information is salient because women receive more prescriptions for opioid medications then men do and they tend to have higher rates of prescription opioid abuse (Back et al., 2011; Darnell & Stacey, 2012).

Research has indicated that opioids are more likely to be prescribed to women and the medications are prescribed at higher doses (Cicero et al., 2009). Several factors contribute to this phenomenon (Darnell & Stacey, 2012):

- Women are at higher risk for developing a variety of chronic pain conditions.
- Women experience higher pain intensities than men.
- Opioids are inadvertently misprescribed for conditions common in women, such as fibromyalgia, osteoarthritis, or headaches, in which opioids are not beneficial.

Concerning opioids, men are seen as having a better response to morphine, but in fact, the medication onset is faster in men. Women do have a response to morphine, but the onset of action is slower. However, women tend to have more side effects, such as nausea and vomiting, from opioid use. Women also have an estrogenic effect that can increase certain types of pain, such as inflammatory pain, and modulate the pain response, whereas certain conditions, such as fibromyalgia, can alter and limit the binding capacity of opioids.

There are some distinct physiologic effects with continued opioid use. Morphine can affect the temperature and the circulating hormone levels due to its action in the hypothalamus. Continued use of morphine can lower the body temperature and inhibit corticotrophin-releasing hormone (CRH) and gonadotropin-releasing hormone (GnRH), which results in decreases in luteinizing hormone (LH), follicle-stimulating hormone (FSH), and ACTH. Conversely, the levels of prolactin and antidiuretic hormones increase (Inturrisi & Lipman, 2010). These changes can affect the fertility of a woman.

When testosterone is affected due to chronic opioid therapy, a condition called *opioid-induced androgen deficiency (OPIAD)* results. With men, erectile dysfunction can occur. When this condition occurs, the pain worsens, depression is common, and efforts to treat the pain become very difficult. This phenomenon can occur in women as well as in men, with the result being progesterone suppression (Inturrisi & Lipman, 2010). Asking male patients on higher dose of long-term opioids about changes in libido or erectile dysfunction should be a part of the ongoing reassessment process.

Research on differences in opioid response between men and women is very scant. Most research is being done on animals, which cannot be compared to real-life use of opioids for pain in humans. Clearly, opioids have physiologic effects on both men and women, but the full understanding behind these differences has yet to be uncovered.

OPIOID MEDICATIONS

The concerns about OUD are affecting patients who use opioids to be more functional and regain a better quality of life. These patients can take opioids at stable doses for long periods of time with no indications of OUD. They are, however, being grouped with those patients who are likely to develop OUD and their prescriptions are being restricted or tapered, creating increased pain and dysfunction.

Educating patients about opioids and using PPAs to guide opioid use is essential for providing a safe climate for patients on opioids. Prescribers also need to receive education and information on how to prescribe safely in their states. Using Risk Evaluation and Mitigation Strategy (REMS) education, offered by the FDA, to provide a baseline of safe practice is becoming more common and can provide the prescriber with needed education.

Today's opioids can be delivered via many routes, including, oral, nasal, sublingual, intravenous (IV), subcutaneous, intrathecal, and rectal. In addition, there are many more formulations of opioids to use for analgesia other than morphine, which was considered to be the best analgesic medication for many years.

The term *opiate* denotes a class of medications derived from the latex sap of *Papaver somniferum*, the opium poppy. The term *opioid* refers to the synthetic or semi-synthetic analogs of this natural substance. Opioids are considered to be any medication that binds to an opiate receptor, most often the mu opioid receptor.

Historically, opium was smoked in China for its euphoric effect and used for pain relief in later years. By the 20th century, opioid use was not only seen as beneficial for treating pain, but had also become problematic as opioid abuse increased. The first two acts the United States passed to control the use of these substances were the Pure Food and Drug Act (1906) and the Harrison Narcotics Act (1914). These were the first two governmental attempts at controlling the use and prescribing of opioid substances. As late as 1970, the federal Controlled Substances Act provided the standard for monitoring, manufacturing, prescribing, and dispensing of opioids and created the five-level division of controlled substances that we use today.

Today, the FDA has issued a mandate that all long-acting (LA) opioids need to have a REMS for prescribers who write prescriptions for the LA opioids and rapid-acting fentanyl medications. These REMS classes provide education on safe prescribing, using PPAs, opioid risk screening, and state monitoring information to get a fuller picture of the individual patient. Some states are considering making REMS education or a course in safe opioid prescribing a requirement for license renewal.

Natural derivatives of opium include morphine, codeine, and heroin. Synthetic analogs, such as fentanyl (Sublimaze) and meperidine (Demerol), were developed much later than the morphine and morphine derivatives as attempts to perfect compounds for better pain relief. These compounds have several common features:

- Their analgelic effects are activated by binding to sites in the body called *mu receptors* to produce analgesia. Mu receptors are found in many places in the body, including the brain, gastrointestinal system, and spinal column neurons.
- Their main action is analgesia.
- Side effects, such as sedation, constipation, and nausea, are common to all members of the drug class.
- They all have the potential for addiction (OUD).

The Various Forms of Opioids

Some opioids are used in their natural form, such as morphine and heroin. Other natural opium alkaloids include codeine, noscapine, papaverine, and thebaine (www.opiates.com). These alkaloids can be further reduced into more common analgesic compounds. The alkaloid thebaine is used to produce semi-synthetic opioid morphine analogs, such as oxycodone (Percocet, Percodan), hydromorphone (Dilaudid), and hydrocodone (Vicodin/Lortab). Other classes of morphine analogs include the 4-diphenylpiperidine, meperidine (Demerol), and the diphenylpropylamine, methadone (Dolophine) (www.opiates.com). Each of these compounds was developed to either increase the analgesic effect or reduce the potential for addiction.

Although all of the opioid substances can be classed as analgesics, they vary in their potency. Each drug in the morphine group has a piperidine ring in its chemical configuration or a greater part of the ring must be chemically present to be classed as a morphian (www.opiates.com).

As mentioned previously, the main binding sites for opioids are mu receptors (Holden, Jeong, & Forrest, 2005). Mu receptors are found in:

- Cortex
- Thalamus

- Periaqueductal gray matter
- Substantia gelatinosa of the spinal cord (Fine & Portnoy, 2007)

Other secondary binding sites include the kappa and delta sites. Kappa sites are found in the brain (hypothalamus), periaqueductal gray matter, claustrum, and the spinal cord (substantia gelatinosa; Fine & Portnoy, 2007). The delta receptors are located in the pontine nucleus, amygdala, olfactory bulbs, and the deep cortex of the brain (Fine & Portenoy, 2007). Recently, an opioid receptor-like site was discovered and called *opioid receptor-like 1 (ORL1)*. The activity at this site is thought to be related to central modulation of pain, but does not appear to have an effect on respiratory depression (Fine & Portenoy, 2007).

When an opioid is introduced into a patient's body, it looks for the binding site that conforms to a specific protein pattern that allows the opioid to bind to the receptor site and create an agonist action: analgesia. At one time, the binding action of opioids was thought to be a simple lock-and- key effect; for example, inject the medication, the medication goes to the receptor binding site, and binds, thus creating analgesia. Today, we know that the process is much more specific and is more sophisticated than a simple lock-and-key effect.

Once the opioid molecule approaches the cell, it looks for a way to bind. On the exterior of each cell are ligands, or cellular channel mechanisms connecting the exterior of the cell with the interior, which convey the opioid molecule into the cell. The ligands are affiliated with the exterior receptor sites and can contain a variety of G-proteins. These G-proteins couple with the opioid molecule and mediate the action of the receptor (Fine & Portnoy, 2007). "One opioid receptor can regulate several G-proteins, and multiple receptors can activate a single G-protein" (Fine & Portnoy, 2007, p. 11). As efforts progress to better identify the process, more than 40 variations in binding-site composition have been identified (Pasternak, 2005). These differences explain some of the variations in patients' response to opioid medications.

The body also has natural pain-facilitating and pain-inhibiting substances. These include:

- Pain facilitating: Substance P, bradykinin, and glutamate
- Pain inhibiting: Serotonin (central), opioids (natural or synthetic), norepinephrine, and gamma-aminobutyric acid (GABA; D'Arcy, 2007).

When these substances are activated or blocked, pain can be relieved or increased. These more complex mechanisms are difficult to clarify, and trying to link them to a specific mechanism of analgesia and opioid effect can be misguided.

CLINICAL PEARL

Starting a patient on an opioid:

- To start a patient on opioid medications, perform an opioid risk screen, get a urine screen, complete and document a PPA, and review the Prescription Drug Monitoring Program (PDMP) in your state.
- Choose a short-acting opioid and start at a conservative dose, that is, the lowest possible effective dose.
- See the patient within 1 month and titrate as needed, monitoring pain relief and side effects.
- Continue to monitor and reassess the patient every 3 months and adjust the plan of care as needed.
- Document all interactions and progress toward the identified goals.

Formulations of Opioid Medications

Opioid medications are very versatile in that they can be given as a stand-alone medication, such as oxycodone, or combined with another type of nonopioid medication such as a nonsteroidal anti-inflammatory drug (NSAID), for example, oxycodone combined with ibuprofen (Combunox) or oxycodone combined with acetaminophen (Percocet). Opioids can be formulated as elixirs (such as morphine [Roxanol]) or as a suppository such as hydromorphone (Dilaudid) suppositories. Because the elixir form can be very bitter, adding a flavoring, which is available at most pharmacies can help the patient tolerate the taste of the medication.

Patients can metabolize medication either very rapidly or very slowly. This can affect the onset and duration of pain relief. The duration of the oral short-acting preparations is usually listed as 4 to 6 hours, but each patient has an individual response and ability to metabolize medications. For example, the duration of action of short-acting morphine may vary between 3 and 7 hours (Quill et al., 2010).

Most of the combination medications are considered to be short acting and the combination of another dose-limited medication, such as acetaminophen, limits the amount of medication that can be taken in a 24-hour period. Those that are combined with acetaminophen follow the recommended daily dose for acetaminophen use to 4,000 mg/d maximum (APS, 2008).

Many opioids are created in LA, sustained-release (SR), and extended-release (ER) formulations that can be dosed every 12 to 24 hours, for example, oxycodone SR (OxyContin) and morphine (Kadian, MS Contin). These ER medications are particularly helpful for patients with chronic pain or when cancer pain is present throughout the day. They are not designed to be used in patients who are opioid naïve, but for those patients who are opioid tolerant and have chronic severe pain daily, and who have been taking the short-acting medications regularly to control their pain.

Some LA opioid medications, such as the fentanyl (Duragesic) patch, have specific short-acting medication requirements before they can be initiated. For example, before initiating the fentanyl 25 mcg/hr patch, to be considered opioid tolerant the patient must have been using a total daily dose of at least 60 mg of morphine, 30 mg of oxycodone, or 8 mg of hydromorphone by mouth per day for 2 weeks prior to patch application (Janssen prescribing information available at www.janssen.com). Fentanyl patches should never be used on opioid naive patients as it can have a fatal outcome. Every patient who uses an ER opioid medication for pain should have a short-acting medication available to take for worsening pain. Referred to as *breakthrough pain*, this is increased intensity of pain that occurs spontaneously, or with increased activity, or from the end-of-dose failure of the LA agent (APS, 2008).

CLINICAL PEARL

Opioid naïve: Patients who are not chronically taking opioid medications on a daily basis.

Opioid tolerant: Patients who take opioid medication regularly for 1 week or longer in the following doses or more (FDA, 2011; National Comprehensive Cancer Network [NCCN] Guidelines, 2011; Stokowski, 2010)

- 60 mg oral morphine/d
- 25 mcg transdermal (TD) fentanyl/hr
- 30 mg oral oxycodone/d
- 8 mg oral hydromorphone/d
- An equianalgesic dose of any other opioid

No matter what type or form of opioid medication is being considered for use, the healthcare prescriber should be aware of the risks and benefits of each medication and weigh the options carefully. A full history and physical examination should be performed. A detailed risk assessment for possible opioid misuse should be done, and ongoing reassessments are needed to highlight any occurrence of problems with opioids or side effects.

Short-Acting Combination Opioid Medications

At recommended doses, short-acting pain medications last for several hours The CDC recommends starting all patients who qualify for opioid therapy on a trial of short-acting opioids at the lowest effective dose (CDC, 2017). For most patients, a short-acting medication is appropriate when pain is less severe and does not last throughout the day or night. Some patients do not have high levels of pain and short-acting opioids may be all that is needed to control the pain. Patients with more severe pain intensities and consistent daily pain require a more complex medication regimen to control their pain effectively.

Most short-acting medications are administered orally as either pills or elixirs. Some patients may have difficulty swallowing pills, but can tolerate an elixir, either swallowed or taken by a sublingual route. Intramuscular (IM) administration of opioids is no longer recommended because the IM route causes irregular absorption and tissue sclerosis. Therefore, most national guidelines have removed the IM administration from their recommendations (APS, 2008; American Society of Pain Management Nurses [ASPMN], 2009; D'Arcy, 2007).

Most short-acting opioid medications are designed for moderate to severe pain intensities. Onset of action is usually 10 to 60 minutes with a short duration of action, that is, 2 to 6 hours (Katz, McCarberg, & Reisner, 2007). Overall advantages of short-acting medications include a synergistic effect if combined with acetaminophen or ibuprofen to improve pain relief and provide a better outcome. However, if the patient has liver impairment, the use of acetaminophen products is not an option.

Common Opioid Medications

Morphine: *Immediate-release morphine (MSIR), Roxanol elixir*

Morphine is the gold standard for pain relief. It is the standard for equianalgesic conversions and has a long history of use for pain control in many different forms and is available in many different forms: pills, elixir, IV, and suppository. It is indicated for severe pain. The biggest drawback of morphine is its side-effect profile. Constipation, nausea/vomiting, delirium, and hallucinations are some of the most commonly reported adverse effects.

Oxycodone-containing medications: *Percocet, Roxicet, Percodan, Oxifast*

Medications containing oxycodone are designed for treating moderate pain. They are commonly used for patients with higher pain intensities and for patients with chronic pain at higher doses. Percocet is a combination medication with 5, 7.5, or 10 mg of oxycodone and 325 mg of acetaminophen. Percodan is oxycodone, you can use higher doses of oxycodone tablets or combined with aspirin. If the patient requires a higher dose of medication for pain control, combining a 5-mg oxycodone tablet with a combined form, such as Roxicet (oxycodone 5 mg/acetaminophen 325 mg), or using a tablet with the dose of 10 mg of oxycodone with 325 mg of acetaminophen will provide additional pain relief, but still maintain the acetaminophen dose at 325 mg. To help patients tolerate the medication without nausea, giving the medication with milk or after meals is recommended (Nursing, 2014).

Hydromorphone: *Dilaudid*

Dilaudid is an extremely potent analgesic designed for use with severe pain. In its oral form, it comes in 2-, 4-, and 8-mg tablets. It also available as a suppository. In IV form, 0.2 mg of Dilaudid is equal to 1 mg of IV morphine. Because of the strength of this medication, it is possible to give small amounts, get good pain relief, and potentially have fewer side effects. It is not available in a combination form with acetaminophen. Therefore, doses can be titrated as needed to achieve adequate pain relief.

Fentanyl transmucosal (Sublimaze): *Actiq, Fentora, Onsolis*

There is no oral formulation for fentanyl. The route of administration is either transdermal (TD), buccal, or IV. When used buccally for breakthrough pain in opioid-tolerant patients, the transmucosal medications can be rubbed or placed against the buccal membrane and absorbed directly into the circulation. Its fast absorption makes oversedation a risk. So it is indicated only for breakthrough pain in opioid-tolerant cancer patients who take opioid medications on a daily basis.

If the entire dose of an Actiq oralet is not used, it should be placed in a child-proof container and disposed of. This medication is not meant to be used for acute or postoperative pain (Nursing, 2014). It is not meant to be used in opioid-naïve patients since serious oversedation can occur (Fine & Portnoy, 2007)

Hydrocodone-containing medications: *Vicodin, Lortab, Norco, Lortab elixir*

Hydrocodone-containing medications are designed to be used for moderate pain. They usually contain 5 to 10 mg of hydrocodone with 325 or 500 mg of acetaminophen. Many patients tolerate the medication very well for intermittent or breakthrough pain. It is available in an elixir form that is very effective and can be used with patients who have difficulty swallowing pills or who have enteral feeding tubes. Norco has a higher dose of hydrocodone per tablet than the other medications listed.

Other Opioid Medications

***Tramad**ol (Ultram, Ultracet)* and Tapentadol *(Nucynta)*

Tramadol and tapentadol are in a unique class of drugs with weak (tramadol) or moderate (tapentadol) mu agonist (opioid-like) properties and a structure similar to tricyclic antidepressantst (TCA; APS, 2008). These drugs were designed for use with moderate pain. Doses should be reduced for patients with increased creatinine levels, cirrhosis, and in older patients. It may increase the risk for seizures and serotonin syndrome (Nursing, 2014). Patients should be instructed to taper off the medication gradually when discontinuing the medication. It should not be stopped suddenly (Nursing, 2014).

EXTENDED-RELEASE (ER) MEDICATIONS: RELIEF FOR CONSISTENT AROUND-THE-CLOCK PAIN

ER medication can give a consistent blood level of medication to provide a steady comfort level. This may increase functionality and improve quality of life, enhance sleep, and let the patient participate in meaningful daily activities. ER medications have a slower onset of action (30–90 minutes) with a relatively long duration of action (up to 72 hours; Katz et al., 2007).

When a patient has pain that lasts throughout the day and the patient is taking short-acting medications and has reached the maximum dose limitations of the nonopioid medication, the prescriber should consider switching the patient to an ER or LA medication. Some of the short-acting medications have an ER formulation, for example, Hysingla, Zohydro, Ultram ER, Oxycontin, Kadian, and MS Contin. Most are pure mu agonist medications, such as morphine, with an ER action that allows the medication to dissolve slowly in the gastrointestinal tract. Some ER medications are encapsulated into beads that allow gastric secretions to enter the bead and force the medication out. Other ER formulations have a coating around an ER plasticized compound that keeps the medication from dissolving too quickly. When a patient begins taking an ER medication, the patient should be instructed on the important aspects of the medication, including:

- ER medications of all types should never be broken, chewed, or degraded in any way to enhance the absorption of the medications. Doing so runs the risk of all the medication being given at one time, with high risk for potentially fatal oversedation. Some ER medications are available in tamper-resistant formulations to decrease the potential for misuse.
- Most ER medications should not be taken with alcohol. Doing so modifies the ER mechanism and allows for a faster absorption of the medication, which can cause potentially fatal oversedation.
- ER medications are not meant to be injected.
- Most ER medications should not be crushed and inserted into enteral feeding tubes. The one exception is Kadian.
- Enteral administration of LA morphine (Kadian) is an option when a 16 Fr or larger gastrostomy tube is present. Kadian ER capsules are filled with pellets. The capsules are opened and mixed into 10 mL of water. This mixture is poured into the gastrostomy tube through a funnel, followed by a 10-mL flush of water (*Web*MD, 2010). Kadian ER pellets may also be sprinkled onto applesauce if the patient can swallow some food. Note that these brand-name formulations are more expensive.

- ER medications are meant to be used on a schedule, not on an "as needed" basis and never for breakthrough pain (APS, 2008).
- If the patient experiences end-of-dose failure several hours before the next dose of medication is due, the intervening interval should be shortened (e.g., every 8 hours instead of every 12 hours) or the dose should be increased (APS, 2008).

When converting a patient from short-acting medications, the rule of thumb is as follows:

- If the medication is the same (oxycodone short acting and oxycodone SR), equivalent doses of the medication can be prescribed. For example, if the patient is taking a 5-mg oxycodone tablet, four tablets per day, he or she can be safely started on oxycodone SR (OxyContin) 10 mg twice a day.
- If switching to a different drug, oxycodone short acting to morphine CR (MS Contin), for example, the daily dose should be calculated using the equianalgesic conversion table and reduced (usually by 30%). To ensure adequate pain relief is maintained, additional doses of breakthrough medication should be prescribed, about 5% to 15% of the total daily dose taken every 2 hours as needed (APS, 2008). Patients should also be informed that they should reserve the short-acting breakthrough pain (BTP) medication for episodes of increased pain, and not use it as an adjunct taken along with the ER medications. Use of the breakthrough medication should be monitored and documented at every visit.

Because these ER medications are potent, the use of tamper-resistant formulas is highly recommended. Some medication now will dissolve into a gum-like substance when one attempts to crush the medication for abuse. This does not allow the opioid component to be used. Other formulas contain a mu antagonist medication, such as naltrexone, that will activate and neutralize the opioid effect of the medication when tampering is attempted.

Methadone: *Dolophine*

Methadone is considered to be an LA medication because it has an extended half-life of 15 to 60 hours (APS, 2008). However, pain relief in the oral form lasts only 6 to 8 hours (Nursing, 2014). Therein lays its danger. If the half-life is long and the pain relief is shorter, dosing must be done carefully to avoid oversedating the patient, which may become apparent only a day or 2 after the doses are given. In general, dose escalation should occur no more than every 5 to 7 days (APS, 2008).

Methadone can be prescribed legally by physicians, nurse practitioners (NPs), and physician assistants (PAs) in primary care for pain relief. However, it is also used for opioid substitution therapy (e.g., methadone maintenance) to control addiction in heroin and other OUD patients. A special license waiver is required to prescribe methadone for addiction management. The addiction program has no connection to prescribing methadone for pain management. However, because there is such risk with this medication, the current recommendation of the APS is that only pain-management practitioners or those skilled and knowledgeable about use of methadone prescribe the drug (Chou et al., 2014; D'Arcy, 2009).

An additional risk factor in methadone use is the potential for QTc interval prolongation. This puts the patient at risk of the potential deadly ventricular arrhythmia torsades de pointes (APS, 2008). Healthcare providers are advised to obtain a baseline EKG for patients who are receiving methadone, with periodic EKG monitoring. At a QTc prolongation of >450, consideration should be given to reducing the dose of methadone or switching to another drug (APS, 2008). Combination of drugs that cause risk of QTc prolongation requires more careful monitoring by clinicians.

Fentanyl Transdermal (TD) patch: *Duragesic*

Fentanyl patches can provide a high level of pain relief and are used for a variety of chronic pain conditions. These patches are the only TD opioid available. The fentanyl TD (Duragesic) patch uses a delivery system that contains a specified dose of fentanyl in a gel formulation. It is designed for use with opioid-tolerant patients and should never be used for acute pain or with opioid-naïve patients.

The fentanyl TD patch should be applied to clean, intact, hair-free skin. It delivers the specified amount of medication for 72 hours, for example, 25 mcg/hr (D'Arcy, 2007). The systemic medication effect begins after the medication depot develops in the subcutaneous fat, which can take from 12 to 18 hours after application (D'Arcy, 2007, 2009). It can also take up to 48 hours for steady-state blood levels to develop; so, when the fentanyl TD patch is initiated, the patient may need additional short-acting pain medication to control breakthrough pain (D'Arcy, 2009).

There are some safety concerns with use of the fentanyl TD (Duragesic) patch. More than 100 patients have died related to fentanyl patch use and misuse. When a TD patch is prescribed for pain relief, education for the patients should include the following:

- **Do not cut the patch.** To do so will result in a dose-dumping effect in which all the medication is released at one time, resulting in an overdose.
- **Do not apply heat over the patch.** Use of heating pads will result in accelerated medication delivery that could result in an overdose.
- **Dispose of the patch properly.** Seal in a baggy with kitty litter or used coffee grounds. Bag the garbage and put it in an outside garbage recep-

tacle immediately. About 16% of the dose remains in the patch after use and an animal or small child could remove the patch and chew it or place it on themselves, resulting in overdose (D'Arcy, 2009). Because there is medication left in the patch, safe disposal is necessary to avoid diversion.

- **Fentanyl patches should only be initiated in an opioid-tolerant patient.** In order to place a 25-mcg fentanyl patch, the patient should be taking one of the following: 30 mg of oxycodone per day for 2 weeks, 8 mg of hydromorphone per day for 2 weeks, or 60 mg of oral morphine per day for 2 weeks (Janssen prescribing information, available at www.Janssen.com).

Rapid-acting fentanyl products for breakthrough cancer pain *Onsolis, Lasanda, Oralets:*

- Fentanyl (Actiq) oralets are a form of rapid-onset fentanyl. These are rubbed against the buccal membrane, thereby releasing the prescribed dose of medication. The oralets come in 200, 400, and 800 mcg. The oralet may be used up to four times per day. Patients must be taught to "paint" the buccal surface with the oralet and keep it in constant motion. They should not "suck" on the oralet as a candy sucker. It takes about 15 to 20 minutes to use the medication. Unused medicine should be dissolved in very hot water. Partially used oralets must be destroyed and not be left lying around, as a child or pet could die from ingesting leftover medicine.
- Fentanyl (Onsolis) buccal film is a small strip that is applied to the buccal membrane that slowly releases the prescribed dose of medication. The starting dose of Onsolis is 200 mcg, which is equivalent to 200 mcg of Actiq.
- Fentanyl (Lasanda) is a nasal spray with a pectin base that has an extremely rapid onset of action, 15 minutes, and is well tolerated by patients. The starting dose of Lasanda is 100 mcg.
- Fentanyl (Fentora) buccal tablet is a dissolvable tablet that rapidly dissolves when placed against the buccal membrane. The starting dose of Fentora is 100 mcg, which is equivalent to 200 mcg of Actiq.

Medications That Are No Longer Recommended

There are two pain medications that are no longer recommended for use because of concerns related to production of toxic metabolites, poor pain relief, or a high profile for side effects.

Codeine-containing medications*: Codeine, Tylenol #3 (codeine 30 mg combined with acetaminophen 325)*

Use of codeine is discouraged. It is effective only for mild pain and causes significant nausea and constipation. In addition, many authors believe that, unlike other opioids, codeine has an analgesic ceiling (meaning that higher doses of the drug do not provide more analgesia). In addition, the number needed to treat is high (11). This means you would see the first effective analgesic effect in the 12th patient who was given the medication for pain relief. About 10% of people lack the enzyme needed to convert codeine to the active metabolite of morphine (APS, 2008).

Meperidine

Meperidine (Demerol) has also fallen out of favor. It is no longer considered a first-line pain medication (APS, 2008; D'Arcy, 2007). Meperidine has a toxic metabolite, normeperidine, that accumulates with repetitive dosing (APS, 2008). This metabolite can cause tremors and seizures. Other drawbacks include the need to use high doses to achieve an analgesic effect that is accompanied by sedation and nausea (D'Arcy, 2007). If meperidine is going to be used, there are certain recommendations to follow:

- Meperidine should never be used in children and infants.
- It should never be used in patients with renal impairment, for example, sickle cell disease, multiple myeloma, or in older patients.
- A potentially fatal hyperpyrexic syndrome with delirium can occur if meperidine is used in patients who are taking monoamine oxidase inhibitors.
- It should never be used for more than 1 to 2 days at doses not exceeding 600 mg/24 hr (APS, 2008).

Mixed Agonist/Antagonist Medications

This class of medications can provide good pain relief for women, but not for men. This difference is the result of a pain pathway that is active in women, but not in men. These medications have both an agonist and antagonist action at various binding sites throughout the body. For this reason, these medications are termed *mixed agonist/antagonist* medications and include the following:

- Buprenophrine (Buprenex injection or sublingual Temgesic, Butrans TD patch)
- nalbuphine (Nubain)
- pentazocine (Talwin)

These medications act at the kappa receptor sites. So the potential for respiratory depression is considered to be reduced. Because these medications have both agonist and antagonist action, they have the potential to reverse the opioid effect of pure opioid agonists such as morphine. If a patient is taking morphine, giving a mixed agonist and antagonist medication will reverse the effect of the morphine and pain relief is lessened. This group of medications also has a high profile for adverse side effects, such as confusion and hallucinations, and has dose ceilings that limit dose escalations (APS, 2008). Use of pentazocine is no longer recommended due its adverse effects.

Buprenophrine is used in chronic pain management. Butrans, a TD buprenorphine patch, has been promoted for use in osteoarthritis and low-back pain. It acts as a partial agonist at the mu receptor sites with antagonist activity at the kappa receptor (Plosker, 2011; Plosker & Lyseng-Williamson, 2012). The risk of respiratory depression with buprenorphine is low, unless used concomitantly with other central nervous system depressants (Plosker, 2011).

The Butrans patch comes in doses of 5, 10, and 20 mcg and is administered once every 7 days (Plosker, 2011; Plosker & Lyseng-Williamson, 2012). The recommended starting dose is 5 mcg/hr. The recommended application sites are the upper outer arm, upper chest, upper back, and side of the chest, with rotation of sites required (Plosker, 2011). In an observational study with 4,263 patients using Butrans (67% being women), initial pain scores of 6.9 on the Numerical Pain Intensity (NPI) Scale were reduced to 2.9 over an 8-week period (Plosker, 2011). In a study with 246 osteoarthritis patients comparing sublingual buprenorphine tablets and Butrans, both medications reduced pain and improved quality of life. The Butrans patch had an analgesic effect for the full 7 days, and it is expected that medication compliance is improved by use of a 7-day medication rather than repeated sublingual dosing, especially in older patients (James, O'Brien, & McDonald, 2010).

SELECTING AN OPIOID

Selecting an opioid for an individual patient can involve a process of trial and error. Each individual has a genetic preference for one or more types of opioids. It is necessary to determine which opioid works best for the patient.

Many patients have tried opioids before for surgery or acute pain from injuries. They may know which one works best and which ones do not work at all. If the patient can provide you with information on the efficacy of pain medications, this information should not be considered drug seeking or an indicator of potential addiction. If the patient has used a medication successfully, starting with one that was effective will in many cases provide the best outcome.

Conversely, if the patient tells you that he or she has tried a medication but it did not work, get more information about when, for what indication, and what doses were tried. In many cases, patients with pain have been underdosed with medications and they consider them as "not working" or ineffective. If the correct dose of medication had been given, the medication could have provided good pain relief. It is always wise to revisit the use of a medication that has been underdosed, using appropriate doses for treating pain, unless there are side effects that would contraindicate the use of the drug.

RISK EVALUATION AND MITIGATION STRATEGIES

Although REMS is a new concept for opioid use, it has been used for years for medications, such as thalidomide, in multiple myeloma treatment so that prescribers have the knowledge to prescribe medications that have been identified with special risk factors. For opioids, LA formulations and newer medications, such as some of the rapid-acting fentanyls, were identified as having higher risks, and so the FDA has asked the manufacturers to develop REMS programs for their medications.

Most REMS programs consist of an educational component that the prescriber must complete successfully to be allowed to prescribe the medication. This has a two-sided effect. One side is the extra education that these prescribers get about the medication they are prescribing. The other side is the need to have an REMS certificate to prescribe these medications, making it easier for the prescriber to use other non-REMS–cited medications, such as short-acting opioids.

In the best scenario, the prescriber can consider that the extra education is helpful in ensuring that these potent medications are prescribed correctly. In the worst-case scenario, REMS may limit the prescribing practices of healthcare providers. Overall, the use of REMS should make prescribing practices safer for both the healthcare provider and the patient.

TREATING THE SIDE EFFECTS OF OPIOIDS

All opioids have the potential for side effects. There is no magic pain medication that does not have the potential for constipation, sedation, or pruritis. When a patient indicates that he or she is allergic to a medication, it is important for the prescriber to determine whether what the patient perceives as an allergy is just an unwanted side effect such as rash or pruritis. Opioids can be used in the presence of side effects, but treatment options to control the unwanted effects or dose reduction to minimize the side effects should be used. One important concept to remember here is that adding a medication that is sedating, such as phenergan, can potentiate sedation from an opioid. Before deciding that an opioid is too sedating, look at all the sedating medications that are being used concomitantly and try to minimize the use of these additional sedating agents.

Constipation

Constipation is a common side effect of opioid use. It is the one effect of which the patient will not become tolerant. Every patient who is prescribed an opioid should take a laxative of some type. Stool softeners are also used to ease bowel movements. Stimulant laxatives are used to counteract the constipation. Combination stool softener/laxatives are available over the counter in most drug stores. Recommended types of laxatives include:

- Senna or senna with stool softener—increases bowel motility
- Bisacodyl—increases bowel motility
- Magnesium citrate 30 mg—a hyperosmolar laxative
- Lactulose—an osmotic laxative
- Sorbitol (easily found in Sorbee candies)—an osmotic laxative
- Methylnaltrexone (Relistor,—approved for opioid-induced constipation for patients with advanced illness or palliative care)—subcutaneous injectable or oral tablets (APS, 2008)

Sedation

Patients may become sedated when opioids are first initiated, but they become tolerant to the effect within a period of 2 weeks or less. If sedation persists or reaches high levels, dose adjustments should be made, so that serious oversedation does not occur. As indicated, sedation occurs most often at the beginning of opioid therapy (D'Arcy, 2007). Patients should be monitored for sedating effects of the opioid and for any additive sedating effects from medications that are sedating, such as antiemetics, sedatives, antihistamines, muscle relaxants, sleeping medications, benzodiazepines, and so forth.

To counteract sedation, stimulants, such as caffeine, dextroamphetamine, methylphenidate, or modafinil, can be used. The medications listed are most often used for patients with chronic cancer pain. Most patients adjust to the sedating effects of opioids within a few weeks at the longest, but the use of caffeine may be recommended for almost any patient.

Pruritis (Itching)

Some patients who begin taking opioids or who are taking high doses of opioids may develop pruritis (itching). The itching is the result of a histamine release and not an indication of a true allergy. The most common way to counteract itch is to use an antihistamine such as diphenhydramine (Benadryl). If itching persists, changing to another opioid may reduce or eliminate this effect.

Delirium/Confusion

Many patients, especially older patients, become confused when they are moved from their usual living situation and put into a new situation, or have surgery and begin taking opioids. For patients with chronic pain, the incidence of confusion or delirium should be minimal. Delirium can be caused by opioids and it is temporary. If the patient becomes delirious, changing the opioid, reducing the dose, or stopping the opioid may provide the needed intervention. Some opioids, such as morphine, have a higher profile for confusion. Changing to another medication, such as low-dose Dilaudid, may provide adequate pain relief and lessen the potential for confusion.

Nausea/Vomiting

Opioids have a high profile for nausea and vomiting. For most opioids, taking the medication with a small amount of food or milk helps to reduce this effect. If the nausea and vomiting do not resolve, using an antiemetic regularly until the effect abates is the best option. Because all antiemetics are sedating, there will be an additive sedating effect when the medications are combined. Recommended antiemetics include:

- Ondansetron
- Phenergan (caution is needed with IV administration; can cause tissue necrosis)
- Reglan
- Meclizine or cyclizine for motion-induced nause
- Scopolamine patches are used for severe cases (APS, 2008)

OPIOID OVERDOSE AND NALOXONE

When a patient with OUD or who is on opioids overdoses and begins to experience respiratory depression, using naloxone (Narcan), an opioid antagonist, either IM or intranasally, can release the opioid from the mu binding sites and restore normal respiratory function. To initiate treatment, give 0.4 mg IV, IM, or subcutaneously (Nursing, 2014). The first dose of medication may not restore full consciousness and may need to be repeated. The medication may only last 4 hours and will need to be repeated if the patient begins to lose respiratory drive.

In some states, such as Virginia, California, and Vermont, coprescribing of naloxone is mandated for patients on high-dose opioids who are considered to be at risk. The coprescribing mandate increased the rate of naloxone prescribing 7.75 times, creating greater availability of naloxone in local pharmacies (Sohn, Talbert, & Huang, 2019).

Educating the patient, family, and significant others about how to use the medication in the case of emergency is an important piece of education for those with chronic opioid use. Prescribing naloxone can be a lifesaving component of the plan of care for a patient who is on long-term opioid therapy and who may be considered to be at risk.

SUMMARY

Opioids are good analgesics when used for the right patient at the correct dose. Some patients with chronic pain can use opioids for many years and show no negative effects. Considering genetics and patient preferences can help find an opioid that will work for the patient. Prescribers should become familiar with the opioids that are offered on their formulary, so that they can use them when appropriate.

To ensure safe opioid prescribing to protect the patient and the prescriber, the CDC guideline recommendations should be observed and the concepts outlined in the FDA's blueprint on prescriber continuing education (FDA, 2012) should be followed. As always, prescribers should stay informed about any opioid-related issues occurring in their states and follow state and national guidelines for prescribing opioids.

TRENDING IN PAIN MANAGEMENT

- Look for new opioids or combinations of opioids that will improve pain relief.
- Look for new techniques in delivery systems that will increase the delivery of the opioid while possibly decreasing side effects.
- Check for the release of medications to replace opioids that target pain-producing substances such as tumor necrosis factor, for example, tanezumab from Pfizer-Lilly.
- Check for state regulation changes requiring the coprescribing of naloxone for patients taking higher dose opioids.

CASE STUDY

Eric is a sanitation worker who lifts large garbage cans daily. He has been taking short-acting opioids as needed for his low-back pain. Recently, he reinjured his back and needed to take his opioid medication regularly, used some muscle relaxers, and participated in a physical therapy program for back patients. His back pain is better,

(continued)

CASE STUDY (*continued*)

he rates it 4/10 with medication, and his strength is better as well. He thinks he can continue with his job if he can take his opioid medication regularly. It is hard for him to stop to take medication every few hours, and he wonders whether there is a better medication available for his pain. His employer is aware of his medication use and monitors his compliance with urine drug screens. He also meets with his company insurance provider to make sure his insurance will cover all of his medications and treatments.

- Eric has been taking opioids for several years and exhibits a low risk for opioid abuse or diversion. Continuing the current opioid is an option, but he is approaching the total daily allowance for the acetaminophen combined with his opioid.
- Considering an ER opioid is also an option. It would provide a more consistent level of pain relief and decrease the number of tablets that Eric needs daily. Unfortunately, Eric's insurance provider will not approve the use of the ER opioid selected. You will need to select a short-acting opioid without acetaminophen for Eric's pain unless you can get an exception approved.
- The national guidelines for low-back pain indicate that opioids are only moderately effective. You discuss options with Eric and he agrees to change his opioid to the one with no acetaminophen and to go to physical therapy to strengthen his back muscles. He also agrees to try a transcutaneous electrical nerve stimulation (TENS) unit for his pain.
- Over the next 3 months, you reduce Eric's opioid dose by small amounts until you reach the point at which his pain is being controlled with the reduced dose. Eric says his pain is still pretty good at 5/10 and he thinks this is the best he has felt in a while.

REFERENCES

American Pain Society. (2008). *Principles of analgesic use in the treatment of acute pain and cancer pain*. Glenview, IL: Author.

American Psychiatric Association. (2013). *Diagnostic and statistical manual of mental disorders* (5th ed.). Arlington, VA: American Psychiatric Publishing,

American Society of Pain Management Nurses. (2009). *Core curriculum for pain management nursing*. Dubuque, IA: Kendall Hunt Publishing.

Bachhuber, M., Weiner, J., Mitchell, J., & Samet, J. (2016). *Primary care: On the front lines of the opioid crisis.* Retrieved from https://ldi.upenn.edu/brief/primary-care-front-lines-opioid-crisis

Back, S. E., Lawson, K. M., Singleton, L. M., & Brady, K. T. (2011). Characteristics and correlates of men and women with prescription opioid dependence. *Addictive Behaviors, 36*(8), 829–834. doi: 10.1016/j.addbeh.2011.03.013

Brown, T. (2018). New attitudes toward pain amid the opioid crisis. *Medscape Nurses*. Retrieved from https://www.medscape.com/viewarticle/893926

Bucheit, T. (2019, October). Expert comment. *Pain Medicine News* p. 18.

Center for Drug Evaluation and Research. U. S. Food and Drug Administration. (2012). Blueprint for prescriber continuing education program. *Journal of Pain and Palliative Care Pharmacotherapy, 26*(2), 127–130. doi: 10.3109/15360288.2012.6800

Centers for Disease Control and Prevention. (2016). CDC guidelines for prescribing opioids for chronic pain. *Mortality and Morbidity Weekly Report, 65*(1), 1–49.

Chou, R., Cruciani, R., Fiellin, D., Compton, P., Farrar, J., Haigney, M., . . . Zeltzer, L. (2014). Methadone safety: A clinical practice guideline from the American Pain Society and College on Problems of Drug Dependence in collaboration with the Heart Rhythm Society. *Journal of Pain, 15*(4), 321–337. doi:10.1016/j.jpain.2014.01.494

Cicero, T., Wong, G., Tian, Y., Lynskey, M., Todorov, A., & Isenberg, K. (2009). Co-morbidities and utilization of services by pain patients receiving opioids medications: Data from an insurance claims database. *Pain, 144*(1–2), 20–27. doi:10.1016/j.pain.2009.01.026

D'Arcy, Y. (2007). *Pain management: Evidence based tools and techniques for nursing professionals.* Marblehead, MA: HcPro.

D'Arcy, Y. (2009). Avoid the dangers of opioid therapy. *American Nurse Today, 4*(5), 16–22.

Darnell, B., & Stacey, B. (2012). Sex differences in long-term opioid use. *Archives of Internal Medicine, 172*(5), 431–432. doi:10.1001/archinternmed.2011.1741

Fine, P. G., & Portnoy, R. (2007). *A clinical guide to opioid analgesia*. New York, NY: Vendome Group.

Green, T. C., Serrano, J. M. G., Licari, A., Budman, S. H., & Butler, S. F. (2009). Women who abuse prescription opioids: Findings from the Addiction Severity Index—multimedia version connect prescription opioid database. *Drug and Alcohol Dependency, 103*(1–2), 65–73.

Holden, J. E., Jeong, Y., & Forrest, J. (2005). The endogenous opioid system and clinical pain management. *AACN Clinical Issues, 16*(3), 291–301. doi:10.1097/00044067-200507000-00003

Inturrisi, C., & Lipman, A. (2010). Opioid analgesicis. In S. Fishman, J. Ballantyne, & J. Rathmell (Eds.), *Bonica's management of pain* (pp. 1172–1180). Philadelphia, PA: Lippincott Wiliams & Wilkins.

James, I., O'Brien, C., & McDonald, C. (2010). A randomized, double blind, double dummy comparison of the efficacy and tolerability of low-dose transdermal buprenorphine (Butrans Seven Day patches) with buprenorphine sublingual tablets (Temgesic) in patient with osteoarthritis pain. *Journal of Pain and Symptom Management, 40*(2), 266–278.

Katz, N., McCarberg, B. & Reisner, L. (2007). *Managing chronic pain with opioids in primary care*. Newton, MA: Inflexxion.

Naprash, H., & Barnett, M. (2019). Decision for opioid prescribing varies by appointment time. *JAMA Network Open, 2*(8). Retrieved from https://jamanetwork.com/journals/jamanetworkopen

National Comprehensive Cancer Network Guidelines. (2011). *National Comprehensive Cancer Network Guidelines: Adult cancer pain.* Retrieved from http://www.nccn.org/professionals/physician_gls/f_guidelines.asp

Nursing. (2014). *Drug handbook*. Philadelphia, PA: Lippincott Williams & Wilkins.

Pasternak, G. W. (2005). Molecular biology of opioid analgesia. *Journal of Pain and Symptom Management, 29*(Suppl. 5), S2–S9. doi:10.1016/j.jpainsymman.2005.01.011

Plosker, G. (2011). Buiprenorphine 5,10,20, mcg/hour transdermal patch. *Drugs, 71*(18), 2491–2509.

Plosker, G., & Lyseng-Williamson, K. (2012). Burenorphine 5,10, 20 mcg/hour patch. A guide to use in chronic non-malignant pain. *CNS Drugs, 26*(4), 367–373.

Quill, T., Halloway, R., Shah, M., Caprio, T., Olden, A., & Storey, J. (2010). *Primer of palliative care*. (5th ed.,). Glenview IL: American Academy of Hospice and Palliative Care.

Sohn, M., Talbert, J., & Huang, Z. (2019). Association of naloxone coprescription laws with naloxone prescription dispensing in the United States. *JAMA Network Open, 2*(6), e196215. https://jamanetwork.com/jamanetworkopen

Stokowski, L. (2010). Opioid-naive and opioid-tolerant patients. *Medscape Today*. Retrieved from http://www.medscape.com/viewarticle/733067_2

U. S. Food and Drug Administration. (2011, October 2). *FDA for health professionals*. Retrieved from http://www.fda.gov

*Web*MD. (2010). *Kadian*. Retrieved from https://www.webmd.com/drugs/2/drug-1509/kadian-oral/details

ADDITIONAL RESOURCES

Cairns, B., & Gazerani, P. (2009). Sex-related differences in pain. *Matauritas, 63*(4), 292–296. doi:10.1016/j.maturitas.2009.06.004

Chou, R., Fanciullo, G., Fine, P., Adler, J., Ballantyne, J., Davies, P., . . . Miaskowski, C. (2009). Opioid treatment guidelines: Clinical guidelines for the use of chronic opioid therapy in chronic noncancer pain. *Journal of Pain, 10*(2), 113–130. doi:10.1016/j.jpain.2008.10.008

Craft, R. (2007). Modulation of pain by estrogens. *Pain, 132*, S3–S12. doi:10.1016/j.pain.2007.09.028

Fillingim, R., & Gear, R. (2004). Sex differences in opioid analgesia: Clinical and experimental findings. *European Journal of Pain, 8*(5), 413–425. doi:10.1016/j.ejpain.2004.01.007

Fine, P. G. (2004). Opioid induced hyperalgesia and opioid rotation. *Journal of Pain & Palliative Care Pharmacology, 18*(3), 75–79.

Institute for Clinical Systems Improvement. (2008). *Assessment and management of chronic pain*. Bloomington, MN: Author. Retrieved from www.guideline.gov

CHAPTER 10

TITRATING, TAPERING, AND CONVERTING OPIOID MEDICATIONS

INTRODUCTION

For patients taking long-term opioids for pain relief, the idea of tapering off the medication or changing the medication can produce anxiety. For patients on opioids, if there is no progress toward goals, there are unmanageable side effects; or if the patient is misusing the opioids or overdoses, tapering off of opioids needs to be implemented.

In practice, if the prescriber determines that a change is needed, the patient may strongly resist the change or continue to take the medication as it was originally prescribed. The patient may truly feel that the pain will return or worsen if the medication is changed or doses are decreased, creating anxiety and fear over any proposed changes. In fact, what actually happens is the pain control is increased and the amount of medication needed to control the pain is less than previously prescribed. Helping the patient to see the benefit of rotating opioids or tapering the medications can help the patient to be more positive about the proposed change. Allowing the patient to be a part of the decision-making process will help with compliance with the process.

When a healthcare provider (HCP) is working with a patient who needs opioid tapering, discontinuation, or rotation, it is likely that he or she has already established a long-term relationship with the patient. Capitalizing on the past positive interactions can reassure the patient that the HCP will not do anything that would be negative for the patient or increase the pain. Reassuring the patient that he or she will have the HCP's support during this time will also give the patient confidence to go forward with the proposed change.

Each patient is a unique individual with a unique genetic composition. There are a large number of binding sites on the mu receptors that allow for opioids to bind in different places in different patients. As early as 2005, Pasternak identified at least 45 subtypes in mu receptor sites. This accounts for the differences we see in patients, one medication does not work despite dose increases, whereas another medication is efficacious at lower doses. The differences in medication action are a function of the patient's genetic and binding affinity for any given medication.

Because there are so many variants in the receptor sites, a condition called *opioid cross-tolerance* can affect the outcome of opioid rotation. In this case, some of the original opioid remains active at the mu receptor sites, while the receptors also respond to the new opioid. This effect will produce a greater potential for sedation or overdose; so careful monitoring during the process is essential.

EQUIANALGESIC DOSING

When a patient is not responding to one medication, another similar medication may prove effective. As stated, the difference in response is due to the patient's genetic preference for one medication over another and the different ways the patient's binding sites respond to the medication. Also, P450 enzymes in the liver are very individual and metabolism rates can also affect the way a medication acts. In this case, changing to another medication may be the answer to better pain control. The way to maintain the patient's pain relief is to change the medication using an equianalgesic conversion.

Equianalgesic dosing can be defined as substituting one medication for another that offers equal pain relief. This also can provide a conversion from one form of the medication, for example, from oral to parenteral. The standard opioid conversion is based on morphine, with 1 mg of parenteral morphine being equivalent to 10 mg of oral morphine. There are a wide variety of conversion calculators available in print and online. Choosing one that is supported by evidence is the best option for the prescriber. Consulting a pharmacist about finding a reputable source is a way to confirm the accuracy of the conversion.

Because equianalgesia is the conversion of one opioid to an equivalent analgesic dose of another opioid based on equivalency charts, becoming familiar with the basic conversion doses helps the prescriber have more confidence in the process. The equianalgesic charts are designed to provide guidance for practitioners who are prescribing for or treating patients on opioid therapy. It may look like a simple exchange to take one medication, see what the equivalent dose is, and then start the new medication, but there are dangers and consequences that make the process challenging.

One of the major pitfalls in the use of an equianalgesic table is that it is based on the potency of the medication. *Potency* is defined as the dose required to produce a given effect (Knotcova, Fine, & Portnoy, 2009). Potency can vary from one individual to another and from one medication to the next. There are external factors that can influence how potent a medication is for a patient, which can skew the results of a comparison.

Equianalgesic tables are based on single-dose trials in healthy volunteers (usually young, adult males). In the past, equianalgesic doses were determined using expert opinion, single-dose studies, and studies in noncancer patients (Shaheen, Walsh, Lasheen, Davis, & Lagman, 2009). it is important to note the change in the population used to determine the dose equivalents. The chronic long-term pain that patients experience is very different than the pain that subjects in the dosing trials experienced. A different type of outcome is expected for a patient with chronic pain than for a much younger patient experiencing a laboratory-produced pain stimulus.

These tables are intended only as an estimation; a precise conversion is not really possible. The conversion is a mathematical comparison that does not take into account all the elements of the patient's presentation, such as comorbidities, genetics, or concomitant medications. The best use of equianalgesic tables is as a guide rather than a conclusive exchange. In a study comparing equianalgesic tables, findings indicate that in some tables, the conversion for oral to parenteral morphine ranged from 2:1 to 6:1, and for oral to parenteral hydromorphone from 2:1 to 5:1 (Shaheen et al., 2009). Once you find a chart that fits your practice, continue to use it consistently, rather than using several for which you have less experience.

For the clinician, this lack of concrete applicability is problematic. Here is where the art and science of pain management meet. The science of pain management provides the structure for an equianalgesic conversion, whereas the art allows the clinician to use his or her clinical experience to then decide on the best dose for the patient. Knowing the patient and the patient's medication history is an important part of a successful conversion. Allowing for additional breakthrough medication can also provide adequate pain relief if the conversion is a bit too conservative than what is needed to maintain sufficient pain relief.

There are many sources for equianalgesic conversion tables. Exhibit 10.1 provides an example of a conversion table. Other sources that can be accessed include:

- American Pain Society (APS, 2008) *Principles of Analgesic Use in the Treatment of Acute Pain and Cancer Pain.* Available at www .ampainsoc.org
- Online opioid analgesic converter available at www.globalrph.com/ narcoticcanv.htm
- Dosing equivalencies from standard medication texts.
- Prescribing information from the package inserts

There are positive and negative aspects of any equianalgesic table. One of the biggest positives is that it simplifies the mathematical conversion required to change from using one medication to another. The medication list usually offers

EXHIBIT 10.1

EXAMPLE OF A CONVERSION

To begin the conversion, calculate the entire 24-hr dose, including any breakthrough medication being used.

This is an example of an opioid rotation conversion from MS Contin to Oxycontin.

Original medication: MS Contin

Dose: MS Contin 120 mg twice per day with Morphine Immediate Release (MSIR) 30 mg every 4 hr as needed for pain (using an average of four tablets per day = 240 mg/d)

Calculate all opioid medications taken within a 24-hr time period, both long- and short-acting opioids.

New medication: Oxycontin

Equianalgesic conversion: MS Contin 120 mg twice per day (240 mg/d) is equal to Oxycontin 80 mg twice per day (160 mg/d).

MSIR 30 mg is equal to oxycodone 20 mg every 4 hrs.

Decrease the new dose by 25% to 50%.

25% = Oxycontin 60 mg twice per day with 15 mg of oxycodone every 4 hrs for breakthrough pain

50% = Oxycontin 40 mg twice per day with 10 mg of oxycodone every 4 hrs for breakthrough pain

Source: Reproduced from D'Arcy (2011). *A compact clinical guide to chronic pain management.* New York, NY: Springer Publishing Company.

conversion of the most commonly used opioid medications and newer medications may not be included. The negatives of these tables, however, are still very significant and include the following (Shaheen et al., 2009):

- There is a failure to standardize a reference opioid.
- Many tables are the product of a single-dose conversion in a laboratory setting with volunteers using artificially produced acute pain.
- There are a wide range of doses given in the table.
- Equianalgesia is compared with short- and long-acting medications not at steady state; therefore, the dose needed may be lower than estimated.
- Computations are used instead of a clinical trial to determine equianalgesic doses.

To use an equianalgesic chart effectively, the prescriber should become comfortable with the conversions and with the clinical results of the conversions. If the patient complains of increased pain after a conversion, the conversion may have been too conservative and the prescriber should consider increasing the baseline dose of the medication while using breakthrough doses of short-acting opioids to supplement pain relief until the pain levels out and a new dose can be confirmed. If the patient becomes too sedated, or has other unmanageable side effects, the prescriber needs to lower the baseline dose until the reaction subsides and continue to monitor and reassess the patient frequently.

CLINICAL PEARL

Equianalgesic dosing is not a precise science. Find a chart that provides a reliable result and adjust the dose according to the patient's response.

USING OPIOID ROTATION TO IMPROVE PAIN RELIEF FOR PATIENTS

Opioid rotation is needed for about 40% of patients with cancer who have advanced disease (Shaheen et al., 2009) and who demonstrate a tolerance to the prescribed opioid; these patients will have a better response to a new opioid. Among those patients who do require a change, about 70% to 80% see an improvement in the balance between analgesia and adverse effects (Mercadante & Bruera, 2006). The rationale for using opioid rotation is to increase the pain relief provided to the patient and/or lessen intolerable side effects such as nausea. The same rationale can be applied to patients with consistent chronic pain and has proven effective in the noncancer pain population.

Patients who complain of decreased efficacy of the opioid do not have improved analgesia with increased doses or who develop intolerable side effects yet still have significant pain, are candidates for opioid rotation. A patient with chronic pain who has been on long-term opioids can benefit from a change and will get better pain control or a lessening of adverse side effects at lower doses of a new medication.

A Cochrane review of the literature on opioid rotation reports that the evidence for opioid switching is largely anecdotal or based on lower level studies (Quigley, 2010) However, the practice has been established in the cancer pain population, where high-dose opioids are used routinely to control pain and opioid rotation is used to improve pain relief. It is also commonly used in the chronic pain population.

For patients with chronic pain, opioid switching offers improved pain relief by increasing opioid response and decreasing unwanted side effects. In a review of the literature on opioid switching, Mercadante and Bruera (2006) reported that clinical improvement is seen in approximately 50% of patients with chronic pain who have a poor response to a specific opioid. Rotating opioids may improve the pain control and decrease fears of having pain that cannot be controlled.

To perform an opioid rotation, first review an equianalgesic chart to determine equivalencies. Then evaluate the following:

- Level of pain
- Level of adverse effects
- Any comorbidities that affect medication choice (such as renal or hepatic impairment)
- Concomitant medications

Extreme care must be used when converting patients from high-dose opioids to another medication in order to avoid overdosing or underdosing the patient and to preserve patient safety throughout the process. If high-dose opioids are being converted, consulting a pharmacist or pain specialist may provide a second opinion that the conversion has been done correctly.

Data on conversions from morphine to hydromorphone or hydrocodone are more available and the results are more predictable. Converting patients from long-acting medications, such as methadone, to a short-acting, fast-onset medication, such as fentanyl, or even making a standard conversion for morphine requires a careful and measured response. Prescribers who are converting patients on fentanyl or methadone should consult a pharmacist or pain specialist because these medications can be very dangerous if calculated incorrectly. Data for the success of such conversions are scant, and using a pharmacist for assistance should be considered.

CLINICAL PEARL

Opioid rotation is defined as a therapeutic maneuver aimed at increasing analgesia while decreasing opioid side effects. It is defined as a change in opioid drug or route of administration with the goal of improving outcomes (Fine & Portnoy, 2009). This includes changing from medications using the same route or maintaining the current medication but changing the route of administration or both (Knotkova, Fine, & Portnoy, 2009; Vadalouca, Moka, Argyra, Sikioti, & Siafaka, 2008).

To avoid an error, issues that should be considered when performing an opioid rotation (Shaheen et al., 2009) include the following:

- Knowledge of opioid pharmacology
- Awareness of the limitations of equianalgesic tables
- Application of the conversion/rotation guidelines
- Tailoring opioid dose to the individual patients and monitoring the response

Because the patient may be more responsive to the new opioid dose, there are some considerations that should be used before completing the conversion. Before implementing an opioid rotation, *best practice guidelines* indicate the following:

- Use an equianalgesic table to calculate the new opioid dose.
- For most opioids other than fentanyl or methadone, use an automatic dose reduction of 25% to 50%. If methadone is the new opioid, reduce the dose by 75% to 90%.
- Exert caution with high-dose conversions (>100 mg morphine equivalents); expert consultation is recommended for these. These conversions may require inpatient monitoring, including serial EKGs.
- Select a dose in the 50% reduction range if the patient is on high-dose opioids, is not a Caucasian, and is elderly or frail.
- Select a dose in the 25% reduction range if the patient is on a low to moderate dose of opioids, is a Caucasian, is under age 60 and reasonably robust, or if the change is from one route to another with the same medication.
- Assess the patient for pain severity or other medical characteristics that would point to a need for higher or lower doses, and decrease or increase the dose by an additional 15% to 30% to increase the chances that the converted dose will be effective or to avoid withdrawal.
- Maintain a schedule of frequent reassessment and monitoring and titrate the dose to maximize outcomes.
- Provide adequate doses for rescue or breakthrough pain, with titration at 5% to 15% of the total opioid dose (Fine & Portnoy, 2009).

Knowing the patient well and understanding how the patient has reacted to opioid medications in the past is part of performing a comprehensive evaluation for an opioid rotation. Because there is the potential for opioid cross-tolerance, use of a conservative approach offering frequent breakthrough medication can help reduce risk during the period of rotation. Monitoring the effect of the new medication is essential. Converting from one problematic opioid to another more successful opioid can provide patients with the pain the relief they need. An example of a simple opioid rotation is provided in Exhibit 10.1.

TAPERING OPIOIDS EFFECTIVELY

Tapering opioids can be an anxiety-producing process for a patient who has been using opioids for an extended period of time. After the idea is broached, the patient may resist, push back, and refuse to cooperate. The patient may tell the prescriber that the medication is the only thing that works for the pain and he or she cannot give it up and endure pain. It may take several visits to convince the patient that there will be benefit to tapering the medication.

The Centers for Disease Control and Prevention (CDC) Tapering Guide recommends considering a taper to reduce doses or discontinue opioids when:

- The patient requests a dose reduction.
- The patient does not have clinically meaningful improvement of pain and function, for example, at least 30% improvement on the three-item pain, enjoyment, general activity (PEG) tool.
- The patient is on dosages higher than or equal to 50 mg morphine equivalents/d without benefit or opioids are combined with benzodiazepines.
- The patient shows signs of substance use disorder, for example, has difficulty controlling opioid use and/or has work or family problems related to opioid use.
- The patient experiences an overdose or other serious adverse event.
- The patient shows early-warning signs for overdose risk, such as confusion, sedation, or slurred speech (CDC, n.d.).

Go slow and offer support and therapies to help the patient through the tapering process. A reduction of 10% per month is a reasonable decrease for a patient who has been taking opioids for over a year. For patients who have taken opioids for weeks or months, a decrease of 10% a week may work (CDC, n.d.). The Veterans Affairs Opioid Taper Decision Tool indicates that a taper of 5% to 20% per month is an acceptable decrease.

Because anxiety or depression is common during the tapering process, offer the patient additional support from counseling or mental health providers. Ask the patient whether he or she would consider using meditation, relaxation, or some form of integrative therapy to better relax. Above all, offer positive affirmations indicating that you feel the patient will be successful. As always, documenting the plan for titrating or tapering is essential, along with documentation of the patient's response to the changes as well as any pain reduction.

Because the patient is undergoing a major lifestyle change, frequent reassessment and monitoring are integral for the success of the taper. A hasty decision to begin a taper or discontinue opioids could result in withdrawal. This will be very distressing to the patient and make him or her want to stop the process. To assess for withdrawal, a tool, such as the Clinical Opiate Withdrawal Tool, can determine the level of withdrawal that the patient is experiencing (Broglio & Matzo, 2018).

Using a medication, such as lofexidine hydrochloride (Lucemyra), can ameliorate the symptoms of withdrawal. If the patient begins to experience nausea, anxiety, agitation, sleep problems, muscle aches, runny nose, sweating diarrhea, vomiting, and drug craving, the patient is experiencing withdrawal. Lucemyra is approved for 14-day use and acts by reducing the release of norepinephrine (Food and Drug Administration [FDA], 2018).

SUMMARY

Changing opioids can be stressful for both patient and the HCP. Learning the best ways to change and taper medications can give the provider a sense of confidence. Knowing that there is a medication to help with any withdrawal symptoms can be reassuring to both patient and provider.

TRENDING IN PAIN MANAGEMENT

- Look for new medications to use to treat withdrawal symptoms in patients who are being tapering or undergoing an opioid rotation.
- Use the new guidelines and decision tools for tapering when engaging in the process with patients.
- Explore using this withdrawal assessment tool (www.tandfonline.com).

CASE STUDY

Suzanne is an oncology patient who has just had a significant abdominal surgery for colon cancer. She was previously treated for lung cancer 5 years ago and has been taking Oxycodone 5 to 10 mg twice a day to control residual chest wall pain. For the new abdominal surgical pain, she needed more opioids, both oral and intravenous. She was converted to an extended-release medication, Oxycontin 20 mg twice per day, to cover her pain, which was lasting throughout the day and night at severe levels of 7 to 8/10. This was barely enough to cover her abdominal pain, bur her healthcare provider did not want to increase her dose, fearing a small bowel obstruction might occur.

(*continued*)

CASE STUDY (*continued*)

After surgery, Suzanne never seems to have adequate pain control. She is not able to take her oral medications, so she has been given a morphine patient controlled analgesia (PCA) set at 1 mg every 10 minutes and has pushed the button 60 times while only getting six doses of medication in the last hour. She is beginning to feel that the PCA is not working, and as she is getting more and more nauseated, she feels like it is not worthwhile to push the button. She would almost rather have the pain than the nausea.

- Suzanne's unrelieved pain is not contributing to a good recovery. Because she cannot take her oral medications, the low-dose morphine PCA is not covering her baseline medication and is not providing enough pain relief to cover her new surgical pain. She will need a continuous rate on her PCA using an equianalgesic conversion to determine this continuous rate. If standard nausea medications do not improve the nausea, Suzanne may need an opioid rotation to another intravenous opioid, which may improve her symptoms.
- When Suzanne is able to take oral medications, she will need to have an increase in her baseline medications with adequate breakthrough medications until her surgical pain lessens to a reasonable level.
- To convert Suzanne to an appropriate oral medication dose, calculate what she is using over a 24-hour period. Add the continuous rate and the PCA demand doses for 24 hours and then use an equianalgesic dose.
- Because the new doses will be higher than her baseline doses, a taper of 10% to 25% will be needed once the pain lessens to a reasonable level. The goal of the taper should be to bring the opioid doses to the lowest possible effective dose.

REFERENCES

American Pain Society. (2008). *Principles of analgesic use in the treatment of acute pain and cancer pain*. Glenview, IL: Author.

Broglio, K., & Matzo, M. (2018). Acute pain management for people with opioids use disorder. *American Journal of Nursing, 118*(18), 2–10.

CDC. (n.d.). *Tapering guide*. Retrieved from www.cdc.gov/taperingguide

D'Arcy, Y. (2011). *A compact clinical guide to chronic pain management*. New York, NY: Springer Publishing Company.

Fine, P., & Portnoy, R. (2009). Establishing "best practices" for opioid rotation: Conclusions of an expert panel. *Journal of Pain & Symptom Management, 38*(3), 418–425. doi:10.1016/jjpainsymman.2009.06.002

Knotkova, H., Fine, P., & Portnoy, R. (2009). Opioid rotation: The science and limitations of the equianalgesic dose table. *Journal of Pain & Symptom Management, 38*(3), 426–439. doi:10.1016/j.jpainsymman.2009.06.001

Mercadante, S., & Bruera, E. (2006). Opioid switching: A systematic and critical review. *Cancer Treatment Reviews, 32*(4), 304–315. doi:10.1016/j.ctrv.2006.03.001

Pasternak, G. (2005). Molecular biology of opioid analgesia. *Journal of Pain & Symptom Management, 29*(5), S2–S9. doi:10.1016/j.jpainsymman.2005.01.011

Quigley, C. (2010). Opioid switching to improve pain relief and drug tolerability. *Cochrane Library, 2010*(11).

Shaheen, P. E., Walsh, D., Lasheen, W., Davis, M. P., & Lagman, R. L. (2009). Opioid equianalgesic tables: Are they all equally dangerous? *Journal of Pain & Symptom Management, 38*(3), 409–417. doi:10.1016/j.jpainsymman.2009.06.004

U.S. Food and Drug Administration. (2018). *FDA approves the first non-opioid treatment for management of opioid withdrawal symptoms in adults.* Retrieved from https://www.fda.gov/news-events/press-announcements/fda-approves-first-non-opioid-treatment-management-opioid-withdrawal-symptoms-adults

Vadalouca, A., Moka, E., Argyra, E., Sikioti, P., & Siafaka, I. (2008). Opioid rotation in patients with cancer: A review of the current literature. *Journal of Opioid Management, 4*(4), 213. doi:10.5055/jom.2008.0027

ADDITIONAL RESOURCES

Centers for Disease Control and Prevention. (n.d.). *Opioid overdose.* Retrieved from www.cdc.gov/drugoverdose

U.S. Department of Health and Human Services. (2019). *Guide for clinicians on the appropriate dosage reduction of long term opioid analgesics.* Retrieved from https://www.hhs.gov/opioids/sites/default/files/2019-10/Dosage_Reduction_Discontinuation.pdf

U.S. Department of Veterans Affairs. (n.d.). *Opioid taper decision tool.* Retrieved from https://vaww.portal2.va.gov/sites/ad/SitePages/home.aspx

CHAPTER 11

OPIOID USE DISORDER, ADDICTION, AND DEPENDENCY

INTRODUCTION

With the ever-increasing misuse and abuse of prescription opioids, the rates of opioid use disorder (OUD)—with addiction being the highest level of OUD—are rising (Box 11.1). People who use prescription opioids coupled with illicit drugs, such as fentanyl and carfentanyl, used alone or mixed with heroin, are experiencing a dramatic increase in overdose deaths.

Between 1999 and 2016, more than 200,000 people died from drug overdose due to prescription opioids (Centers for Disease Control and Prevention [CDC], 2017). On average, 46 people die every day from overdoses related to prescription opioids, with 46% of opioid overdose deaths in 2016 involving a prescription opioid (CDC, 2017). This equates to 116 people dying every day from an opioid (National Center for Drug Abuse Statistics, 2019). The medications that are most commonly abused are methadone, oxycodone products, and hydrocodone products (CDC, 2017; Center for Drug Evaluation and Research, U.S. Food and Drug Administration [FDA], 2012).

Where do people get these medications as they are prescribed for pain to patients who need the medication? The FDA (2018) indicates that the most common source (53%) of prescription opioids used for abuse is a friend or relative who has an opioid prescription, gotten either through medication sharing or theft (Volkow & McLellan, 2016). The second most common source (35%) is a physician's prescription.

CLINICAL PEARL

Educating patients about the danger of sharing or taking medications from friends or relatives is crucial for patient safety.

BOX 11.1

DIFFERENCE BETWEEN MISUSE AND ABUSE OF AN OPIOID

Misuse: Use of an opioid medication for conditions other than pain, for example, sleep or using an opioid from an old prescription for a new complaint

Abuse: Use of an opioid for the feeling of pleasure or getting high, not for pain relief (CDC, 2012)

What does this mean for the healthcare providers who prescribe opioids? Some statistics on overdose deaths can provide insight into who the patients with the biggest risks are:

- The overdose rates from prescription opioids were highest in people aged 25 to 54 years.
- Using 2016 data, the overdose rate for men was 6.2 compared to 4.3 in women.
- Overdose rates were highest among non-Hispanic Whites and American Indian or Alaska natives.
- States with the highest death rates from prescription opioids were West Virginia, Maryland, Maine, and Utah (CDC, 2017).

For prescribers using opioids for pain relief in their patients with chronic pain, looking at the data can provide some insight into which patients might need more screening and monitoring. Statistics show us that roughly 21% to 29% of patients who are prescribed opioids for chronic pain misuse them, whereas 8% to 12% of these patients develop an OUD (National Institute of Mental Health [NIMH], 2019).

This means that the majority of patients who are prescribed opioids do not develop an OUD. However, data suggest that those patients who take higher doses of opioids (>100 morphine milligram equivalents [MME] of morphine) over longer periods of time are at a higher risk of developing an OUD or overdosing (Volkow & McLellan, 2016).

CLINICAL PEARL

If opioids are being used for pain management, to reduce the risk of OUD and overdose, limit the time that opioids will be used and decrease the amount being prescribed to the lowest possible dose.

The abuse of synthetic opioids, such as fentanyl, which is 50 times more powerful than heroin and 100 times more potent than morphine, and carfentanyl, a powerful opioid with a strength 10,000 times more powerful than morphine, has caused an increase in overdose deaths (CDC, 2017). The source of these drugs is illicit production, often not in the United States, with the rates of United States fentanyl prescriptions remaining stable. Fentanyl products are often mixed with heroin or cocaine to enhance the effect. However, the onset of fentanyl is very rapid and users often overdose, given the short onset time and lack of quality control in the illicit drugs.

WHO IS THE OPIOID ABUSER IN YOUR PRACTICE?

Opioid abusers and misusers come from all patient demographics. They include not only younger people, but also extend into older population groups. Teenagers and people with mental health disorders have a higher risk for drug use and development of an OUD (National Institute on Drug Abuse [NIDA], 2018). The use of alcohol or marijuana can also indicate that the patient may be a candidate for developing an OUD. Of note, 23% of heroin users develop chronic opioid addiction disease (American Society of Addiction Medicine [ASAM], 2015)

In a study of over 50,000 patients aged 12 to 25 years, 27.5% of the respondents indicated prescription opioid use in the past year (Hudgins, Porter, Monuteaux, & Bourgeois, 2019). Data on opioid misuse indicated that of those in the adolescent group (12 to 17 years of age), 3.8% reported opioid misuse and in the older age group (18 to 25 years of age), 7.8% reported opioid misuse. When this group was queried about the source of the opioids, most of them reported that a family member or a friend provided the opioid (55.7%). Other sources of opioids cited were the healthcare system (25.4%) and other means (18.9%). When looking at gateway substance use, prior cocaine use was reported by 35.5%, hallucinogens by 49.4%, heroin by 8.7%, and inhalant use by 30.4%. Tobacco use was reported by 55.5%, alcohol by 66.9%, and cannabis use by 49.9%; respondents indicated frequent use of all three (Hudgins et al., 2019).

Older patients also have increased risk for overdose and death and can misuse and abuse opioids as well. As a group, older patients have a number of painful conditions, such as osteoarthritis, that can be incapacitating. Although older patients tend to try self-treatment, such as over-the-counter medications, they also use alcohol as a way to decrease pain. Prescribers who are treating older patients with painful conditions should assess the use of alcohol and attempt to get a good idea of just how much the patient is drinking related to pain. As a general rule of thumb, it is wise to assess alcohol consumption in all patients, including those in the older patient group.

Age-related physical changes cause changes in the way the body processes opioid medications. These include:

- Decreased renal clearance
- Decreased hepatic function
- Higher ratio of fat to lean muscle mass
- Decreased serum protein levels
- Reduced first-pass metabolism (D'Arcy & Bruckenthal, 2011)

As opioid clearance is lessened, overdose can result. The patient may not have intended to take too many pills, but may have forgotten just what he or she took and when they were taken; therefore, his or her cardiac or renal function decreases, causing oversedation. There is also a risk of a medication–medication drug reaction causing increased sedation. The patient will also need to stop using alcohol as the added sedation can potentially be fatal. Medications used to induce sleep can also increase the risk of oversedation and cause the patient to be foggy, resulting in falls or poor judgment.

CLINICAL PEARL

To use opioids in older patients, decrease the dose by 50% and carefully monitor the patient for any unwanted adverse effects such as sedation and confusion (CDC, 2012).

Gender Differences

In a study of 29,906 assessments from national treatment centers, the researchers tried to determine whether there were any gender-specific tendencies that would predispose women to abuse prescription opioids. The study findings indicated that the positive correlates were:

- Problem drinking
- Age less than 54 years
- Inhalant use
- Residence outside of the western U.S. census region
- History of drug overdose (Green, Serrano, Licari, Budman, & Butler, 2009)

In this study, more women than men reported abusing opioid prescription drugs, and women abusers were less likely to report a pain problem as the reason for opioid abuse (Green et al., 2009). Women in this study also reported obtaining the opioids they abused, aside from their own prescriptions, from friends, family, or acquaintances, rather than using a drug dealer (Green et al., 2009).

In specific drug-related data, issues for drug use in women include the following:

- Women are particularly vulnerable to the reinforcing and hormonal effects effects of stimulant drugs , with estrogen increasing the effect and progesterone decreasing the feeling of "high."
- Women tend to have more serious mental illness as a comorbid condition.
- Women abuse more prescription opioids than men, with abuse being more common among younger women.
- Women are prescribed more opioids than men, and they reported that their first source of opioids was a prescription provided by a healthcare provider.
- Women use less heroin than men and tend to inject the drug less often than men.
- Women tend to mix sedatives, opioids, and other drugs.
- Men are more likely to use marijuana than women.

Men are interested in the pleasurable aspects of nonmedical use of prescription drugs, whereas women more often misuse medications to deal with negative emotions (Back, Lawson, Singleton, & Brady, 2011). Women also experience a telescoping effect, during which the time from authorized use to abuse is shortened as compared to men. Women also engage in the aberrant behavior of medication hoarding more often than men, and use other types of medications, such as sedatives, to enhance the effect of prescription medications (Back et al., 2011). Polysubstance abuse and nonuse of treatment options are common for both men and women (Back, Payne, Simpson, & Brady, 2010). Looking at preference, long- and short-acting oxycodone seems to be favored by men who abuse opioids, whereas women tend to prefer hydrocodone, tramadol, and codeine.

OPIOID USE DISORDER

The fear of OUD and addiction is not just something that affects patients. Fear of addicting patients is also a very real concern for nurse practitioners and caregivers.

In a survey of 400 nurse practitioners who were asked about the biggest barrier to prescribing opioids, the largest group of respondents said cost was the biggest barrier to opioid prescribing, whereas the number two and three responses indicated a fear of increased regulatory oversight and addiction (D'Arcy, 2009).

The *Diagnostic and Statistical Manual of Mental Disorders*, Fifth Edition (*DSM-5;* American Psychiatric Association, 2013) outlines the criteria for substance use disorders (SUDs). SUDs include alcohol abuse, tobacco abuse, and opioid abuse, with addiction being considered the highest level of OUD. In order for a patient to be classified as having an SUD, the main criteria include:

- Hazardous use
- Social/interpersonal problems related to use
- Neglect of roles of obligations to use.

Additional criteria include:

- Cravings
- Withdrawal
- Tolerance
- Use of larger amounts/ more frequent use
- Repeated attempts to quit/control use
- Much time spent using
- Physical/psychological problems related to use
- Activities given up to use (Hasin et al., 2013)

Using the *DSM-5* (APA, 2013) criteria to determine an OUD highlights red flags that prescribers can use. If the patient has lost his or her job, wants more and more opioids with stable pain, keeps trying to quit using opioids but cannot, the patient is demonstrating characteristics of OUD. At this point, the patient should be sent to an addiction specialist, psychologist, or treatment facility to implement measures to taper the patient from opioids and institute methadone or suboxone treatment.

Physiology of OUD: Addiction

The ASAM defines *addiction* as a "*chronic, relapsing brain disease characterized by compulsive drug-seeking behavior and drug use despite harmful consequences*" (ASAM, 2015). Physiologically, some patients have a latent chronic addictive disease that can be triggered by any type of opioid (ASAM, 2015). This definition highlights the fact that addiction is a brain disease that cannot be cured, and that relapses should be expected.

CLINICAL PEARL

Patients with a history of addictive disease are prone to relapse. Therefore, monitoring these patients more carefully, performing urine screens, and being aware of any red flags, such as repeated requests for additional pain medications or repeated dose increases, are necessary precautions.

Addiction is governed by the neural pathways that also govern reward and pleasure. Opioids have both a direct and indirect effect on these centers within the brain. The centers that are most involved are the mesocorticolimbic dopamine system, which originates in the ventral segmental section of the brain and extends into the nucleus accumbens, amygdala, and prefrontal cortex (Ballantyne, 2007). Activation of this neural area by opioids can produce euphoria and reinforce reward-seeking behaviors. The fear of withdrawal also tends to stimulate continued drug taking (Ballantyne, 2007).

Continued use of a drug, such as heroin, increases the body's desire for the drug as reward and pleasure follow drug use, creating reward-related learning and memory (Kircher et al., 2011). As drug use continues, there is a dopaminergic release from the ventral tegmental area (VTA) to the mesocorticolimbic system, which causes a cascade of cellular and molecular changes that lead to neuroplastic changes in the neural system, reinforcing the learning pattern and memory for reward-seeking behavior (Kircher et al., 2011). Addiction creates a vicious cycle of drug use, creating physiologic changes that increase desire for more drugs, leading to continued use.

At the same time, neuroadaptations and cellular changes are taking place that make relapse more likely. Patients who are in withdrawal or abstinence from drugs, such as heroin, have a stress response and hormonal activation that can lead to compulsive drug use (Kircher et al., 2011). The stress response can cause the release of excessive levels of norepinephrine, ACTH, corticotrophin-releasing factor (CRF), beta-endorphin, cortisol, vasopressin, and dynorphin (Kircher et al., 2011). These physiologic changes make it difficult to control pain in these patients, and opioid requirements may be higher than expected.

Long-term opioid use for chronic pain presents a different situation in which prescribers may be more reluctant to continue to prescribe opioids for the residual chronic pain. In the past, prescribing for chronic pain followed the cancer-pain model, and it is just in the past few years that more focus on the long-term outcomes of continued opioid prescribing have been evaluated. Many healthcare providers also fear readdicting a patient who has stopped using illicit drugs but who has a history of illicit drug use. It is wise to consider that in a primary care practice, the prevalence of true addiction in patients using opioids for pain relief is low, meaning that the majority of the patients do well (Fishbain, Cole, Lewis, Rossamoff, & Rosamoff, 2008). Each patient's pain and opioid use needs to be carefully monitored over the course of long-term opioid therapy and doses should be reduced as low as possible.

Healthcare providers cannot give opioids to patients to support addiction, but they can prescribe opioids to treat pain. Patients who have a history of addiction are at risk for readdiction when opioids are used to treat pain. These patients need to have pain relief, but should be made fully aware of the consequences and both the risks and benefits. For an addicted patient, a team approach to pain management is needed using clinicians skilled in addiction, such as psychologists, counselors, addiction specialists, and pain-management specialists. No matter what the patient's status, each patient deserves adequate pain control.

Dependency is often confused with addiction. *Physical dependence* is defined as a state of adaptation that is manifested by a class-specific withdrawal syndrome that can be produced by:

- Abrupt cessation of the drug
- Rapid dose reduction
- Decreasing blood levels of the drug and/or on administration of an opioid antagonist (American Academy of Pain Medicine, American Pain Society, American Society of Addiction Medicine (2001; D'Arcy, 2011)

All patients with pain who take opioids longer than 7 to 14 days become dependent on the medication. This only means that if the opioids are suddenly stopped or the dose is decreased rapidly, a withdrawal syndrome will occur. This condition manifests as shaking, chills, pain, nausea, vomiting, or diarrhea. *All addicted patients are dependent on their opioid substance, whereas all dependent patients are not addicts.* The focus on treating a patient with long-term opioids is to treat pain, not fuel addiction. Knowing the difference between the two ensures that opioid-dependent patients will not be categorized as addicts.

Tolerance occurs when one of the effects of the opioid, such as sedation, nausea, or pain relief, decreases despite dose escalations and manipulations. This is exemplified by the patient who says that taking more medication does not decrease the pain. It is a natural occurrence of long-term use and does not indicate addiction. Some patients also have a high metabolic rate causing them to use medications at a faster rate than others. Conversely, some patients have a slower metabolism and medications last longer in these patients.

Universal Precautions

Universal precautions is a term often used in infectious disease practices to indicate the minimum level of precaution needed for all patients to avoid infection or contamination. In pain management, *universal precautions* means using accepted standards and guidelines to minimize the risk of opioid prescribing (Gourlay, Heit, & Almahrezi, 2005). It is not possible to assess all risks when prescribing opioids, so applying the minimum level of precautions to all patients utilizing opioids is recommended. Some elements from the guidelines include (Gourlay et al., 2005):

- Make a diagnosis using an appropriate differential
- Psychological assessment, including the risk of addictive disorders
- Informed consent
- Treatment agreement
- Pre- and postintervention assessments of pain level and function
- Appropriate trial of opioid therapy with or without adjunctive medication
- Reassessment of pain score and level of function
- Regular assessment of the four A's of pain medicine: analgesia, activities of daily living, adverse effects, and aberrant behaviors
- Periodic review of pain diagnosis and comorbid conditions, including addictive disorders
- Complete documentation that addresses all elements of assessment, medications, and treatment indications such as pain

SCREENING FOR OPIOID ABUSE AND IDENTIFYING ABERRANT DRUG-TAKING BEHAVIORS

Prescribers who provide long-term opioids to patients with pain have a variety of screening tools that they can use to monitor the risk inherent with opioid use, the occurrence of aberrant behaviors, and compliance with opioid agreements. Behaviors that are considered to be aberrant include (Fine & Portnoy, 2007):

- Hoarding medications
- Taking someone else's medication for pain
- Requesting a specific drug or dose
- Increasing drug doses without a prescription
- Drinking more alcohol when in pain

- Smoking more cigarettes when in pain
- Using opioids to treat other symptoms

These dysfunctional behaviors are aimed at increasing pain relief, but are less predicative of addiction. Behaviors that are more predictive of addiction include (Fine & Portnoy, 2007):

- Concurrent use of illicit drugs
- Stealing or selling prescription drugs
- Injecting oral medications
- Obtaining medications from nonstandard sources such as street dealers

Tools for Screening

Screening tools used prior to and during opioid use should not be considered lie detectors. These tools should be used to identify patients who are at risk of developing aberrant behaviors or who have a higher potential for addiction if long-term opioids are used. Sometimes simple questions, such as those listed here, can give an idea of the patient's potential for addictive behavior or willingness to engage in illegal activity (Kircher et al., 2011):

- Are you a smoker?
- Do you have a personal or family history of alcoholism?
- Have you ever used marijuana?
- Have you ever purchased medications off the street?
- Have you ever been in a substance use treatment program?

There are several other simple screening tools that can help identify patients at risk for difficulty with long-term opioids. These tools are not meant to rule out the patients with a positive screen from getting prescriptions for opioids to treat their pain; instead they are meant to indicate when more care and careful monitoring are needed.

The CAGE questionnaire uses a set of questions centered on alcohol use. The higher the number of positive responses, the greater the likelihood that the patient has a drug or alcohol abuse disorder. The CAGE questions are:

- Have you ever tried to ***c***ut down on your alcohol or drug use?
- Have people ***a***nnoyed you by commenting or critiquing your drug or alcohol use?
- Have you ever felt bad or ***g***uilty about your drinking or drug use?

- Have you ever needed an *e*ye opener first thing in the morning to steady your nerves or get rid of a hangover?

The TRAUMA Screen uses personal injury as a measure of risk for abusing opioids. If the patient has two or more positive answers, there is a high potential for abuse. The questions of the TRAUMA Screen include:

Since your 18th birthday, have you:

- Had any fractures or dislocations to your bones or joints excluding sports injuries?
- Been injured in a traffic accident?
- Injured your head, excluding sports injuries?
- Been in a fight or been assaulted while intoxicated?
- Been injured while intoxicated?

For some patients, using a simple screen provides enough information to rule out any potential opioid-related issues. For other patients, there is a need for more complex screening tools that can identify the magnitude of risk for the patients when opioids are used for pain relief. In a study of 48 patients who attended a pain clinic but were discontinued from opioid therapy for aberrant behavior, a psychologist interviewed these patients and patients completed three complex assessment tools: the Screener and Opioid Assessment for Patients with Pain-Revised (SOAPP-R), the Opioid Risk Tool (ORT), and the Diagnosis, Intractability, Risk, and Efficacy Inventory (DIRE). The clinical interview part of the study protocol had the highest sensitivity for predicting aberrant drug-taking behaviors (0.77). The tool with the highest sensitivity rating for predicting aberrant drug-taking behaviors was the SOAPP-R (0.72), followed by the ORT (0.45) and DIRE (0.17; Moore, Jones, Browder, Daffron, & Passik, 2009).

Using a more complex tool can help identify those patients who will develop aberrant behaviors or are at higher risk for misuse or abuse of opioids.

- The SOAPP-R uses a 14-item self-report format to assess for abuse potential. This is a reliable and valid measure in which a score of 8 or greater indicates a high risk of misuse or abuse.
- The ORT screens for aberrant behaviors in patients using long-term opioids. It has a simple five-item yes/no format for self-report. Questions center on the patient's personal and family history of drug use; age; any history of preadolescent sexual abuse; and the presence of any psychological disease such as depression, obsessive-compulsive disorder, schizophrenia, or bipolar disease. Each question has several subsections for specific substances or disease states. Scores of 0 to 3 are

considered low risk, scores of 4 to 7 moderate indicate risk, and a score of 8 and above indicates high risk.

- The DIRE score is a clinician-rated scale based on questions in four categories: diagnosis, intractability, risk, and efficacy. The categories are then broken down into further divisions: psychological, chemical health, reliability, and social support. A score of 14 and above indicates that the patient is a good candidate for opioid therapy and those with lower scores are not considered good candidates.
- Current Opioid Misuse Measure (COMM) is a 17-item self-report tool used to identify aberrant drug-related behaviors for patients on long-term opioid therapy. This tool is to be used once opioid therapy has started. The COMM uses questions that can identify emotional/psychiatric issues, evidence of lying, appointment patterns, and medication misuse and noncompliance (D'Arcy, 2011; Passik, Kirsch, & Casper, 2008).

Copies of these tools are available online(www.painedu.com). These tools are meant to be used as a part of a comprehensive treatment plan and not as a sole measure of suitability for opioid therapy.

TREATING A PATIENT WHO HAS A HISTORY OF OUD FOR PAIN

Patients who have a history of opioid abuse deserve to have their pain treated. The question remains, what is the best way to treat their pain, yet avoid readdicting the patient to opioids?

The Agency for Healthcare Research and Quality (AHRQ; 2012) recommends the following guidelines for treating pain in patients in recovery from SUDs:

- Perform a full assessment to include pain intensity, psychiatric comorbidities, functional level, and screening for SUD.
- Develop a treatment plan.
- Integrate pain and comorbidity treatments.
- Treat initially with nonopioids and nonpharmacological methods.
- Treat with opioids only after a careful risk/benefit analysis.
- Add an addiction specialist to the team.
- Taper or discontinue failing opioid treatment or other treatment.
- Monitor and manage aberrant drug-related behavior.

- Establish relationships with drug testing laboratory staff and addiction specialists.

In addition, all pertinent information needs to be well documented and entered into the patient's formal record.

Patients with OUD or those who are in recovery are often undertreated for pain (Prater, Zylstra, & Miller, 2002). This practice is understandable, as practitioners are afraid of legal issues and readdicting the patient if using opioids in a patient with an addiction history. However, undertreating the pain in these patients can have dire effects, such as relapse and suicide (Prater et al., 2002). The detailed documentation that is required can also be burdensome for a busy practitioner.

One method used to provide both pain relief and addiction treatment is medication-assisted therapy (MAT). The Substance Use Disorder Prevention that Promotes Opioid Recovery and Treatment (SUPPORT) for Patients and Communities Act was signed into law on Oct 24, 2018. This Act allows nurse practitioners to prescribe buprenorphine for OUD treatment (Moore, 2019). These nurse practitioners take special courses and have a waiver attached to their licenses to show they are qualified to practice MAT. Each practitioner may provide MAT treatment for 100 patients.

In practice, the patient is put into mild withdrawal and buprenorphine is substituted for the opioid. As doses become stable, the patient uses buprenorphine as treatment for addiction, just as methadone was used years ago.

In the United States, there are not enough treatment facilities for patients with OUD. Using nurse practitioners (NPs) in primary care practices can augment the availability of treatment for these patients. This can be especially true for NPs practicing in rural areas with a few resources. If a practice wishes to add MAT to its therapies, counseling support for the patients and coverage for emergencies must be provided.

SUMMARY

Each practice is individual in the way opioids are used by each provider. Patient agreements, patient education, and practice patterns are decided by the members of the practice. Provider education on opioid use and OUD and how to treat patients with OUD or a history of OUD is essential. Opioid use for chronic pain will continue and patients with OUD will continue to have pain. Knowing how to work with these patients and developing a level of comfort with the practice will go a long way in making sure that all patients get adequate pain management.

TRENDING IN PAIN MANAGEMENT

- Look for improved tools to screen patients for opioid risk.
- Some primary care providers are providing MAT using suboxone. These providers have additional education in treating patients with OUD and require a license waiver to practice in this area.

CASE STUDY

Stella, 35, is married and has three children. She comes from a very conservative home, where strict social standards were enforced. She was often told what young ladies did and did not do. Her husband comes from a similar background. Three years ago, Stella fell down a steep embankment while hiking on a vacation and sustained multiple fractures. She spent months in rehab and is finally able to walk. She has residual pain, which she rates as severe with prolonged activity. She rates her pain at 4/10 to 8/10 depending on the day and how much activity she has at work and at home. She has been consistently using Vicodin to get through the day. Her healthcare provider has tried many different times to move Stella to a nonopioid medication, but Stella tells her it is the only thing that works.

What Stella has not told the healthcare provider is that she sees several other doctors for the same complaint. She also "borrows" medication from her family members when she runs low and uses some sedatives and sleeping medication to augment the effect of the opioid. She regularly uses alcohol at night to take the edge off her pain. Her husband is alarmed at her increased medication use; it is becoming harder for Stella to perform at work and at home. Her husband suspects that Stella uses many more pills than she admits to. He sees her get so sedated at times that he is worried that she won't wake up. What is happening to Stella?

- Like many patients, Stella started using opioids to relieve acute pain from trauma. Failing to taper off opioids after her injury and to move to a nonopioid for further pain relief has resulted in a greater dependence on medications to control her pain and an OUD.
- Stella's family background makes it harder for Stella to admit she is abusing her medications. The prescriber should be using the state's Prescription Drug Monitoring Program (PDMP) to see whether Stella is getting medications from a number of providers, since Stella is not going to be a honest reporter. Once the multiple prescriptions are found, the prescriber should enforce the patient–provider agreement (PPA) that they signed and begin to taper Stella's opioids to the lowest possible level.

(*continued*)

CASE STUDY (*continued*)

- In addition to tapering her opioids, the healthcare provider should add nonopioid options, such as physical therapy, yoga, or a transcutaneous electrical nerve stimulation (TENS) unit to help with pain control. Stella should also see a psychologist for OUD to help her develop better coping mechanisms for her pain.
- Patient education is key for Stella to understand that using sedatives or alcohol with opioids to reduce pain is a dangerous practice. Stella's husband should be taught what is expected of Stella as her plan of care changes. He should also be given a naloxone prescription to use in case Stella relapses.

REFERENCES

Agency for Healthcare Research and Quality. (2012). *Taken from the National Guideline Clearinghouse*. Retrieved from http://www.guideline.gov

American Academy of Pain Medicine, American Pain Society, & American Society of Addiction Medicine. (2001). *Definitions related to the use of opioids for the treatment of pain*. Retrieved from http://www.painmed.org/productpub/statements/pdfs/defintiion.pdf

American Psychiatric Association. (2013). *Diagnostic and statistical manual of mental disorders* (5h ed.). Arlington, VA: American Psychiatric Publishing.

American Society of Addiction Medicine. (2015). *Opioid addiction disease 2015 facts and figures*. Retrieved from www.ASAM.org

Back, S., Lawson, K., Singleton, L., & Brady, K. (2011). Characteristics and correlates of men and women with prescription opioid dependence. *Addictive Behaviors, 36*(8), 829–834. doi:10.1016/j.addbeh.2011.03.013

Back, S., Payne, R., Simpson, A., & Brady, K. (2010). Gender and prescription opioids: Findings form the national survey on drug use and health. *Addictive Behaviors, 35*(1), 1001–1007. doi:10.1016/j.addbeh.2010.06.018

Ballantyne, J. (2007). Opioid misuse in oncology pain patients. *Current Pain and Headache Reports, 11*(4), 276–282. doi:10.1007/s11916-007-0204-6

Centers for Disease Control and Prevention. (2017). *Prescription opioid overdose data*. Retreived from https://www.cdc.gov

Center for Drug Evaluation and Research. U. S. Food and Drug Administration. (2012). Blueprint for prescriber continuing education program. *Journal of Pain and Palliative Care Pharmacotherapy, 26*(2), 127–130. doi:10.3109/15360288.2012.680013

D'Arcy, Y. (2009). Be in the know about pain management. *Nurse Practitioner, 34*(4), 43–47. doi:10.1097/01.npr.0000348322.40151.2f

D'Arcy, Y. (2011). *A compact clinical guide to chronic pain*. New York, NY: Springer Publishing Company.

D'Arcy, Y., & Brukenthal, P. (2011). *Safe opioid prescribing for nurse practitioners*. New York NY: Oxford University Press.

Fine, P., & Portnoy, R. (2007). *A clinical guide to opioid analgesia*. New York, NY: Vendome Group.

Fishbain, D., Cole, B., Lewis, J., Rossamoff, H., & Rossamoff, R. (2008). What percentage of chronic non malignant pain patients exposed to chronic opioid analgesic therapy develop abuse/addiction and or aberrant drug related behaviors? A structured evidence based review. *Pain Medicine*, *9*(4), 444–459.

Green, T., Serrano, J., Licari, A., Budman, S., & Butler, S. (2009). Women who abuse prescription opioids: Findings from the addiction severity index-multimedia version connect prescription database. *Drug and Alcohol Dependence*, *103*(1–2), 65–73. doi:10.1016/j.drugalcdep.2009.03.014

Gourlay, D., Heit, H., & Almahrezi, A. (2005). Universal precautions in pain medicine: A rational approach to the treatment of chronic pain. *Pain Medicine*, *6*(2), 107–112. doi:10.1111/j.1526-4637.2005.05031.x

Hasin, D. S., O'Brien, C. P., Auriacombe, M., Borges, G., Bucholz, K., Budney, A., . . . Schuckit, M. (2013). DSM-5 criteria for substance use disorders: Recommendations and rationale. *American Journal of Psychiatry*, *170*(8), 834–851. doi:10.1176/appi.ajp.2013.12060782

Hudgins, J., Porter, J., Monuteaux, M., & Bourgeois, F. (2019). Prescription opioid use and misuse among adolescents and young adults in the United States: A national survey study. *PLOS Medicine*, *16*(11), e1002922. doi:10.1371/journal.pmed.1002922

Kircher, S., Zacny, J., Apfelbaum, S., Passik, S., Kirsch, K., Burbage, M., & Lofwell, M. (2011). Understanding and treating opioid addiction in a patient with cancer pain. *Journal of Pain*, *12*(10), 1025–1031. doi:10.1016/j.jpain.2011.07.006

Moore, D. (2019). Nurse Practitioners pivotal role in ending the opioid epidemic. *Journal for Nurse Practitioners*, 15(5), 323–327. doi:10.1016/j.nurpra.2019.01.005

Moore, T., Jones, T., Browder, J., Daffron, S., & Passik, S. (2009). A comparison of common screening methods for predicting aberrant drug-related behavior among patients receiving opioids for chronic pain management. *Pain Medicine*, *10*(8), 1426–1433. doi:10.1111/j.1526-4637.2009.00743.x

National Center for Drug Abuse Statistics. (2019). Retrieved from https://www.drugabuse.gov

National Institute on Drug Abuse. (2018). *Drugs, brains, and behavior: The science of addiction*. Washington, DC: Author.

Passik, S., Kirsh, K., & Casper, D. (2008). Addiction-related assessment tools and pain management instruments for screening, treatment planning, and monitoring compliance. *Pain Medicine*, *9*(Suppl. 2), S145–S166. doi:10.1111/j.1526-4637.2008.00486.x

Prater, C., Zylstra, R., & Miller, K. (2002). Successful pain management for the recovering addicted patient. *Primary Care Companion to the Journal of Clinical Psychiatry*, *4*(4), 125–131. doi:10.4088/pcc.v04n0402

Volkow, N., & McLellan, A. (2016). Opioid abuse in chronic pain-Misconceptions and mitigation strategies. *New England Journal of Medicine*, *374*(13), 1253–1263. doi:10.1056/nejmra1507771

ADDITIONAL RESOURCES

Cotto, J., Davis, E., Dowling, G., Elcano, J., Staton, A., & Weiss, S. (2010). Gender effects on drug use, abuse, and dependence: A special analysis of results from the National Survey on Drug Use and Health. *Gender Medicine, 7*(5), 402–413. doi:10.1016/j.genm.2010.09.004

D'Arcy, Y. (2010, August). How to manage pain in addicted patients. *Nursing, 40*(8), 60–64. doi:10.1097/01.nurse.0000383898.65472.8f

Slevin, K., & Ashburn, M. (2011). Primary care physician opinion survey on FDA opioid risk evaluation and mitigation strategies. *Journal of Opioid Management, 7*(2), 109–115. doi:10.5055/jom.2011.0053

Substance Abuse and Mental Health Services Administration Office of Applied Studies. (2009). *Results from the 2008 National Survey on Drug Use and Health: National findings* [NSDUH Series H-36. HHS publication no. SMA-09-4434]. Rockville, MD: US Department of Health and Human Services.

PART III

Essentials for Safe Prescribing

CHAPTER 12

SAFE PRESCRIBING FOR PATIENTS AND PRACTICE

INTRODUCTION

Safe prescribing is more a way of life rather than a concept. Recent data suggest that more than 50% of opioid prescriptions are written by primary care providers (Breuer, Cruciani, & Portnoy, 2010). This means the exposure for prescription misuse or abuse is great for a large number of healthcare providers.

Each practitioner who is prescribing opioids needs to ensure that the patient understands how to use opioid medications safely and that the way the opioids are prescribed conforms to recognized safe prescribing practices.

Healthcare practitioners should be familiar with what constitutes safe opioid prescribing. This includes:

- Being aware of what the state requires for a legal prescription.
- Using national guidelines, such as the Centers for Disease Control and Prevention (CDC) guidelines, to inform their practice, for example, limiting the number of days or medication amounts on prescriptions.
- Performing and documenting a complete history and physical exam to establish a diagnosis and treatment plan.
- Using an opioid screening tool to assess risk and implement a patient–provider agreement (PPA) for patients on opioid therapy before beginning treatment with opioids.
- Using the state's prescribing databases to monitor patient prescriptions and personal practice.
- Beginning opioids on a trial basis and explaining the parameters of opioid use to the patient.
- Knowing the signs and symptoms of opioid diversion, misuse, and abuse and addressing any issues with the patient (D'Arcy & Brukenthal, 2011).

- Obtaining a urine drug screen before beginning an opioid trial and using urine drug screens randomly as a monitoring precaution.

CLINICAL PEARL

When prescribing opioids, following clear office polices from the beginning demonstrates that you will maintain appropriate boundaries.

Being knowledgeable about the elements of safe prescribing can help a practitioner be sure that their prescribing practice is within the recommended national guidelines and follows the state in which they practice. It also provides the patient with medication management that will provide safe pain relief .

CLINICAL PEARL

Although taking time to ensure safe prescribing seems to be time-consuming, the ramifications of not using safe prescribing practices are too significant to ignore.

ELEMENTS OF A PRESCRIPTION

Most primary care practitioners are aware of the key elements of writing a prescription; yet, there are some who fail to make sure that all elements of the prescription are included. In the past, prescribers used prescription pads that made manual prescription writing more of a chore and allowed a greater chance of someone adulterating a prescription. Using a handwritten prescription allowed manipulation of numbers, such as a 1 being turned into a 7, or removal of the medication information with nail polish remover, allowing the patient to write in different medication information. Today, the electronic medical record (EMR) makes generating a prescription a simpler process. However, the prescriber needs to ensure that all the salient information is correctly entered to get a safe prescription.

The elements of a safe prescription include:

- Date of issue
- Patient's name and address
- Practitioner's name, address, and drug enforcement agency (DEA) registration number

- Drug name, strength, and dosage form
- Quantity prescribed
- Directions for use
- Number of refills
- Manual signature of the prescriber if using a paper prescription; if using an EMR, the prescription is signed digitally (D'Arcy, 2011).

PRESCRIBING CONTROLLED SUBSTANCES ELECTRONICALLY

In June 2010, the DEA issued the final rule allowing electronic prescribing of controlled substances (EPCS; www.deadiversion.usdoj.gov/ecomm/e_ex/index.html). States have been slowly implementing rules to allow or require EPCS, and effective from January 2020, Walmart requires electronic prescriptions at all of its locations (www.nethealth.com/walmartepcs2020). Regulations on EPCS are evolving. Knowing the regulations in your state is essential, such as, is EPCS allowed or required? Know how to access the EPCS for your EMR system.

Prior to electronic data interchange, the authenticity of a prescription was proven by possession of a prescription pad with a duplicate copy or embedded security features similar to those on currency, so as to offset counterfeit prescriptions. These techniques could be circumvented. The EMR provides greater prescription security.

The widespread use and evolution of EMRs has introduced standard information technology (IT) access controls to the process of prescribing medications. Users gain access to their terminal and the electronic record by using unique account names and increasingly complex passwords to prove their identity. For some drugs, the DEA requires more rigorous authentication known as *multi-factor authentication (MFA)*. MFA requires the use of more than one of something you have (token), something you know (password), or something you are (biometric). This enhanced security control reduces the likelihood that an account with privileges to prescribe sensitive medications could be compromised.

When a prescription is written for a controlled substance, the prescriber must be registered with the DEA in both the state in which the prescriber practices and the federal DEA. Each prescription must have the practitioner's state DEA number listed. This information will generate entries into the state database, so practitioners can check on their own practices.

Consider this example:

Jane is a primary care nurse practitioner who writes opioid prescriptions for a small number of patients with chronic pain. Her patients are very com-

pliant and she has never discovered any discrepancies in her state reports. However, upon returning after a leave of absence she discovers that an opioid prescription was written for a patient in her name while she was on maternity leave. She was not in the office and did not write the prescription. She must now try to track the prescription in the patient record and inform the state database that this was not her prescription. In all probability, the state database will start an investigation into who wrote the prescription and how it was generated.

There are also some dangerous practices that should not be used when writing an opioid prescription:

- Do not postdate a prescription.
- Do not sign a prescription and allow another person to fill it in.
- Do not give a patient a set of sequential prescriptions. Some types of medications such as those for attention deficit disorder (ADD) commonly used by college students can be prescribed as a set of three prescriptions with dates that are clearly indicated at 30-day intervals. The prescriptions can only be filled on the date indicated. For students who are away at college this eliminates a trip home for each medication refill (D'Arcy, 2011).

The final part of the prescribing process is to make sure the patient understands how to use the medication and has received education about each medication, its side effects, and interactions. Documenting the process is crucial not only to track the medications being used, but also to ensure that all legal aspects of the prescribing practice have been followed.

USING NATIONAL PRESCRIBING GUIDELINES

The U.S. Food and Drug Administration (FDA) and the CDC have written guidelines that help healthcare providers standardize opioid prescribing. Some of the guidelines provide general information as well as specific recommendations for using opioids. The CDC guidelines, in particular, give recommendation about how long a prescription should be written for acute pain (no longer than 7 days) and opioid amounts (<50 morphine milliequivalents [MME] preferred). The following is a list of guidelines that can inform opioid use:

- Center for Drug Evaluation and Research, U.S. Food and Drug Administration (2012): *Blueprint for Prescriber Continuing Education Program*
- Chou (2009): *Clinical Guidelines for the Use of Chronic Opioid Therapy in Noncancer Pain*

- Federation of State Medical Boards of the United States (2004): *Model Policy for the Use of Controlled Substances for the Treatment of Pain*
- Haergerich and Chou (2016): *CDC Guideline for Prescribing Opioids for Chronic Pain*
- The Joint Commission (2018): *Facts About Pain Management*

URINE SCREENS

Urine screens are essential for monitoring how the patient is using opioid medications. A screen can also indicate any deviation in the prescribed use, for example, bingeing or use of any nonprescribed medications or substances. There are two different types of tests:

- Point of care (POC): This is usually performed in the clinic using the standard collection technique. Care should be taken to ensure that the urine being collected is coming from the patient and, if needed, observing the patient is an option. This test provides information on the class of medication detected, but not specific medications or substances, for example, anxiolytic, opioid, and so forth. It cannot detect synthetic opioids such as fentanyl. Know which tests are on your point of care (POC) list. The advantage is a quick turnaround time for the results.
- Gas chromatography (GC): This test uses a urine sample collected at the clinic site and tested in a laboratory setting using the chromatography technique. It can identify exactly which substance or medication is present, for example, morphine, fentanyl, or cannabinoids. It can detect synthetic opioids. Information is specific enough to be used in court. It can be used to confirm results of a POC test. Turnaround is longer, but the results will be more specific. As always, using two tests increases costs and may not always be needed.

Federal workplace urine testing requires testing for marijuana, cocaine, opioids, methamphetamine, amphetamines, and phencyclidine. There are formal cutoff levels that are designated as acceptable and unacceptable levels of the substances (Moeller, Lee, & KIssack, 2008). Most workplace testing is done as point of care with GC used as needed for confirmation. To ensure tests conform to regulations, contact the place of employment to confirm what testing is needed. The key to success when using urine screening is to build a rapport with the patient and know what parameters your specific laboratory is using. The use of random urine screens should be listed and discussed with the patient as part of the PPA. Telling the patient that you will always be honest and that you expect to reciprocate with honest information can establish a good foundation for the process.

Primary care clinics often have a set schedule for urine testing of patients on opioid therapy. Some do the test once or twice a year, whereas others are less structured. The key is that the test should be random. A test is also indicated if red flags, such as aberrant behavior, are seen. Patients should not be able to opt out of a urine screen. Once requested, the screen should be performed; if the patient refuses, opioid prescribing can be stopped.

CLINICAL PEARL

Patients may feel they are being singled out or targeted when a urine sample is requested. Requesting a urine screen does not mean there is a lack of trust; it should be presented as a part of normal opioid medication management (Haegerich & Chou, 2016).

Interpreting the results of a urine drug screen can be difficult when an unexpected result occurs. If the screening test is negative for the prescribed medication or if an illicit or unexpected result occurs, it is wise to hold off on a decision and reserve judgment until a conversation about the results takes place with the patient. For example:

Sean is a college student who was in a traffic accident over the summer. He is using low-dose opioids to aid his physical therapy. The healthcare provider has mentioned tapering Sean off of his opioids. At his next urine screen, the prescribed opioid shows up. There is also a positive result for an anxiolytic that has not been prescribed to the patient. When asked about the anxiolytic, Sean responds that he became nervous about tapering the opioids and his friend gave him a few alprazolam (Zanax) to calm him down. This leads to a discussion about the dangers of combining sedative medications and a review of the PPA. Sean is told to never do this again. A slow taper of the opioids is started and Sean is reassured that his provider will help him if unmanageable pain returns.

CLINICAL PEARL

Before requesting a urine screen, ask the patient when he or she last took the medication. This allows the patient to tell you whether they have taken the medication before the screening results are reported.

With each urine screen, there is the possibility of a false-positive or a false-negative result. If an unexpected result occurs on a POC test, the sample can be sent for confirmation with GC testing to confirm the original result. Document the rationale for the second test in the patient's record.

False-positive results for opioids can be confirmed with GC testing and may be the result of cross-contamination or cross-reactivity in the initial laboratory test or the use of some quinolone antibiotics. Cocaine may show a false-positive result if topical cocaine is used as a topical anesthetic for dental procedures or coca leaf tea is ingested (D'Arcy, 2011).

CLINICAL PEARL

Misinterpretation of a urine drug screen can have devastating effects for a patient who may be documented as being in violation of the PPA. It is appropriate to call the laboratory toxicologist if you are unsure of the final results (Hudspeth, 2016).

Diversion is always a possibility when a negative result comes back when a positive result is expected. False-negative results can have several sources that are not related to diversion and should be considered. Some patients may binge on their medications in the first weeks after the prescription if filled, leaving them with no medication prior to the urine screen. When this occurs, a serious conversation about how to use the opioid medication is needed. A reassessment of the pain is to be made to make sure the patient is receiving adequate medication to control his or her pain.

False-negative results can also occur if the patient is a rapid metabolizer or the level of the medication was too low to detect (D'Arcy & Bruckenthal, 2011).

The detection of drugs or medications relies heavily on the patients themselves: The patient's physical condition, hydration, dosing, metabolism, body mass, and urine pH, as well as the duration of use and a drug's particular pharmacokinetics (Olsen, 2008), may affect the test result. Most drugs remain in a patient's system for 1 to 3 days.

Some common drugs that can be detected after use are:

- Heroin (48 hours)
- Hydromorphone (2 to 4 days)
- Methadone (3 days)
- Morphine (48 to 72 hours)
- Oxycodone (2 to 4 days)
- Cocaine (2 to 4 days)
- Amphetamine (48 hours)

- Marijuana (single use = 3 days; daily use =10 to 15 days; Moeller et al., 2008)

Some drugs are detected as metabolites, such as heroin being detected as morphine.

Manipulating urine is an easy process, and patients who know their sample is contaminated will try to alter the results. Substances that can be used to change results are liquid drain cleaner, chlorine bleach, liquid soap, ammonia, hydrogen peroxide, lemon juice, and eye drops. There are also commercially available solutions used to adulterate urine, such as glutaraldehyde sodium or potassium nitrate, peroxide or peroxidase, and pyridinium chlorochromate (PCC; Moeller et al., 2008).

When a patient adulterates a urine specimen to avoid detection of a nonprescribed substance, a serious conversation should take place with confirmatory testing done on a sample taken from the patient. An exit from opioid prescribing may be indicated at this point.

CLINICAL PEARL

Within 4 minutes of collection, each urine specimen should be inspected prior to testing for a clear yellow color and temperature. Temperature should be between 32°C to 38°C, and the pH should range between 4.5 and 8.0.

TECHNIQUES THAT PROMOTE SAFE PRESCRIBING

Each primary care practice has its own set of policies and procedures. Following the procedures provides support for decisions made about opioid prescribing. Many clinics have regular staff meetings during which practice questions can be addressed.

Joining your professional organization is a good way to keep in touch with current practice issues. The American Association of Nurse Practitioners (www.aanp.com) and the American Association of Physicians Assistants (www.aapa.com) have special interest groups for pain in which clinical experts can answer questions and provide information to other members. State and local organizations can also be a good source of information on what is happening locally with prescribing practices.

Using experts in other fields, such as a psychiatrist, psychologist, or pain specialist, can provide confidence in prescribing practices. Referring a patient to one of these specialties is not considered a failure, but a good way to ensure that prescribing practices are on track with guidelines and current practice.

SUMMARY

Safe prescribing is an essential element of primary care practice. Using safe prescribing can provide the patient with safe medication management and ensure that the prescriber is following the regulations and rules that surround medication prescribing.

TRENDING IN PAIN MANAGEMENT

- If caring for patients from adjoining states, look for prescription databases that allow prescribers to access information from additional databases.
- Look for changes in the CDC and FDA guidelines that focus more on needs of chronic pain patients who are opioid dependent.

CASE STUDY

Ryan is a new primary care provider working in a practice with several other providers and is seeing a wide variety of patients. Most of his patients do not require any opioids, but he has several patients who transferred into the practice on opioids. He also has a small cohort of patients on low-dose opioids who are very compliant.

He has both a state and federal DEA number and is very protective about using his prescriptive authority. Recently, he received a notification from the state DEA that he was prescribing a large amount of opioids to one of his patients. When he reviewed the patient's record, he found several prescriptions for antibiotics and one for blood pressure medications, but no opioid medications.

Because he was a new practitioner, he liked to keep a copy of all of his prescriptions. When he asked the DEA agent for the prescription number, he realized that the original prescription was for an antibiotic, not for an opioid. He was shocked to think that his patient had adulterated the prescription to get opioids. The DEA now knows the problem was not with Ryan, but with his patient. Ryan is concerned and wonders how he can keep this from happening again.

- With the old-style prescription pads, patients can remove the original written information with nail polish remover and a new prescription can be written. Patients can also change a "1" to a "7," so writing out numbers can help make sure the prescription is filled for the right amount of medication.

(*continued*)

CASE STUDY (*continued*)

- Always documenting the prescription information in the patient's record can provide a written record of what was given to the patient.
- Checking your own prescribing information in the state database periodically can make sure no one is misusing prescriptions or doctor shopping for opioids.

REFERENCES

Breuer, B., Cruciani, R., & Portnoy, R. (2010). Pain management by primary care physicians, pain physicians, chiropractors, and acupuncturists: A national survey. *Southern Medical Journal. 103*(8), 739–747.

Chou, R. (2009). Clinical guidelines for the use of chronic opioid therapy in noncancer pain. American Pain Society. *Journal of Pain, 10,* 113–130.

D'Arcy, Y. (2011). *A compact clinical guide to women's pain management*. New York, NY: Springer Publishing Company.

D'Arcy, Y., & Bruckenthal, P. (2011). *Safe opioid prescribing for nurse practitioners*. New York, NY: Oxford University Press.

Federation of State Medical Boards of the United States. (2004): *Model policy for the use of controlled substances for the treatment of pain.* Retrieved *from* at www.fsmb.org/pdf/2004_grpol_controlled_substances.pdf

Haegerich, D., & Chou, R. (2016). CDC guideline for prescribing opioids for chronic pain United States, 2016. *Morbidity and Mortality Weekly Report, 65*(1), 1–49.

Hudspeth, R. S. (2016). Safe opioid prescribing for adults by nurse practitioners: part 1. patient history and assessment standards and techniques. *Journal for Nurse Practitioners, 12*(3), 141–148. doi:10.1016/j.nurpra.2015.10.012

Moeller, K., Lee, K., & KIssack, J. (2008). Urine drug screening: practical guide for clinicians. *Mayo Clinic Proceedings, 83*(1), 66–76. doi:10.4065/83.1.66

Olsen, K. (2008). *Interpretation of Opiate Urine Drug Screens. Health partners: Institute of medical education.* Retrieved from http://www.lmehealthpartners.com

The Joint Commission. (2018). *Facts about pain management. Retrieved* from www.jointcommission.org/pain_management.pdf

U.S. Food and Drug Administration. (2012). *Blueprint for prescriber continuing education program.* Retrieved from www.fda.gov/downloads/Drugs/drugsafety/informationDrugClass/UCM277916.pdf

CHAPTER 13

REGULATORY CONSIDERATIONS IN PAIN MANAGEMENT

INTRODUCTION

Opioid prescribing is one aspect of clinical practice that has stirred up a great deal of professional discussion. The opioid "epidemic" and overdose statistics have created a climate of opiophobia, a fear of opioids. There is no doubt about the serious nature of opioid prescribing today. The fact that 46 people die every day from overdoses of prescription opioids is a strong stimulus to decrease opioid prescribing (Centers for Disease Control and Prevention [CDC], 2017a).

The fear of regulatory investigation of individual practices has added to the fear of prescribing a class of medications that has a long history of being used to relieve pain. Not only are the prescribers concerned about opioid use, but the patients are also concerned about developing an opioid use disorder (OUD). Primary care providers can help diffuse the situation by becoming educated about opioid prescribing and, in turn, educating their patients about the risks and benefits (Andrews & Mortensen, 2017).

The pros and cons of using opioids have been discussed, considered, and reconsidered, and, in some cases, the cons have won. Some practitioners have found constraints on opioids and regulations on practice to be so onerous that they have stopped prescribing opioids. When this happens, it denies patients one of the better ways to treat pain when pain is severe and continuous.

Some experts have stated that opioid overprescribing was fueled by the "pain as the fifth vital sign" campaign. The intention of the campaign was appropriate: Treat pain effectively. However, the idea was misinterpreted and some practitioners felt they were being pressured into prescribing opioids at higher levels to make sure pain was relieved when pain intensity ratings were high. The outcome of using pain as the fifth vital sign was studied using 300 randomly selected visits with 15 providers in a general medicine clinic. The findings indicated that pain treatments were no different after the pain campaign was initiated than before (Mularski et al., 2006). In the patient group, 79 patients who had significant pain did not receive the recommended care; of these patients, 22% had no pain documentation, 27% had no reassessment documented, and 52% had no new therapy offered to help relieve the pain (Mularski et al., 2006). The final outcome being that a well-intentioned effort at focusing on pain hoping to get better relief for patients was not successful in changing practice.

The focus has changed to treating pain effectively with the lowest possible opioid dose for the shortest possible time (CDC, 2017b). This position has led to patients with chronic pain on long-term opioid therapy being taken off opioids. Nether approach has produced the desired results and the CDC is providing more information about the intent of the new guidelines, so that chronic pain patients do not suffer needlessly (Dowell, Haegerich, & Chou, 2019).

The Center for Drug Evaluation and Research of the U.S. Food and Drug Administration's (CDC, 2012) Blueprint for Prescriber Continuing Education Program has not had better luck. Five years after the educational programs were implemented, it was unclear as to whether opioid prescribing practice had improved (Brooks, 2020). An FDA senior executive stated that the FDA has tools that could mitigate opioid risks more effectively by controlling opioid prescribing, manufacturing, and distribution (Brooks, 2020).

So, overall, most national interventions to control opioid prescribing and opioid misuse and abuse have failed at some level. The Veterans Affairs (VA) program to make pain the fifth vital sign, the CDC guidelines, and the FDA Blueprint have all fallen short of the expected outcomes of improved pain management and safe prescribing. Unfortunately, national guidelines, such as those of the CDC, have led to some patients being undertreated for pain or inappropriately tapered off of their opioids. Looking at these programs and documents, it is helpful to use the positive aspects rather than focus on the negatives. Learning about the guidelines can give the prescriber a better idea of what is appropriate and recommended for his or her patients.

THE CDC AND THE FDA

The CDC and the FDA have responded to reports of opioid overdose and deaths with efforts to reduce opioid prescribing and the amount of opioid prescribed in each prescription. Each organization has very good intentions and is hoping that the interventions outlined will be helpful in fighting the growing opioid epidemic. Practitioners who prescribe opioids need to understand the guidelines, recommendations, and educational requirements.

The CDC (2017a) developed an evidence-based consensus guideline for prescribing opioids for chronic pain. The goal of the guideline was to reduce the quantity of opioids in the U.S. that could be diverted for abuse and misuse. The aim was to create a safe opioid-prescribing climate for both patients and prescribers.

Using the guideline for safe prescribing and documenting as outlined here is important so as to comply with regulations. Some of the key elements of the CDC guideline (2016) include:

- Begin pain management using nonopioid medications and integrative strategies such as cognitive behavioral techniques or physical therapy. Use opioids only if the benefit outweighs the risks.
- Prior to beginning opioid therapy, establish realistic goals for pain and function. The opioid therapy should only continue if there is demonstrable progress.
- Document a risk/benefit discussion with the patient.
- Opioid therapy should be initiated with short-acting (immediate-release) opioids only.
- Opioids should be started at the lowest possible dose and prescription amounts should be limited to doses of no more than or equal to 50 morphine milliequivalents (MME) per day. A maximum dose should be no more than 90 MME per day with careful documentation to justify the need for the higher level.
- Because long-term opioid use can begin with acute pain treatment, clinicians should be judicious when prescribing opioids for acute pain. For acute pain, prescription amounts should be limited to a 3-day supply with a maximum of a 7-day supply.
- A reassessment of opioids' benefits and harms should take place within 1 to 4 weeks of starting opioid therapy or when doses are increased. For longer therapy, reassessment should take place every 3 months or more frequently as needed. Combination therapy with integrative techniques is encouraged.
- At the onset of therapy, the risk/benefit analysis should incorporate any risks for overdose and the use of naloxone, the use of high-dose opioids, the use of benzodiazepines with opioids, or any history of OUD or overdose.
- Utilizing the state Prescription Drug Monitoring Program (PDMP) for patient compliance with opioids should begin with the initial opioid prescription and continue at least every 3 months or as needed with each prescription.
- Urine drug screens should be done at the onset of the opioid prescription and at least annually.
- Avoid prescribing opioids and benzodiazepines at the same time.
- For patients with an OUD, the clinician should offer or arrange medication-assisted therapy (MAT) with buprenorphine or methadone (CDC, 2017a).

CLINICAL PEARL

The CDC recommendations do not apply to active cancer patients and palliative care or hospice patients at the end of life.

The FDA Blueprint (2012, 2018) is focused on educating clinicians about safe opioid prescribing. It supports elements, such as appropriate use of immediate-release and extended-release opioids, using screening tools and urine screens, plus advocating for the use of patient–provider agreements (PPAs). Educational programs based on the FDA Blueprint have been developed for clinicians to help them to understand what is expected for practice to be considered safe. An important element of the FDA Blueprint is educating the patients about their medications, expectations of opioid therapy, and proper disposal of medications once they are no longer needed.

Combining the efforts of the FDA and the CDC provides the healthcare provider who is prescribing opioids with a firm foundation in what constitutes safe practice. There are other guidelines that address opioid use, such as the American Pain Society Opioid Guidelines for Treating Chronic Pain (Chou et al., 2009). All guidelines can be accessed by using the society and organization websites:

- APS: www.aps.org
- CDC: www.cdc.gov
- FDA: www.fda.gov

MAINTAINING A SAFE PRACTICE

Prescribing practices are governed by federal and state laws and nursing and medical boards and, in some cases, pharmacy boards. These groups determine what is allowed within each state for prescribing and, for the Drug Enforcement Administration (DEA), what licensure is required for prescribing opioid medications. It is important to stay up to date on any changes in state or federal laws to ensure compliance with practice recommendations.

CLINICAL PEARL

Maintaining a safe practice is in the hands of the practitioner. Choosing to be compliant with clinic policies and national guidelines, maintaining both federal and state licenses, and completing documentation help demonstrate appropriate practice.

Should a prescriber be unlucky enough to receive a complaint from the DEA or state board, documentation is the best defense. If clinicians lack the needed documentation, it will be as if any undocumented conversations and decisions made never existed. It cannot be stressed enough that complete documentation will provide the best defense for a formal complaint.

If the complaint involves opioid prescriptions, documentation on when and how often the PDMP was reviewed will be crucial. Patients can alter prescriptions, so checking the PDMP for the prescriber's prescription history can catch a forgery early. Inordinately large amounts of opioids in prescriptions will alert pharmacists and anyone reviewing the PDMP that there is a problem.

SUMMARY

Record keeping and documentation are time-consuming. Attending educational programs also takes time away from a busy clinic day. However, the negative consequences of not doing these are serious and damaging.

TRENDING IN PAIN MANAGEMENT

- Look for new changes and revisions to the current CDC guidelines.
- Stay informed about your state's PDMP review requirement. Some states are now making PDMP review mandatory at each visit.
- Look for changes in required education on pain management. More and more states are making pain-management education mandatory for license renewal.

CASE STUDY

Robert is a new nurse practitioner practicing in an urban primary care practice. He has been working in the practice for 6 months. His patient panel includes a group of opioid-dependent chronic-pain patients and some cancer survivors who have chronic pain and use opioids for pain relief.

This week, Robert was due for a 6-month review of his practice by the clinic manager and a senior nurse practitioner (NP). The two reviewers noted that on several occasions, Robert had failed to document that a PPA had been completed and the PDMP had been accessed before opioids were prescribed. When Robert reviewed the two charts, he found that he had done the PPA and a PDMP review, but he failed

(*continued*)

CASE STUDY (*continued*)

to document it. As a new NP, he was having trouble managing his large patient load and, in turn, had overlooked two important elements for documentation.

The reviewers told Robert that he would need to complete a late entry for these patients. They also felt it would be best for both the clinic and Robert to continue to review his charts for an additional 6 months to make sure that he was following all the safe prescribing principles that were needed. They also expected him to complete the FDA Blueprint risk evaluation and mitigation strategy (REMS; FDA, 2018) education in the next 6 months.

Robert was embarrassed that his documentation had been found lacking. He was also very glad that he had the support of his peers to make sure that it did not happen again.

- As a new NP, Robert got caught up in doing clinical practice. He had let his documentation take second place and he needed to take the time to make sure his documentation reflected what he was doing with his patients.
- Robert never again failed to use the PDMP program, and he documented it each time he did so. He now realized there was valuable information being provided that he needed for his practice.
- His documentation practice changed and he consistently entered the patient's data and any conversations they had into the medical record. His reviewing physicians did a spot check and felt that Robert's documentation had improved dramatically.

REFERENCES

Andrews, R., & Mortensen, E. M. (2017). Opioids and substance abuse: Education or just regulation. *Journal of General Internal Medicine, 32*(10), 1067–1068. doi:10.1007/s11606-017-4137-4

Brooks, M. (2020). *No proof FDA strategy to mitigate opioid risks is working*. Retrieved from https://www.medscape.com/viewarticle/923312_print

Center for Drug Evaluation and Research. U. S. Food and Drug Administration. (2012). Blueprint for prescriber continuing education program. *Journal of Pain and Palliative Care Pharmacotherapy, 26*(2), 127–130. doi: 10.3109/15360288.2012.680013

Centers for Disease Control and Prevention. (2017a). *Guidelines for prescribing opioids for chronic pain*. Retrieved from https://www.cdc.gov

Centers for Disease Control and Prevention. (2017b). *The current drug overdose epidemic in the United States: Executive summary. Annual Surveillance Report of Drug Related Risks and Outcomes.* Retrieved from https://www.cdc.gov/drugoverdose/pdf/pubs/2017-cdc-drug-surveillance-report.pdf

Chou, R., Fanciullo, G., Fine, P., Adler, J., Ballantyne, J., & Davies, P. (2009). Clinical guidelines for the use of chronic opioid therapy in chronic noncancer pain. *Journal of Pain, 10*(2), 113–130. doi:10.1016/j.jpain.2008.10.008

Dowell, D., Haegerich, T., & Chou, R. (2019). No shortcuts to safer opioid prescribing. *New England Journal of Medicine, 380*, 2285–2287.

Mularski, R. A., White-Chu, F., Overbay, D., Miller L, Asch, S. M., & Ganzini, L. (2006). Measuring pain as the 5th vital sign does not improve quality of pain management. *Journal of General Internal Medicine, 21*(6), 607–612. doi:10.1111/j.1525-1497.2006.00415.x

U.S. Food and Drug Administration. (2018). *FDA's opioid analgesic REMS education blueprint for healthcare providers involved in the treatment and monitoring of patients with pain.* Retrieved from www.fda.com

ADDITIONAL RESOURCE

Hudspeth, R. (2011). Avoiding regulatory complaints when treating chronic pain patients with opioids. *Journal of the American Academy of Nurse Practitioners, 23*, 515–520. doi:10.1111/j.1745-7599.2011.00666.x

CHAPTER 14

IDENTIFYING AND TREATING OPIOID WITHDRAWAL

INTRODUCTION

Anyone who takes opioids for any length of time is at risk of becoming addicted to them, but almost all patients who take opioids for pain longer than several weeks will become dependent on them (Case-Lo, 2017). This includes short-term use such as postoperative pain management in the recovery period.

Dependence should not be confused with addiction, which is also called *opioid use disorder (OUD)*. All patients who take opioids become dependent on them as time progresses. This just means that the body has adjusted to the medications and that sudden cessation will cause withdrawal. Addiction (OUD) is in a different category that requires a *Diagnostic and Statistical Manual of Mental Disorders,* Fifth edition (*DSM-5*; American Psychiatric Association, 2013) diagnosis and has very different diagnostic criteria. When opioids are ingested regularly, there are several physical adaptations that take place.

- *Dependence* simply means that when a patient takes opioids regularly, the patient's body becomes physiologically accustomed to the daily doses. The body adapts to the regular consumption and when the opioids are rapidly discontinued or an opioid antagonist is used, the body reacts by going into withdrawal. Withdrawal is caused by a rapid decrease of the drug in blood levels.
- *Addiction (OUD)* is a disease that is caused by a variety of physiologic changes coupled with psychosocial and environmental causes. It is a chronic disease with no cure and has a high potential for relapse. Patients with an OUD have little control over their drug use and will continue to take drugs even though they know they are harming themselves.
- *Pseudoaddiction*: A patient with pseudoaddiction is really displaying a response to undertreated pain. The patients are not being given enough medication to control their pain and the medication does not control the pain for a long enough period of time. They may be seen as "clock watchers" or "drug seeking." However, once their pain is adequately treated, the behaviors disappear.

All patients who take opioids long term for chronic pain will become dependent on them. If these patients stop their opioid use suddenly, opioid withdrawal occurs. The patient will be more symptomatic if doses are higher or if the duration of drug use is longer. Neonates who are exposed to opioids before birth will go into withdrawal within hours or days following birth (Prunty & Prunty, 2016). This syndrome is called *neonatal abstinence syndrome (NAS).*

Opioid withdrawal is a natural effect of sudden cessation of opioids. The body responds by producing a variety of physical changes such as nausea, abdominal pain, vomiting, piloerection, restlessness, or diarrhea. These effects are uncomfortable, but fatalities are rare.

Patients who are taking opioids for pain can put themselves into withdrawal for a variety of reasons:

- Taking too many opioids at the beginning of the prescription period so medication runs out before the end of the prescription period
- Diverting the opioids, resulting in no medication for the patient
- Inability to take the prescribed opioids due to an illness
- Stopping opioids suddenly without tapering
- Use of a mixed agonist–antagonist medication, such as buprenorphine, in an opioid-dependent patient
- Use of a reversal agent, such as naloxone, for treating overdose or oversedation
- Entry into a formal detoxification program using buprenorphine during induction

Whatever the cause, withdrawal is an uncomfortable condition and patients with severe symptoms often seek help in the ED, where they can get intravenous (IV) opioids and medications that relieve the withdrawal symptoms. Patients in withdrawal need support and help with symptom management. Being nonjudgmental with the patients provides a good basis for setting up a treatment plan after the withdrawal has resolved.

Patients with mild withdrawal symptoms may feel like they have the flu. These patients may have muscle aches, abdominal pain, nausea, or vomiting. Because they assume they have the flu, they go to see their primary care provider.

The primary care provider can help sort out the cause of the perceived illness by adding a question or two to the usual assessment questions such as, "I see you have chronic low-back pain, can you tell me about what you use to treat it?" or "Do you take any opioids for your chronic low-back pain?" A positive response to opioid use can lead to "When did you take your last dose of medication?" If the patient has not been taking the medication for several days, a trial of the patient's opioid may resolve the flu-like symptoms.

When a patient with mild withdrawal is seen in primary care and the symptoms have resolved, it is time to reeducate the patient about how to use opioids. Determining the reason why the patient stopped opioids is important. If the patient stopped the opioids because the patient did not like the way they made him or her feel is one thing. But if the patient stopped the opioids because he or she ran out of the medication, the issue is more serious and requires a discussion about how the patient is using the opioids, any unrelieved pain, or possibly medication diversion. If insurance coverage has stopped, that is another type of problem, requiring more of a formulary or cost solution.

CLINICAL PEARL

Patients who are taking or using opioids daily can end up in withdrawal if admitted to the hospital for treatment of a non-opioid–related condition. Trauma and surgery often involve opioid use, but cardiac irregularities or infections have no indication for opioids and they may not be ordered. The patient should be honest and reveal the opioid use to avoid withdrawal.

IDENTIFYING WITHDRAWAL

Withdrawal is the body's natural response to the sudden elimination of an opioid. It can occur with prescription medications as well as illicit drugs. Opioid withdrawal differs from other types of withdrawal because management and treatment goals are different.

The onset of withdrawal can occur soon after the medication or drug is stopped. Some common onset and duration times are presented in Table 14.1.

These data are for the initial withdrawal time period. Medications like methadone, hydrocodone, and oxycodone can have a secondary withdrawal period that can last up to 6 months with milder symptoms (Prunty & Prunty, 2016).

If the patient has a history of OUD, relapse is always possible. Addiction is a chronic relapsing disease that has no cure. Helping a relapsing patient through a period of withdrawal is challenging. The healthcare provider will not only be treating the withdrawal symptoms, but also dealing with readdiction and the patient's failure to maintain his or her recovery. If the patient has a 12-step sponsor, using the support that can be offered will be important to the final steps of recovery. The care plan for this type of patient may involve inpatient treatment and detoxification.

TABLE 14.1 **Common Withdrawal Onset and Duration Times**

	ONSET OF WITHDRAWAL (HRS)	DURATION OF WITHDRAWAL (D)
Buprenorphine	6–24	7
Fentanyl	3–5	4–5
Heroin	6	8–10
Hydrocodone	8–12	5–14
Methadone	24–96	10–14
Morphine	8–12	7–10
Oxycodone	6–12	7–14

Source: Data from Prunty, L. & Prunty, J. (2016). Acute opioid withdrawal: Identification and treatment strategies. *U.S. Pharmacist, 41(11), HS2–HS6.* Retrieved from https://www.uspharmacist.com/article/acute-opioid-withdrawal-identification-and-treatment-strategies

PHYSIOLOGY OF WITHDRAWAL

The physiology of withdrawal starts with how opioids bind in the human body. Most opioids bind at the mu sites located throughout the body, for example, brain, spinal cord, gastrointestinal (GI) system. There are some secondary binding sites that are located outside of the brain, for example, the delta and kappa sites are located in the spinal cord. Medications like buprenorphine bind to the kappa sites, unlike the pure opioid agonists, such as morphine, which bind exclusively at the mu sites. If a patient is on a pure opioid agonist like morphine, hydrocodone, or oxycodone, giving the patient a medication that is a mixed agonist–antagonist like buprenorphine will block and reverse the effects of the opioid and cause withdrawal.

In the brain, opioids bind to the mu sites in the limbic system, which controls emotions such as relaxation or pleasure (Case-Lo, 2017). The part of the brain that triggers withdrawal is the locus coeruleus, found at the base of the brain (Shah & Hueker, 2019). The neurons in the locus coeruleus have an increased number of opioid receptors. These neurons are also noradrenergic. These noradrenergic neurons activate the limbic system and the cerebral and cerebellar cortexes (Shah & Hueker, 2019). The noradrenergic activity in locus coeruleus neurons, an opioid-linked mechanism, is the prime cause of the symptoms of opioid withdrawal (Shah & Hueker, 2019). Other areas of the brain that contribute to withdrawal include the gray matter and the nucleus raphe.

CLINICAL PEARL

Withdrawal from opioids is individual to each patient. The length of time opioids have been used as well as the dose are factors in the severity of withdrawal symptoms. Withdrawal symptoms may be worsened if the patient has been taking benzodiazepines.

Patients who stop taking opioids, run out of opioids, or divert their opioid medications will experience the onset of withdrawal in a very short period of time. Once the withdrawal symptoms start, they gradually worsen. For some patients who have not been on opioids for a long period of time and are taking smaller doses, providing their prescribed opioid can help lessen the withdrawal symptoms. For patients who have been on high-dose opioids for an extended period of time, withdrawal is a more serious condition that may merit admission to a hospital for IV medications for nausea and vomiting, and clonidine to reduce anxiety and control symptoms.

After the withdrawal resolves, the discussion about what precipitated the event needs to take place. Some patients inadvertently put themselves into withdrawal by not knowing enough about their opioids and how to take them appropriately. Other patients go into withdrawal by selling the medications on the street or binge dosing at the beginning of the prescription period. No matter what the cause, patient education is needed. For diversion and bingeing behaviors, a decision about tapering the opioids off is needed with a referral to an addicition specialist, pain specialist, or psychologist, with an option for methadone or buprenorphine treatment.

Clinical Opiate Withdrawal Scale

Using a standardized tool to assess withdrawal can help identify withdrawal and the severity of the symptoms being experienced by the patient. Opioid withdrawal can be categorized as mild, moderate, moderately severe, and severe (Case-Lo, 2017). The Clinical Opiate Withdrawal Scale (COWS) can help identify which withdrawal symptoms are problematic and the severity of each symptom.

The COWS is a clinician-administered, pen-and-paper instrument that rates 11 common opiate withdrawal signs or symptoms (Wesson & Ling, 2003). Using the summed score of the 11 items, the clinician can use the score to assess the patient's level of opioid withdrawal and can make inferences about the level of physical dependence on opioids (Wesson & Ling, 2003). It was tested using opioid-dependent volunteers and found to be both reliable and valid (Tompkins et al., 2009).

The tool consists of 11 symptoms:

- Resting heart rate
- Sweating
- Restlessness
- Pupil size
- Bone or joint aches
- Runny nose or tearing
- Gastrointestinal (GI) upset
- Tremor
- Yawning
- Anxiety or irritability
- Gooseflesh skin

Each category is scored using a rating of 0 to 5, with 0 being none and 5 being present, severe, or constant. Summing the scores allows the clinician to rate the withdrawal as mild (5–12), moderate (13–24), moderately severe (25–36), and severe (more than 36).

Opioid withdrawal scales have been used since the mid-1930s (Wesson & Ling, 2003). Since that time, new tools have been developed and existing scales have been revised. There are other scales that can be used to determine the severity of the patient's withdrawal, such as the Clinical Institute Narcotic Assessment (CINA), but the COWS is more prevalent in clinical practice. It is often used to determine the stage of withdrawal in patients who are undergoing buprenorphine induction in a substance use disorder (SUD) treatment clinic. A copy of the COWS tool can be downloaded (www.asam.org/docs/default-source).

TREATING WITHDRAWAL

There are a variety of medications that can be used to treat withdrawal. Some medications for mild symptoms include acetaminophen, nonsteroidal anti-inflammatory drugs (NSAIDs) such as ibuprofen, loperamide for diarrhea, and Visteril or Atarax for nausea. Hydration is important and patients should drink 2 to 3 L of water daily, and vitamin supplementation with vitamin B and vitamin C is indicated (Shah & Hueker, 2019).

Methadone and buprenorphine are opioids that can reduce withdrawal symptoms and drug cravings. As a mixed agonist–antagonist, buprenorphine should only be started after the patient begins to experience withdrawal symptoms. Using the COWS tool can help measure the severity of the withdrawal symptoms.

For more severe cases, adding clonidine to the recommendations for treating mild withdrawal is indicated. Clonidine can help ease anxiety, cramping, and muscle aches and is usually part of a regimen for a hospitalized patient. Using opioids, such as buprenorphine and methadone, as needed is also indicated (Shah & Hueker, 2019).

Clonidine can reduce the severity of withdrawal symptoms by 50% to 75% (Case-Lo, 2017). It is used for inpatient treatment to reduce muscle aches, tearing, runny nose, cramping, anxiety, chills, insomnia, tremors, vomiting, and diarrhea. The side effects of clonidine include drowsiness, dizziness, and low blood pressure. Blood pressure should be monitored, and clonidine should be stopped if blood pressure falls below 90/50 mmHg (Shah & Hueker, 2019).

The newest medication approved for symptom management in the early period of inpatient opioid discontinuation is lofexidine (Lucymera). In two studies with opioid-dependent patients using placebo control, lofexidine reduced the severity of opioid withdrawal symptoms (Alam, Tirado, Pirner, & Clinch, 2020). Lofexidine is a nonopioid medication that acts as an agonist at the central alpha2-adrenergic presynaptic receptors, creating a suppressive effect on noradrenergic hyperactivity (Alam et al., 2020). Dosing adjustment is required for patients with renal or hepatic disease. Side effects include dizziness, orthostatic hypotension, insomnia, hypotension, and bradycardia (Alam et al., 2020).

Treatment Options

- Muscle and joint pain: For mild symptoms, use acetaminophen or NSAIDs such as Aleve and ibuprofen
- Diarrhea: Loperimide (antidiarrheal medication)
- Vomiting: Visteril or Atarax (antiemetic medications)
- Anxiety: Clonidine, meditation, or relaxation
- Itching: Atarax or Benadryl

Adult Medication Dosing for Use in Inpatient Settings

Methadone

- Days 1 to 4: 30 mg
- Days 5 to 8: 35 mg
- Day 9: 30 mg
- Day 10: 25 mg

- Day 11: 20 mg
- Day 12: 15 mg
- Day 13: 10 mg
- Day 14: 5 mg
- Day 15: 0 mg (World Health Organization [WHO], 2009)

Buprenorphine

- Day 1: 6 mg
- Day 2: 8 mg
- Day 3: 10 mg
- Day 4: 8 mg
- Day 5: 4 mg (WHO, 2009)

Clonidine

See Table 14.2 for clonidine dosing during withdrawal.

TABLE 14.2 Clonidine Dosing Information

	MORNING (MCG)	EARLY AFTERNOON (MCG)	NIGHT (MCG)
Day 1	150	150	150
Day 2	150–300	150–300	150–300
Day 3	150–300	150–300	150–300
Day 4	75	75	75
Day 5	75	Nil	75

Source: From World Health Organization (2009). *Clinical guidelines for withdrawal management and treatment of drug dependence in closed settings.* Geneva, Switzerland: Author.

Lofexidine (Lucemyra) for use in acute opioid detoxification

- Initial dose: 0.54 mg orally four times per day during the period of peak withdrawal
- Dosing should be guided by symptoms and side effects
- Frequency of dosing: Every 5 to 6 hours

- Maximum daily dose: 2.88 mg/d
- Maximum duration of therapy: 14 days (Drugs.com, 2018)

Nonpharmacologic Techniques

- Relaxation and meditation
- Discourage exercise and physical activity
- Encourage rest
- Defer counseling and psychological therapies until active withdrawal is over

CLINICAL PEARL

Pregnant women should not undergo withdrawal. Withdrawal in pregnancy can result in miscarriage and birth defects (Shah & Hueker, 2019).

SUMMARY

There is no doubt that opioid withdrawal is a physically and psychologically painful experience. Many people continue taking opioids rather than go through the withdrawal process. The risk of overdose increases if the patient relapses after discontinuing opioid use and tries to take their usual high dose of opioid. This can result in death.

Using medications to help ease the patient through the withdrawal process is very helpful. Studying opioid withdrawal physiology can provide new and unique physical targets for the development of new drugs (Rehni, Jaggi, & Singh, 2013). Targets for development include receptors, such as calcitonin gene-related peptide receptors (CGRP) and *N*-methyl-D-aspartate (NMDA) receptors. New areas of study include second messengers such as nitric oxide synthase, cytokines, arachidonic acid metabolites, and corticotropin releasing factor (Rehni et al., 2013).

Overall, reassuring patients that there are ways to lessen the side effects of withdrawal can help them decide to forego opioids. For some patients, opioids can provide a means of pain relief that allow them to have a better life with increased function. For patients not in that category who try to stop opioids and go into withdrawal, the experience may be so negative that they continue using opioids. It is to be hoped that the new drugs and new approaches can help minimize the negative effects of withdrawal.

TRENDING IN PAIN MANAGEMENT

- Watch for new medications to treat withdrawal symptoms using unique physiologic targets.
- Watch for the development of new or revised tools that can better diagnose the elements of withdrawal.

CASE STUDY

Sally is a 45-year-old patient who is seen in the ED for severe abdominal pain and vomiting. She rates her pain as 8 out of 10. She is slightly obese, holding her abdomen, and states she has been experiencing the abdominal pain for several days. She says she does not know what caused the pain, but it seems to be increasing. She has not been able to eat for 3 days and feels this may be adding to her abdominal pain. She is admitted to the hospital, kept on nothing per os (NPO) status, and given IV fluids and antiemetic medications. She is not given any opioids since the hospitalist is concerned she may have a bowel blockage and opioids would make it worse. A full abdominal pain workup is ordered to determine the possible cause of her abdominal pain.

When you, a hospitalist, interview Sally in her hospital room, she seems to be more comfortable because her nausea has stopped. As you review her medical history, which includes diabetes, high blood pressure, and obesity, Sally tells you she forgot to mention that she has low-back pain. When you ask what she was taking for the pain, she says she takes extended-release morphine 40 mg twice per day. She says it works for her pain and she has been taking it for 2 years. When you ask her when she took her last dose, she tells you she ran out of medication and her last dose was taken 1 week ago.

It is now fairly obvious that the cause of Sally's abdominal pain is opioid withdrawal. Once the opioid is restarted, her symptoms resolve. She is able to go home, but the questions still remain: How was the opioid use overlooked in the ED and why did Sally run out of her medication?

- Sally seems oblivious to the fact that by stopping her medication she put herself into withdrawal. Whoever was prescribing her opioids failed to educate her about what would happen if she suddenly stopped her medication.
- Why did Sally run out of her medication? Sally says she was moving and was lifting and carrying large boxes. Because her pain increased, she took more medication. She had not done it before to the extent she did it this time. In the past, she only took a pill or two extra between prescriptions.

(*continued*)

CASE STUDY (*continued*)

How did Sally get admitted to the hospital and receive a full abdominal pain workup?

- ED staff are trained to deal with trauma, strokes, and heart attacks. Abdominal pain falls low on the priority list. Sally was seen by a brand-new hospitalist who did not realize that Sally was in withdrawal because she did not mention her opioid prescription on the medication list.
- The hospitalist should inform the patient's primary care provider about her admission. Sally will need to follow up with primary care and this will provide an opportunity for education and a review of Sally's patient–provider agreement (PPA). She will also need more careful monitoring to avoid reoccurrence of her withdrawal. In the end, she may need to be titrated off of her current opioids and either taper off opioids entirely or go for buprenorphine or methadone treatment.

REFERENCES

Alam, D., Tirado, C., Pirner, M., & Clinch, T. (2020). Efficacy of lofexidine for mitigating opioid withdrawal symptoms: Results from two randomized, placebo controlled trials. *Journal of Drug Assessment, 9*(1), 13–19. doi:10.1080/21556660.2019.1704416

Case-Lo, C., (2017). *Withdrawal from opiates and opioids*. Healthline. Retrieved from www.healthline.com/health/opiate-withdrawal

Prunty, L., & Prunty, J. (2016). Acute opioid withdrawal: Identification and treatment strategies. *U.S. Pharmacist, 41*(11), HS2–HS6. Retrieved from https://www.uspharmacist.com/article/acute-opioid-withdrawal-identification-and-treatment-strategies

Rehni, A. K., Jaggi, A. S., & Singh, N. (2013). Opioid withdrawal syndrome: emerging concepts and novel therapeutic targets. *CNS and Neurological Disorders, 12*(1), 112–125. doi:10.2174/1871527311312010017

Shah, M., & Hueker, M. (2019). *Opioid withdra*wal. NCBI Bookshelf. Treasure Island, FL: Stat Pearls.

Tompkins, A., Bigelow, G., Harrison, J., Johnson, R., Fudala, P., & Strain, E. (2009). Concurrent validation of the Clinical Opiate Withdrawal Scale (COWS) and single item indices against the Clinical Narcotic Assessment (CINA) opioid withdrawal instrument. *Drug and Alcohol Dependence, 105*(1–2), 154–159. doi:10.1016/j.drugalcdep.2009.07.001

Wesson, D. R., & Ling, W. (2003). The clinical opiate withdrawal scale. *Journal of Psychoactive Drugs, 35*(2), 253–259. doi:10.1080/02791072.2003.10400007

World Health Organization. (2009). *Clinical guidelines for withdrawal management and treatment of drug dependence in closed settings*. Geneva, Switzerland: Author.

ADDITIONAL RESOURCES

American Academy of Pain Medicine, American Pain Society & American Society of Addiction Medicine. (2001). *Definitions related to the use of opioids for the treatment of pain*. Retrieved from http://www.painmed.org/productpub/statement/pdfs/definition.pdf

D'Arcy, Y., & Brukenthal, P. (2011). *Safe opioid prescribing for nurse practitioners*. New York, NY: Oxford University Press.

Gowing, L., Ali, R., White, J., & Mbewe, D. (2017). Buprenorphine for managing opioid withdrawal. *Cochrane Database of Systematic Reviews, 2*(2). doi:10.1002/14651858.CD002025.pub5

CHAPTER 15

MANAGING PATIENTS ON OPIOID THERAPY

INTRODUCTION

Once a patient begins an opioid trial, the primary care practitioner needs to set up a monitoring plan. Monitoring parameters are outlined in the patient–provider agreement (PPA) and follow the recommendations of the Center for Drug Evaluation and Research of the U.S. Food and Drug Administration (FDA) Blueprint (2012).

Each clinic should have a policy pertaining to using opioids for its patients. Compliance with these policies can help maintain safe prescribing for both the prescriber and the patient.

Current recommendations include telling the patient that the use of opioids is being started as a trial to see whether there is any improvement in pain or increase in functionality. By telling the patient the medication is a trial, it reinforces the fact that if there is no benefit, the medications will be stopped. If the medication is stopped, other types of therapy or other medications will be tried.

CLINICAL PEARL

Following clinic policies and national recommendations provides support for practice. Clear and enforced boundaries are an important part of monitoring successful opioid use.

Documentation of the care plan is also very important. The plan itself should be documented in the patient's chart, so that there is a frame of reference for anyone seeing the patient while the primary provider is unavailable. Test results and patient discussions should also be included in the documentation. If the documentation is lacking, proving to insurance companies or regulatory agents that discussions occurred and demonstrating that the plan of care is being followed will be very difficult for the healthcare provider.

- The plan itself should include the parameters listed in the PPA for refills, urine screening, and follow-up visits.
- The medication and the dose should be clearly identified in the plan.

- The diagnostic workup that is the basis for the medication should be listed in the plan.
- Results of all tests, including the opioid risk screening, and the results of the state's Prescription Drug Monitoring Program (PDMP) should be fully documented in the plan.
- All discussions with the patient and family and all decisions should be recorded in the plan of care.

Monitoring patients is as important as prescribing drugs for them. If monitoring fails, both the patient and the prescriber are at risk, both safety-wise and legally. With opioids, failing to monitor the patients and how they are using their opioids can result in a tragic and fatal ending.

MONITORING THE PATIENT ON OPIOIDS

For primary care providers, monitoring a patient on opioids can be time-consuming, but it is one of the most worthwhile aspects of using opioids with patients. Using a PPA can help eliminate some of the issues that can arise with opioid prescribing, such as requests for early refills or urine screens that reveal unprescribed substances were used.

A PPA outlines all the aspects of the opioid trial. The Centers for Disease Control and Prevention (CDC) guideline recommendations endorse the use of a PPA with all patients being started on an opioid trial. The PPA is a document that outlines the responsibilities of the patient as well as the provider.

- A PPA includes information regarding the patient's willingness to comply with the PPA, as indicated by the signature of both the patient and the healthcare practitioner.
- The PPA can also serve as nformed consent.
- This list includes the medication, dose, and how to use the medication. It also includes a discussion of adverse effects such as constipation, nausea, or sedation.
- The PPA stipulates that only one provider should prescribe opioids, usually the primary care provider. No other healthcare provider is to write prescriptions for opioids for the patient.
- The PPA states that no early refills or sharing of medications is allowed.
- It includes use of random urine screens as needed. The PPA also indicates what the repercussions will be if a nonprescribed substance shows up in the urine screen. It also includes what will happen if the

prescribed medication does not show up in the urine screen. An exit strategy can be included here.

- A PPA includes a discussion of the risk of addiction.
- By signing the PPA, the patient commits to coming to all follow-up appointments.
- In the PPA, the provider commits to providing care for the patient while the patient is on opioids, and if the opioids need to be stopped, the provider will continue to care for the patient and offer alternate methods of pain management.

How well are primary care providers doing with using PPAs for patients on opioids? In a study of resident and attending physicians, 54% of the residents and 42% of the attending physicians had PPAs with their patients (Khalid et al., 2015). Urine screen percentages were a bit higher, with 58% of the residents and 63% of the attending physicians using urine drug screen testing (Khalid et al., 2015).

Early refill requests are problematic for many practices. In a study of residents and attending physicians, residents were more likely to supply two or more early refills (42%) compared to attending physicians (32%; Khalid et al., 2015). The resident patient population included a higher percentage of new patients, young males, and those who were on Medicaid, creating a higher potential for red-flag behavior.

Overall, the study indicated that both residents and attending physicians were only partially compliant with the guideline recommendations for monitoring patients on opioids. This lack of compliance demonstrates the need for further education for providers on the benefits of monitoring patients on opioids and the risks of not following monitoring recommendations.

Using the PDMP regularly to monitor opioid prescribing can be very helpful in getting documentation that can find patient misuse very early on. Forty-nine states have developed drug- monitoring programs. Missouri is the only state that does not have a state monitoring program. In the United States, 27 states mandate the use of the PDMP (PDMP Training and Technical Assistance Center, n.d).

Using PDMPs offers clear benefits. The rate of registration for prescribers of opioid prescriptions is still only 33% and not all registered users consistently use the program. Incentives that have been suggested to increase the use of PDMPs are pay for performance, malpractice discounts, and immunity from liability for prescribers who consistently use the programs (Haffajee, Anupam, & Weiner, 2015).

Educating the patient on the dangers of opioid misuse and abuse is an important part of the care plan (Box 15.1). Family and friends are the biggest source of nonprescribed opioids (FDA, 2016). Sharing opioids offers significant risk for adverse effects and the patient may not realize the implications.

Taking an opioid prescribed for pain for sleep is considered opioid misuse, and teaching patients not to use opioids for sleep unless the problem is pain related

BOX 15.1

DIFFERENCES BETWEEN OPIOID MISUSE AND OPIOID ABUSE

- Opioid misuse: Use of a prescribed medication other than intended, that is, using a pain medication for sleep rather than pain relief
- Opioid abuse: Use of a prescribed medication for a purpose other than pain, that is, using a pain medication for its euphoric effect (U.S. Food and Drug Administration [FDA], 2018)

Source: Center for Drug Evaluation and Research, *U.*S. Food and Drug Administration. (2012). Blueprint for prescriber continuing education. *Journal of Pain and Palliative Care Pharmacotherapy, 26*(2), 127–130. doi: 10.3109/15360288.2012.680013

can help the patient better understand the role of opioids. There are many different ways to enhance sleep, rather than just using the opioid prescribed for pain.

Opioid misuse is a serious issue. Getting illegal drugs or opioids from illicit sources is a good indication of a substance use disorder (SUD), which requires intervention from a specialist skilled in addiction treatment. Primary care practitioners should not be treating these patients for pain, unless they are licensed to provide treatment with suboxone or methadone. The amount of monitoring required by these patients is cost prohibitive, and most primary care practitioners cannot afford the time in their schedules and are not trained to treat these patients.

One way to get more information about the patients is to ask the medical assistant (MA) or registered nurse (RN) in the clinic what he or she has observed. Often, patients will tell the staff things that they do not share with the healthcare provider. Also, the MAs and RNs are in a position to observe the patient and note behaviors that are not congruent with the patient's reports.

MEDICATION MANAGEMENT

When a patient is taking opioids for pain, the patient requires careful monitoring and focused medication management. Learning to reassess patients for appropriate opioid use and discuss opioid use at each visit can help detect problems early. Using the state PDMP program faithfully at each visit can help spot any deviation from the PPA and also look for any medication–medication interactions. In many cases, there are several healthcare providers prescribing medications for any one patient and one may not know what the other is prescribing.

If there are violations detected in the PDMP, the patient will need to provide information about the violation. Is the patient doctor shopping or procuring medication from other medical or nonmedical sources? If there is opioid misuse or abuse, the healthcare provider needs to determine what actions should be taken.

Early refill requests require action on the part of the healthcare provider. Patients will often call the clinic stating they need more pain medication as they have used all the medication they received or, in some cases, they will demonstrate aberrant behaviors related to losing medications. Patients who drop medications into the toilet repeatedly, report medications as stolen without having a police report for the theft, or who say they just lost the pill bottle or the prescription are sending up red flags that require investigation.

CLINICAL PEARL

When seeing a patient who has been on opioids for any length of time for the first time, it is not incumbent on the healthcare provider to give the new patient an opioid prescription. For a new opioid-dependent patient, getting medical records, doing an opioid risk screen, getting a urine screen, and reviewing the supporting documents for diagnosis are essential.

Pill counts can be a way to see how the patient is using his or her medications. The patient brings their medications to the clinic and a physical count of the pills is done. This is a rather antiquated way to determine compliance, but it can provide reinforcement that the medication needs to be taken as prescribed. If the pill counts are off and too many pills are missing, the healthcare provider needs to discuss the discrepancy and determine what happened to the missing pills. If the patient says their pain was not controlled and they took extra medication, a reassessment of the care plan will need to be done and, in some cases, an increase in medication is needed.

CLINICAL PEARL

Be aware that there are fake pills being sold on the Internet that look just like real medications. When doing a pill count, make sure that all the pills look alike. If there are questions, ask a pharmacist to look at the pills to determine whether any of them are fake.

If a decision is made to stop opioids, the pills need to be tapered. Reassuring the patient that you will continue to offer support can make the taper less of an issue. Tell the patient you will continue to offer care for their medical needs, but you will not prescribe opioids any longer.

Most patients who have been taking opioids for any length of time are reluctant to give up the one thing they see as controlling their pain. They can become anxious and angry. Maintaining a calm and reassuring demeanor while explaining how the taper will progress can help diffuse the situation.

A recommended taper progression includes the following (Box 15.2):

- Calculate the 24-hour medication usage.
- Calculate the new daily dosage by decreasing the amount by 25% to 50%; 10% reduction is acceptable for a fragile patient.
- Over a period of 3 days, decrease doses to last a week or two depending on how robust the patient is and how long the patient has been taking opioids.
- For higher doses and for patients who have been on opioids for a long period of time, a slow taper over weeks or months is recommended.
- Monitor the patient for any signs of withdrawal, that is, nausea, vomiting, and abdominal pain, and provide medications as needed; it may be necessary to slow the taper (CDC, 2017).

If the patient fails the taper and cannot reduce the medication, referring the patient for buprenorphine or methadone treatment is recommended. This can be done by referring the patient to a pain-management expert who can help with the taper and a new program of new medication management.

Aside from PPA violations, tapering may be needed for other reasons. A patient with pain may be able to have surgery to correct the problem and can then be tapered off of the opioids after surgery. Some patients have side effects that they cannot tolerate, or some patients just decide that they do not like opioids and wish to stop them.

BOX 15.2

EXAMPLE OF A TAPER PROGRESSION SCHEDULE: DECREASE DOSE EVERY 2 WEEKS

Current dose: oxycodone 100 mg/d
  8–10-mg tablets
  4–5-mg tablets for breakthrough pain
25% taper—new dose: oxycodone 75 mg/d
  6–10-mg tablets
  3–5-mg tablets for breakthrough pain
Second taper: 25% oxycodone 75 mg/d
  4–10-mg tablets
  3–5-mg tablets for breakthrough pain

Coverage Issues

Most clinics have a call schedule, meaning one provider will cover the patients during nights and weekends. Providing clear documentation of the patient's care plan will allow the covering provider to make an informed decision about medication use.

Nurse practitioners (NPs) and physician assistants (PAs) often see patients in follow-up care for physicians who have seen the patient during the primary visit and then transition the care to the NP and PA staff. The attending physician usually sets up a plan of care for the patient.

What can an NP or PA do when they feel the pain-management plan is not correct for the patient, with too little, too much, or the wrong type of opioid prescribed? There are several options open to the NP or PA:

- Have a discussion with the attending provider to determine what factors influenced the decision about opioid use. The attending provider may know something that is not included in the chart.
- Tell the attending provider that you are not comfortable with providing too little medication for controlling the pain or too much medication for the identified pain complaint. Ask what can be changed for the patient.
- If the plan of care has not been fully supported, such as no low-back workup even though a diagnosis of low-back pain is being used to support opioid use, explain that you will need to do more testing to be comfortable continuing to prescribe opioid medications.
- If the attending provider continues to ask you to prescribe outside of the national guideline recommendations, offer the provider a copy of guidelines. The prescriber may not be aware of newer information. In the end, you may have to transfer the patient back to the attending provider for pain management.

CLINICAL PEARL

If you are not comfortable prescribing opioids for a patient whom you are seeing in follow-up, remember that it is your license that is at stake. If regulatory agents question your prescribing patterns and find they are outside of the national recommendations, you may risk losing your license, especially if there has been a fatality related to opioid use.

SUMMARY

The role of provider education in monitoring patients using opioids cannot be underestimated. An educated provider is aware of what is required for monitoring and is prepared to address red flags if they occur.

The importance of the PPA is also underestimated. Using a PPA can protect both the patient and the provider if problems occur with opioid therapy. In order to make opioid therapy a safe and effective practice, using a PPA can provide support for the practice.

TRENDING IN PAIN MANAGEMENT

- Look for changes in the number of states that require a PDMP review during the patient visit.
- Look for changes in documentation requirements so that you can remain current.

CASE STUDY

Ester is a 56-year-old patient who has been on opioid therapy for 2 years. She has degenerative joint disease that failed to respond to nonsteroidal anti-inflammatory drugs (NSAIDs) and steroid injections, and she has stopped going to physical therapy because it increases her pain. She is depressed and anxious because she cannot seem to get her pain under control so that she can become more functional. She tells you, "I am only 56 years old, but I feel like I am 100. Isn't there something you can do to help me? Maybe I need an increase in pain medication." She is taking oxycodone 13 mg twice per day. In her clinic urine screen 3 months ago, the screening result came back negative for oxycodone. The confirming gas chromatography screening result showed very low levels of oxycodone in her sample. A discussion with the patient revealed that she had been taking two tablets of her medication at times, so she had to ration her medication in the weeks before her appointment. She agreed to return to the prescribed medication regimen with no further independent dose escalations. You ask her to return in 4 weeks for a follow-up appointment.

At her appointment, she provides a urine sample. You note on the PDMP that she has started to see another provider for depression. When the urine screen results return, there is positive result for a benzodiazepine that you did not prescribe for her. You ask her to return to the office for a discussion.

(*continued*)

CASE STUDY (*continued*)

At this appointment, she reveals she is very anxious about her continuing pain. She tells you nothing seems to work to control that pain. She is depressed and frustrated. She admits she went to another healthcare provider who gave her a prescription for a benzodiazepine and offered her a prescription for oxycodone, which she declined. She did not realize how serious it was to use a benzodiazepine medication with her opioids.

At this point, there have been several violations of her opioid agreement. She is not benefiting from the opioid therapy because she is no closer to reaching her goal of adequate pain relief. You carefully explain to Ester that you have to stop prescribing opioids for her. You will continue her care for her other health problems, but you will need to taper her off of opioids. She will need to see a psychologist for help with her anxiety and depression. You also tell her that you will make a referral to a pain specialist who can help her with her pain. Ester is not happy, but she understands that she needs more help to manage her pain.

- The first red flag for Ester was her unauthorized dose escalation. Because she agreed to take her medication as prescribed, the healthcare provider hoped that the issue was resolved.
- Ester needed more frequent and careful monitoring. The second urine screen was definitely indicated and revealed continuing problems with medication use.
- In fact, Ester may not have been getting enough pain medication to control her pain. A change in the medication dose may have resolved the problem.
- Ester could have gotten into serious problems combining a benzodiazepine with an opioid. Her past behavior reveals she takes more medication than needed at times. She could have easily become oversedated, with tragic results.
- Ester may be a good candidate for buprenorphine therapy. It can potentially control her pain better and ease some of her anxiety about "nothing" helping her pain.
- Careful monitoring is essential for Ester. Her pain is chronic and will continue to be a presence in her life. Helping her to manage her preoccupation with the pain and incorporate ways to better manage pain, depression, and anxiety will, in the end, be the best solution for her pain management.

REFERENCES

Center for Drug Evaluation and Research. U. S. Food and Drug Administration. (2012). Blueprint for prescriber continuing education program. *Journal of Pain and Palliative Care Pharmacotherapy, 26*(2), 127–130. doi: 10.3109/15360288.2012.680013

Centers for Disease Control and Prevention. (2017). *Common elements in guidelines for prescribing opioids for chronic pain.* Retrieved from https://www.cdc.gov/drugoverdose/pdf/common_elements_in_guidelines_for_prescribing_opioids-20160125-a.pdf

Haffajee, R., Anupam, J., & Weiner, S. (2015). Mandatory use of prescription drug monitoring programs. *Journal of the American Medical Association, 313*(9), 891–892. doi:10.1001/jama.2014.18514

Khalid, L., Liebshutz, J., Xuan, Z., Dossabhoy, S., Kim, Y., Crooks, D., . . . Lassu, K. (2015). Adherence to prescription opioid monitoring guidelines among residents and attending physicians in the primary care setting. *Pain Medicine, 16*(3), 480–487. doi:10.1111/pme.12602

PDMP Training and Technical Assistance Center. (n.d). Retrieved from http://www.pdmpassist.org/content

U. S. Food and Drug Administration. (2018). *The FDA opioid analgesic REMS education blueprint for healthcare providers involved in the treatment and monitoring of patients with pain.* Retrieved from www.FDA.gov

CHAPTER 16

MAKING REFERRALS AND USING A PERSONAL NETWORK FOR PAIN MANAGEMENT

INTRODUCTION

As more pain management is being provided by primary care clinicians, ready access to clinicians who can provide support and address the complex variables that impact pain can improve outcomes. Using a team approach addressing the biopsychosocial aspects of pain is recommended in many pain guidelines (Chou et al., 2007; Dowell, Haegerich, & Chou, 2016; Owen et al., 2018). Making a quality referral makes the process smoother for you, the consultant, and the patient. You may create your own team network of professionals in the community or work with a team in your facility or health system.

> **CLINICAL PEARL**
>
> Where and when to refer a patient will depend on the patient, your practice, and your personal preferences and skills.

TEAMWORK AND RELATIONSHIPS

The team approach to managing pain is supported by many healthcare organizations. The Health and Medicine Division (of the National Academies of Sciences, Engineering, and Medicine) blueprint for relieving pain (Institute of Medicine [IOM], 2011) states that the patient should be part of the team and care should be coordinated by primary care (Steglitz, Buscemi, & Ferguson, 2012). There are many ways to coordinate care; to perform this task in a busy primary care practice requires following established processes that build referrals and communication with consultants into clinic workflow.

The International Association for the Study of Pain (IASP) recommends system coordination and "a biopsychosocial approach to assessment and management that involves a team of healthcare professionals working closely together within a non-hierarchical framework" (IASP, 2011).

Johnson describes desirable models of care for chronic pain as individualized to include improving the patient's well-being by using all available avenues, including lifestyle, psychological intervention, and nonpharmacological approaches; he also notes that the World Health Organization promotes multidisciplinary teams that work with patients, empowering them to improve their self-efficacy (Johnson, 2019). As the clinician with the best overall perspective of the patient, primary care providers are optimally positioned to coordinate complex care.

Positive relationships are an important component of quality healthcare. This includes relationships with patients and with other clinicians. This is especially important when addressing patients with complex constellations of symptoms and diseases. Taking the time to establish, nurture, and expand a network of relationships with clinicians skilled in the myriad disciplines that can impact pain is essential.

This team can be formed with members of your facility or can include members of your local community, and, through use of technology, even those across the country or the world. Having processes and workflows in place will make referral or consultation simpler. Although it takes time to create these processes, the resources can be useful for all patients in primary care.

PAIN-MANAGEMENT TEAMS

How to Create Your Team

The multiple factors that contribute to chronic pain benefit from different perspectives. Maintaining an active lifestyle, developing self-care, especially with regard to mental health, and improving quality of life for everyone can be difficult and be a bigger challenge for people with pain. When thinking about referrals, consider options beyond classic physical therapy (PT) or surgery and incorporate integrative therapies like acupuncture or community-based lifestyle support, for example, a recreational center walking program. If you work in a health system, become familiar with the consultation services and other resources available within the system. These may include behavioral health, PT, surgery, nutrition, and coaching. Reach out to departments and learn about the services they offer, how to refer someone to them, and the response time for referrals. Establishing these relationships supports your ability to advocate for your patients.

Consistently taking patients' biopsychosocial factors into account can improve pain management. "The majority of the medical evidence supports a biopsychosocial model of pain that integrates physical, emotional, social and cultural variables" (IOM, 2011). Primary care clinicians have an overall perspective of the patient; including other disciplines to provide therapies provides additional skills to enhance outcomes.

Positive relationships are an important component of quality healthcare. Taking the time to establish and then nurture and expand this network of relationships with clinicians skilled in the myriad disciplines that can impact pain is essential. This is especially important when addressing patients with complex constellations of symptoms and diseases.

CLINICAL PEARL

The network you create to support patients with pain may also be useful for other patients in a primary care practice.

Having a personal relationship with support staff or clinicians in another office who can provide the expertise your patient needs, streamlines the process, making it easier for you to make referrals. These relationships evolve over time; as with any organism, a referral network either grows or deteriorates.

CLINICAL PEARL

Maintaining a comprehensive list of clinicians available to provide support to your patients and having a process in place to contact them improves your clinic workflow.

Start with a "wish list" of team members from the myriad choices offered in the "Specific Pain-Management Referrals" section. Start with people you are familiar with, physical therapists, behavioral health, orthopedists, and so forth. Then look for the biggest gaps. Do you frequently wish you could provide support for patients with depression? Look within your system or community, who is known to be approachable? Who do colleagues choose for referrals? Who is available for appointments?

How you develop the network depends on your personal style. For some people, reaching out is uncomfortable; as with any other challenging task, the more you practice, the more the skill becomes part of your repertoire. You may think you do not have time to create this network. Think of it like creating macros for the electronic health record (EHR), it is an investment that pays over and over. There are many formal and informal strategies for personally interacting with clinical colleagues. Attend professional meetings in your specialty area and outside your discipline. Attending a pharmacology or naturopathy conference can provide a new perspective and the opportunity to meet other clinicians. Attend professional meetings that may be outside your comfort zone. At a PT conference, you will see evaluation and management through a different lens and may interact with PTs. Take a class at the community center in yoga, Pilates, fitness, and walking; while participating, consider how this could be useful for some patients.

CLINICAL PEARL

As you develop your network, one personal contact can lead to another.

Challenges

You may have limitations of time, or Accountable Care Organization and insurance network restrictions; learn the rules and optimize what you can. A rural location may limit access to specialists, but there are many talented clinicians available in rural areas.

Create a file with names, addresses, websites, email addresses, and phone numbers of key clinicians and staff; if you are given a private number, protect it and use it judiciously. The file can take the form of a spreadsheet, contact list, or notebook—whatever fits your workflow. You may need to add an insurance category to make the list workable for all your patients.

MAKING REFERRALS

How to Refer

Writing the referral: If the referral is incorporated into your EHR, know what the final document looks like. Is it providing the recipient with easy access to relevant information? Does it contain too much information with too little relevance? If necessary, create a process for easily and securely sending the relevant information.

CLINICAL PEARL

A referral should be concise and complete, easily read by the recipient or staff without having to wade through superfluous information.

Use a referral form that includes the important information and provides a starting point for the consultant. This makes the process easier for the patient and the consultant and helps the consultant provide the services you need.

A referral should include:

- A brief summary of your concerns or specific request, for example, a procedure
- A copy of the most recent office note

If the following information is not easily accessible in the office note, put it on the form:

- Past medical history and comorbidities
- Current medication list
- Imaging: Some clinicians only want the report, whereas surgeons and interventionists generally want to see images that have been created; if digital access is not available, have the patient take a copy of the images to the appointment
- Relevant labs, other tests
- Insurance demographics

When referring a patient with pain, consider the purpose of the referral. If you are asking for assistance in identifying the pain generator or for a nonsurgical intervention, consider pain management, physical medicine, or PT. The pain specialist can recommend or order imaging if needed to identify the pain generator. If you are referring to pain management, indicate whether you are asking for consultation regarding your current treatment plan, or for evaluation and treatment. Refer to a surgeon if you think surgery is the next step.

When to Make a Referral

Emergent: If the patient has red flags indicating an emergency, such as saddle anesthesia, loss of bowel or bladder control, or an imminent mental health crisis

Urgent: New onset of profound pain or mental health challenge that requires intervention

Early: Use all available resources to impact pain. Guidelines encourage use of PT and behavioral therapy (Centers for Disease Control and Prevention [CDC], 2016) before prescribing opioids. Morlion describes the importance of awareness of psychosocial factors and early intervention to avoid the progression of acute to chronic pain (Morlion et al., 2018). Owen et al. (2018) advise remembering the impact of psychosocial factors on the risk of chronic pain and recommend consideration of referral when opioids are being considered.

For an ongoing treatment plan:

- If the patient is not improving, refer them for assistance in identifying the pain generator or alternative treatment.
- If the patient or family has known psychosocial challenges, refer sooner

rather than later to avoid chronification. The CHANGE PAIN Chronic Advisory Board consensus statement describes chronification as “the process of transient pain progressing into persistent pain” (Morlion et al., 2018).

- When diagnosis requires care beyond what you can provide, or the patient would benefit from adjunctive therapy to support your pain-management plan, a referral is needed. Options are as diverse as PT, surgery, behavioral health, chiropractic care, or yoga.
- Refer the new or established patient if they are on a dose of opioids that you do not feel comfortable maintaining. There are patients with conditions that require sufficient opioid dosing to maintain function. Obtain consultation regarding the most appropriate management for the patient regarding dosing, determine whether taper is indicated, whether the current plan is appropriate, or what alternative treatments are available.
- Refer when a patient does not progress as expected: Perhaps the initial treatment plan did not impact pain or the patient is not able to follow or is uninterested in your plan. A different clinical recommendation could provide an alternative or support your recommendation.
- When you are not able to identify a pain generator or when symptoms are not consistent with physical findings, you may refer to PT, surgery, or a pain specialist.
- Refer when a patient needs a particular intervention, for example, a spinal injection or acupuncture.
- Refer the patient when they have been stable and then develop new symptoms or increased pain.
- Refer the patient when they have made gains and plateaued and are ready to take the next steps. Occupational therapy (OT), PT, Pilates, an individual workout program, or behavioral health may help the patient improve their ability to manage the pain.
- Health coaching can be useful for making lifestyle changes; it can also be a bridge for patients who are not willing to pursue behavioral health.
- Changes in function, pain intensity, or quality may signal deterioration of a chronic problem or onset of a new problem.

Developing Your Referral Network

The list for clinicians with expertise in impacting pain is long. Your list will be tailored to your patient population, geographic location, and practice setting. It may include licensed and unlicensed individuals. It can be helpful to develop various options that are accessible to patients. When considering who to put on your referral list, consider the following: Which (if any) third-party payers cover their services? Do they bill insurance or are they cash only? If cash is required, do they provide a superbill? Can your patients cover out-of-network costs?

The CDC guidelines (Dowell et al., 2016) recommend considering community resources for patients, in addition to traditional medical settings. For example, an uninsured patient with limited resources who is able to exercise independently with minimal guidance could benefit from the community gym or a yoga or Pilates studio. When referring to these facilities, you want to know the attitude, caliber, and capabilities of the people providing the services.

Always think of patient's individual needs when creating a treatment plan. The Health and Medicine Division (of the National Academies of Sciences, Engineering, and Medicine) blueprint advocates for individualized approaches to managing pain (IOM, 2011). Collaborating on patient care is personal; working with clinicians who share your perspective and support your care is a gratifying experience. As a primary care clinician, you know patients beyond their pain diagnosis; you can tailor the patients' treatment experience by matching them with clinicians with the skills and approaches that the patient can embrace.

Licensing and certification of healthcare professionals provides information regarding their baseline qualifications. Professionals like yoga teachers are unlicensed, but adhere to professional association criteria. For all referrals, know the reputation of providers in your community; what are people known for: skills, interpersonal interactions, willingness to collaborate?

Consider the qualities and qualifications of clinicians for your referral network. Choosing a yoga instructor is an example that you can use to develop your personal rubric (see Table 16.1).

The list that follows is not exhaustive, but offers a starting point to begin looking around your community to identify individuals and disciplines that can support you in providing the best pain management for your patients:

- Pharmacist and compounding pharmacist: Consult on medications, medication interactions, dosing, and so forth
- Social services: Consult on domestic violence, homeless services, detox/addiction programs, and suicide support. Do you have access to a psychiatric ED?
- Movement—PT and OT: Know the consultant's specialty and the populations they work with, for example, joint replacement, preventive care, rehabilitation or work hardening, neurological care, sports, Yoga, Pilates, Qi Gong

- Behavioral health—prescribers and therapists
- Surgeons, pain specialists—both medical and interventional
- Other medical providers, including dentists, neurologists, rheumatologits, gastroenterologists, physical medicine and rehabilitation therapists
- Community health or recreation centers

Other Things to Consider

When you make a referral, do your patients improve? Do patients feel part of the treatment planning? Do they feel heard by the consultant?

TABLE 16.1 How to Choose a Yoga Instructor

Training	Multiple levels available, (minimum to maximum: 200-hr, 500-hr, Master Teacher, Yogi Raj)
Credentials	YA is a registry of qualified schools that acknowledges levels of training. It is not a licensing group. "IYT" denotes specific advanced training.
Specialties	Anatomy; restorative yoga; prenatal yoga; condition-specific yoga, such as osteoporosis, cancer, trauma; yoga for teens; IYT
Experience	Years of teaching and populations served: studio classes, private classes, community classes
Presence	Does the teacher present as calm, balanced, vital?
Motivation	What is the teacher's passion? Understand the teacher's purpose in teaching.
Cost	Fees for community or group programs vary (private fees $80–200/hr)
Style	• Hatha: Most common style taught; movement is linked with breath • ISHTA • Iyengar: Focus is on alignment, with props used for support • Ashtanga: Demands strength • Yin and restorative: Slow, gentle movements • Kundalini: Emphasis is on increasing breath capacity and absorption of breath (not appropriate for chronic or acute illness) • Power or hot: High level of fitness required
Choosing a yoga approach	**Beginner or individual with health conditions:** ISHTA, Yin, Restorative, Gentle, Chair, Therapeutic **Fitness/mobility needed:** Ashtanga, Iyengar, Vinyasa, Power/hot, Kundalini

ISHTA, Integrative Science of Hatha, Tantra, and Ayurveda; IYT, integrated yoga therapy; YA, Yoga Alliance.

Source: Used with permission from Deirdre Breen, Master Yoga Teacher–ISHTA lineage, AHC, NBC-HWC.

Are appointments available in a timely manner or is the waitlist months long? If the wait is long, can a phone consult move the diagnostic evaluation forward while waiting for the appointment?

Create an urgent list, where you refer patients with red flags. Your default may be to the ED; it is also useful to have an alternative that could be more specific to the urgency:

- Behavioral health: Suicidal ideation, profound depression or anxiety, family crisis/domestic violence
- Sudden onset of pain that would benefit from an injection

Tips

- Find out how busy the clinicians on your list are and who has room to accept new patients.
- Know what conditions the clinicians manage and which ones they prefer.
- Find one or two people who have extensive connections in the local community who you can contact for recommendations or referrals.
- Patient preference: Allopathic or integrative, payer coverage for therapies, local availability, and so on

SPECIFIC PAIN-MANAGEMENT REFERRALS

Physical Therapy

PT is a key component of pain management and is included in the CDC and the American College of Physicians (ACP) guidelines (Chou et al., 2007; Dowell et al., 2016). "Physical Therapists are movement experts who improve quality of life through prescribed exercise, hands-on care, and patient education" (American Physical Therapy Association, 2019). PTs work in hospital systems and independent practices. A physical therapist can benefit patients who need help with minor or major physical complaints. They have varied approaches and skills. Some PTs have advanced training and certification in biomechanically based manual therapy. You will find not only generalists and others who have had generalist training, but also specialty in musculoskeletal, neurological, cardiopulmonary, and others; they may prefer to work with specific populations such as children, elderly, or sports persons.

Physical therapists can establish a clinical diagnosis and develop a plan of care. When referring a patient, you can indicate "evaluate and treat," and the consultant will return a report containing the findings and care plan. If you have a specific concern, you can include a specific treatment plan if you have identified a particular course of treatment you are requesting. Including PT early in treatment provides the patient with access to the assessment and intervention skills of a therapist and shows the patient the importance of movement.

CLINICAL PEARL

When prescribing PT, include a home exercise program (HEP) from the beginning to promote the idea that the patient is a part of the team. Reinforce the importance of the HEP at follow-up visits.

Behavioral Health

Many disciplines can provide behavioral health support. Availability will depend on your location and patient insurance coverage. You will have fewer options in rural or remote areas than in academic centers. Telehealth technology offers more behavioral health options. Psychiatrists and psychiatric-mental health nurse practitioners (PMHNPs) can prescribe medication, and some do therapy. Psychologists and counselors, such as clinical social workers, licensed professional counselors, or marriage and family counselors, do individual and group therapy. Some behavioral health clinicians offer biofeedback. Cognitive behavioral therapy (CBT) is recommended in the ACP guidelines (Chou et al., 2017). Titles of professionals can vary among states. Pain psychologists receive specific postgraduate training in pain management; the American Association of Pain Psychology (AAPP, 2019) membership is open to all health professionals and offers multiple resources on its website. Consider referral to behavioral health for assistance with difficult anxiety, depression, or other mental issues, including addiction.

Clinicians Who Manage Pain With Medication, Procedures, or Surgery

Pain specialists include dentists, APRNs, physician assistants (PAs), MDs, and DOs. All can diagnose and prescribe medication. Interventional pain specialists are generally board certified after completing a fellowship. They provide interventions, including spinal and joint injections, nerve blocks, and spinal cord stimulation. Some limit their practices to interventions only, whereas others also provide consultation regarding medication management. Orthopedists and neurosurgeons evaluate and perform surgical procedures, including inserting spinal cord stimulators. Pain practices may employ nurses, physical and behavioral health therapists, and various physician specialties, including neurologists, physical medicine specialists, interventionists, and APRNs and PAs. Each of these clinicians can help in identifying a pain generator and creating a treatment plan.

Integrative Clinicians

Integrative therapies are being used by more and more people across the United States. People turn to these practices to improve wellness and to manage pain. Some patients welcome integrative referrals, whereas others are not interested. Using therapies that are congruent with patients' preference and beliefs can enhance their participation.

Yoga

Extensive research is emerging on the effectiveness of yoga in managing pain (Chang, Holt, Sklar, & Groessel, 2016; Deepeshwar, Tanwar, Kavuri, & Budhi, 2018). Yoga instructors are trained, but not licensed. The Yoga Alliance is a national database of approved yoga programs; yoga teachers register with this database. Although the database does not represent certification, it identifies a yoga teacher's location, levels of training, and years of experience. It is important that you know the skills of any yoga teacher you will refer to, especially if you are referring a patient with any physical limitations (e.g., cardiac, neurological, developmental, or musculoskeletal). Because yoga is potentially very valuable for your patients and training and approaches vary, it is important to take time to research local yoga teachers and identify those with the skills and interest to work with patients in pain. In addition to providing movement, core integration, stability, and flexibility, a skilled yoga teacher provides a mindful/meditative environment, which can be very therapeutic. Mind–body connection and incorporation of purposeful breathing are key components of yoga practice and can be very helpful for patients managing chronic pain. Table 16.1 lists the criteria to assist you in evaluating a yoga instructor. An excellent way to evaluate a yoga studio is to use these criteria to form an opinion as you take a class, speak with the instructor, while considering the needs of a patient with pain.

Naturopath

The National Institutes of Health (NIH) National Center for Complementary and Integrative Health offers a resource page containing information on naturopathic practitioners (NCCCIH, 2017). Naturopaths use many different approaches, including herbs and supplements, stress reduction, lifestyle changes, and homeopathy. In some states, naturopathic physicians prescribe medication. Formal education for the doctor of naturopathy (ND) is 4 years of postgraduate education in a naturopathic medical school. Traditional naturopaths receive training in a variety of disciplines and may not be eligible for licensing in some states. Licensure requirements and scope of practice for naturopaths vary from state to state; details for each state can be found on the American Association of Naturopathic Physicians website (American Association of Naturopathic

Physicians, 2020a). A map detailing the state regulations regarding naturopathic practice, including insurance reimbursement, is available (American Association of Naturopathic Physicians, 2020b).

If you have a patient who prefers supplements and/or nonpharmaceutical approaches, a naturopathic physician can provide consultation on pain management. Some people consult naturopaths in addition to or in lieu of allopathic clinicians.

Chiropractors

The National Center for Complementary and Integrative Health at NIH describes chiropractic medicine as a treatment that often includes manual therapy, including spinal manipulation, that emphasizes the body's ability to heal itself (NCCIH, 2019). Licensure requirements and scope of practice for chiropractors vary from state to state. ACP guidelines state that spinal manipulation is moderately effective for subacute or chronic low-back pain (Chou et al., 2017).

LIFESTYLE/WELL-BEING REFERRALS

The biopsychosocial aspect of pain provides many opportunities to impact patient suffering and improve quality of life. Encouraging participation in a gym or yoga class can provide social interaction in addition to physical activity. Nutrition impacts inflammation, risk of chronic disease, and obesity. Nutritionists or health coaches can assist with improving dietary choices and provide support for your recommendations.

Creating a rubric like the one outlined in Table 16.1 can help you to make appropriate community referrals. Know your local resources. Large health systems or community centers may offer wellness programs, including nutrition information, movement classes, socialization, or coaching. These programs can be very useful for patients who have mild pain or who would benefit from the resources available as adjuncts to more traditional medication and PT approaches.

CLINICAL PEARL

Ask patients and clinicians who their go-to person is for a given problem and seek that person out.

WORKING WITH A NETWORK

After you make the referral and the patient is being treated, ongoing communication between yourself and the consultant is useful. As a primary coordinator of the patient's care, it is helpful for you to know how things are progressing in PT or with the pain specialist. It is also useful for the specialist to hear from you if you find the patient is not progressing or the patient or specialist reports challenges. Maintain open communication using the form that works best for you: phone, fax, or sharing EHR notes.

SUMMARY

There are many people who have the skills needed to assist primary care in impacting the biopsychosocial components of pain. The team you create may or may not be part of the facility where you practice; even if you work within a large system, there may be interventions available outside that system that could benefit your patient.

To create this team requires effort that really does pay off. There is art to this; it evolves as you meet new people, team members retire, and your patient population changes. The Health and Medicine Division (of the National Academies of Sciences, Engineering, and Medicine) and others are validating the importance of both patients and primary care providers leading the pain-management team. When looking at a patient with pain, consider all factors, including living situation, stressors, and resources, that can make the pain worse or better.

TRENDING IN PAIN MANAGEMENT

- Possible expansion of the Centers for Medicare & Medicaid Services (CMS) and other payers' coverage of integrative therapies, including acupuncture
- Expanded use of health coaches
- Increase in behavioral telehealth applications

CASE STUDY

Marie is a 70-year-old woman who is slightly obese with borderline diabetes and mild osteoarthritis (OA) of both hands and the right knee; she works part-time as a substitute teacher. Marie has been complaining of low-back pain that sometimes shoots into her legs and gets worst when standing; it has been increasing over the past 6 months. She has been reluctant to attend PT, and ibuprofen is not helping.

(*continued*)

CASE STUDY (*continued*)

Lumbar spine x-rays demonstrate moderate lumbar stenosis at all levels.

- You explain the mechanics of the back and natural progression of stenosis, that pain will not spontaneously resolve, but there are things she can do to improve her quality of life and improve her pain.
- You explain the importance of core activation for overall health and stability and to manage the stenosis. You advise Marie that a conservative plan would be to have 4 to 6 weeks of PT and then evaluate her response. If this does not reduce her pain, you can order a lumbar MRI and refer her for pain management for evaluation of an epidural steroid injection.
- You write a referral to a PT practice that you know has a good program for teaching home exercise programs (HEPs) that patients can implement and that your patients with stenosis have reported as helpful. In the referral, you ask the PT to evaluate and treat, including addressing the lumbar stenosis and right knee pain.
- You tell Marie that PT is necessary to help her get stronger and that when she is able, she could progress to participation in Pilates or yoga, with a focus on stability, not flexibility; flexibility may increase, but it is not the primary goal. This will allow Marie to be active. Tell her you are very familiar with the teachers in some studios, and that the environment will be safe and welcoming. Offering community exercise as the next step can help Marie feel less like she is entering the healthcare system and won't get out.
- You tell her about a local mall-walking group that meets every morning and suggest she consider joining this group a few weeks after she starts PT.
- You schedule follow-up 1 month after Marie begins PT and advise her that you will discuss possible referral to pain management and MRI if needed. You advise her that epidural steroid injections may provide some improvement, but they would be much more effective if combined with PT, where she will learn core activation and leg strengthening to improve her posture and ability to optimize her situation. You also advise that the injection may make her more comfortable to be able to fully participate in PT, but it is the PT that will get her on the road to strength.
- You remind Marie that it is good news that she has the ability to impact her pain herself, and that clinical services are there to support that.

REFERENCES

American Association of Naturopathic Physicians. (2020a). *Principles of naturopathic medicine*. Retrieved from https://naturopathic.org/page/PrinciplesNaturopathicMedicine

American Association of Naturopathic Physicians. (2020b). *Regulated states and regulatory authorities*. Retrieved from https://naturopathic.org/page/RegulatedStates

American Association of Pain Psychology. (2019). *American Association of Pain Psychology*. Retrieved from https://aapainpsychology.org

American Physical Therapy Association. (2019). *About physical therapists (PTs) and physical therapist assistants (PTAs)*. Retrieved from https://www.choosept.com/AboutPTsPTAs/Default.aspx

Centers for Disease Control and Prevention. (2016). *Welcome to CDC stacks*. Retrieved from https://stacks.cdc.gov/view/cdc/38025

Chang, D. G., Holt, J. A., Sklar, M., & Groessl, E. J. (2016). Yoga as a treatment for chronic low back pain: A systematic review of the literature. *Journal of Orthopedics & Rheumatology, 3*(1), 1–8.

Chou, R, Deyo, R., Friedly, J., Skelly, A., Hashimoto, R., Weimer, M., . . . Brodt, E. D. (2017). Nonpharmacologic therapies for low back pain: A systematic review for an American College of Physicians Clinical Practice Guideline. *Annals of Internal Medicine, 166*(7), 493–505. doi:10.7326/M16-2459. Retrieved from https://www.ncbi.nlm.nih.gov/pubmed/28192793

Chou, R., Qaseem, A., Snow, V., Casey, D., Cross, J. T. Jr., Shekelle, P., & Owens, D. K. (2007). Diagnosis and treatment of low back pain: A joint clinical practice guideline from the American College of Physicians and the American Pain Society. *Annals of Internal Medicine, 147*(7), 478. doi:10.7326/0003-4819-147-7-200710020-00006

Deepeshwar, S., Tanwar, M., Kavuri, V., & Budhi, R. B. (2018). Effect of yoga based lifestyle intervention on patients with knee osteoarthritis: A randomized controlled trial. *Frontiers in Psychiatry, 9*, 180. doi:10.3389/fpsyt.2018.00180

Dowell, D., Haegerich, T. M., & Chou, R. (2016). CDC guideline for prescribing opioids for chronic pain—United States, 2016. *Morbidity and Mortality Weekly Reports, 65*(1), 1–49. doi:10.15585/mmwr.rr6501e1

International Association for the Study of Pain. (2011). *Desirable characteristics of national pain strategies*. Retrieved from https://www.iasp-pain.org/Advocacy/Content.aspx?ItemNumber=1473

Institute of Medicine (US) Committee on Advancing Pain Research, Care, and Education. (2011). *Relieving pain in America: A blueprint for transforming prevention, care, education, and research*. Washington, DC: National Academies Press. https://www.ncbi.nlm.nih.gov/pubmed/22553896

Johnson, M. I. (2019). The landscape of chronic pain: Broader perspectives. *Medicina, 55*(5), 182. doi:10.3390/medicina55050182

Morlion, B., Coluzzi, F., Aldington, D., Kocot-Kepska, M., Pergolizzi, J., Mangas, A. C., . . . Kalso, E. (2018). Pain chronification: What should a non-pain medicine specialist know?" *Current Medical Research and Opinion, 34*(7), 1169–1178. doi:10.1080/03007995.2018.1449738

National Center for Complementary and Integrative Health. (2017). *Naturopathy*. U.S. Department of Health and Human Services. Retrieved from https://nccih.nih.gov/health/naturopathy

National Center for Complementary and Integrative Health. (2019). *Chiropractic*. U.S. Department of Health and Human Services. Retrieved from https://nccih.nih.gov/health/chiropractic

Owen, G. T., Bruel, B. M., Schade, C. M., Eckmann, M. S., Hustak, E. C., & Engle, M. P. (2018). Evidence-based pain medicine for primary care physicians. *Baylor University Medical Center Proceedings, 31*(1), 37–47. doi:10.1080/08998280.2017.1400290

Steglitz, J., Buscemi, J., & Ferguson, M. J. (2012). The future of pain research, education, and treatment: A summary of the IOM report 'relieving pain in America: A blueprint for transforming prevention, care, education, and research.' *Translational Behavioral Medicine, 2*(1), 6–8. doi:10.1007/s13142-012-0110-2

CHAPTER 17

SPECIALTY POPULATIONS

INTRODUCTION

In 2012, the U.S. Food and Drug Administration (FDA) began focusing on educating healthcare providers about opioid prescribing. In what came to be known as the *Risk Evaluation and Mitigation Strategies (REMS)* education program, thousands of healthcare providers were educated on opioids, pain assessment, monitoring of patients on opioids, and specialty populations, such as children and the elderly, when more care with prescribing was indicated.

Pain management for children, elderly persons, and pregnant women requires extra care because of differences in metabolism, body mass, ability to clear medications, and risks to the fetus. Considering all available options, including nonpharmacologic, over-the-counter, and prescription medications—opioid and nonopioid—offers many options for pain relief in these specialty populations. There are risks and benefits to consider when using or avoiding any pain-management approach.

Elderly patients require care and planning when opioids are prescribed. Careful assessment and monitoring are essential to ensure that the patient receives adequate pain relief and that adverse events, such as sedation, delirium, and constipation, are reduced or eliminated.

Treating children with opioids is a source of controversy. Although infants and children of all ages should have adequate pain relief, opioids are usually reserved for those patients who have a cancer diagnosis, heavy-trauma patients, or those with a highly painful chronic illness such as sickle cell disease. The fear of creating an opioid use disorder (OUD) in a child is very real, and parents are fearful that opioid use in childhood can lead to an OUD in later life.

The FDA also identified pregnant women and women of childbearing age as a patient population that requires special monitoring. Using opioids in women of childbearing age who could accidentally become pregnant while on opioids and inadvertently expose a fetus to opioids means that all young women will need education about opioid use and pregnancy. For women who are already pregnant, using opioids during pregnancy can result in an abstinence syndrome in the newborn, the baby is born dependent on opioids, resulting in withdrawal after birth.

Patients with a distant history of OUD also face barriers to pain management. These are patients who abused opioids or used illicit drugs in the past. Now, later in life, they are in need of pain management for a chronic condition or surgery. Many healthcare providers are skeptical about the need for higher doses of medications to control pain or of readdicting these patients if opioids are used. One absolute fact is that the patient is entitled to adequate pain relief. These patients do require higher doses of opioids because their prior misuse has changed their pain physiology permanently. Educating healthcare providers about how to treat these patients for pain can help facilitate adequate pain relief for this patient population.

THE OLDER PATIENT

The elderly patient population is an obvious choice for special care when opioids are being used. They are not a one-size-fits-all group in which one 65-year-old patient is the same as the next. Some older patients in their 80s may be healthier than another patient who is 65, depending on comorbidities and lifestyle.

Most practitioners tend to attempt to avoid opioids and use nonopioid medications coupled with nonmedical techniques such as massage, transcutaneous electrical nerve stimulation (TENS), and heat or ice. For some patients, this strategy works well. Nonopioid medications also have a risk profile. Nonsteroidal anti-inflammatory drug (NSAID) medications, for example, present renal risks. The current recommendation for NSAIDs is the lowest dose possible taken for the shortest period of time. In addition, patients with hypertension are not candidates for NSAID use. Acetaminophen can impact liver function, so older patients with decreased liver function should not take acetaminophen or should reduce doses as recommended. For other patients with more severe consistent pain, more complex methods are needed and can include the use of opioids.

Unfortunately, pain in the elderly is often left untreated or undertreated (Cavalieri, 2007; D'Arcy, 2010; Quinlan-Colwell, 2012). The rationale for this undertreatment of pain revolves around fears of opioid use in the elderly, where adverse events can cause significant difficulties with the pain management. Opioids can be used with the elderly; this population just requires more monitoring, lower doses, and regular reassessment.

A large portion of the world population is aging. As a global population, the number of patients who are over 65 years of age is expected to reach 71 million by 2030, compared to 35 million in 2000 (Lavan, Gallagher, & O'Mahoney, 2016). Life expectancy is also increasing. By 2050, the increase is expected to be 10 years, and by 2080, the over-80 population is expected to double (Lavan et al., 2016). In the United States, it is estimated that by 2050, there will be 82 million Americans over 65 years of age (U.S. Census Bureau, 2001, cited in Quinlan-Colwell, 2012). The majority of these patients will be using primary care as the source of their healthcare needs, which includes pain management.

As life expectancy and the number of elderly patients increase, primary care will see increasing numbers of patients who report daily pain of all types. Not only will they have pain, they will also need complex management of their multiple chronic conditions such as diabetes, high blood pressure, and osteoarthritis. Some of these conditions also create neuropathic pain, such as neuropathies from diabetes or postherpetic neuralgia.

The most common types of chronic pain for older patients include (D'Arcy, 2010):

- Back pain (28%)
- Arthritis and joint pain (19%)
- Headache and migraine (17%)
- Knee pain (17%)
- Shoulder pain (7%)

As a group, elderly patients have many types of conditions and chronic illnesses that predispose them to pain. It is estimated that 25% to 50% of community-dwelling elders have chronic conditions that create daily pain (Cavalieri, 2007). In long-term-care facilities, the rates of pain are higher, estimated to be between 45% and 80% (Cavalieri, 2007). Because there is a high incidence of pain in this population, it would seem that more attention and focus should be placed on pain management for the elderly. Unfortunately, the opposite is more common. Kaye, Baluch, and Scott (2010) indicate that in a study of nursing home patients, 66% of the patients had pain and, in 34% of these patients, the pain was undetected by the treating physician.

Why do older patients have more untreated and undertreated pain? Some reasons have been identified. Communication with older adults can often be impaired by physical limitations such as vision and hearing disabilities (D'Arcy, 2010). Cognitive impairment also can complicate pain assessment in the elderly (Kaye et al., 2010; Periyakoil, 2018). Use a comprehensive approach to pain assessment that includes different types of assessment tools developed for patients with cognitive impairment, such as the Pain Assessment in Advanced Dementia (PAINAD) Scale, and add other disciplines to the case, such as psychologists to assess for depression and anxiety, which are common with chronic pain (Kaye et al., 2010).

CLINICAL PEARL

Before performing an assessment on an older patient, make sure that all assistive devices, such as hearing aids and glasses, are in place. The patient cannot give you the answer you want if he or she cannot see or hear you.

Patients with dementia are difficult to assess and require a pain assessment tool such as the PAINAD assessment scale. These types of tools look at behavior and function to ascertain the presence of pain and can give an indication of the intensity of pain. Restlessness in a demented patient can be an indicator of pain. Providing pain medication for a demented patient with a painful condition, such as a hip fracture, requires frequent observation and reassessment to see whether the patient becomes calmer and less restless. If the patient becomes more relaxed, less anxious, and has a better functional ability, the pain medication has been helpful. If the patient is still anxious, frustrated, and agitated after pain medication, a trial of other medications and interventions is indicated.

Older patients may expect to have pain as they age. They consider it a part of old age. Or in some cases, older patients want to be "good" patients and feel that complaining about pain would make them seem demanding. Whatever the reason, older patients should be told that there are ways to treat their pain, which will give them a better quality of life.

CLINICAL PEARL

Older patients can hide pain well. Observing the patient when he or she does not know you are watching can reveal pain behaviors such as guarding, limping, or favoring a leg.

In some cases, opioids are indicated for pain relief in the elderly. Older patients can tolerate opioids in reduced doses, with frequent reassessment and careful monitoring for adverse events. The Centers for Disease Control and Prevention (Haegerich & Chou, 2016) recommends reducing opioid doses in the elderly to 50% of the usual starting dose. Older patients have physiologic differences that make the processing of medications more complex.

As aging causes the patient's body to change, the patient's perception of pain may change as well. Patients may not feel a cut or burn in the same way they did when they were younger.

As the patient ages, changes in the deep tissues of the body may affect the pain experience and how pain is perceived (Quinlan-Colwell, 2012). The fact that older patients have skin and tissue changes may alter the way superficial pain is felt. Factors that can influence the way that older patients experience pain include:

- Age-related changes in the nociceptive system
- Pain tolerance may decline with aging
- Studies have found elevated heat and electrical pain thresholds among older patients (Quinlan-Colwell, 2012)

There are some physical changes that are expected with aging, but not all patients age in the same way and at the same time. Just by virtue of being older, organs have been used for many years. Kidney and liver function is impacted, causing medications to clear the body at a slower rate. Some of the changes affecting drug metabolism include the following:

- Increases in mu opioid receptors, coupled with a slowed gastrointestinal motility, increases the potential for constipation.
- Kidney mass decreases by 25% to 30% between the ages of 30 and 80. This causes a decrease in renal excretion function, so that doses of medications that are renally excreted need to be adjusted to avoid toxicity.
- Because of decreased renal function, drug elimination and excretion are reduced by 10% for each decade after the age of 40.
- Body fat to lean muscle mass changes as patients age, with older patients having more fat and less muscle.
- Poor nutrition can affect the amount of protein available to help medications bind. If protein stores are low, medications have to compete for protein-binding sites, creating the potential for one or more of the medications rendered ineffective (D'Arcy, 2010; Quinlan-Colwell, 2012).

Prescribing opioids for older patients requires frequent reassessment for efficacy and the presence of adverse events. The use of opioids should be limited to those patients who have severe consistent pain, where the benefit outweighs the risk—as with any patient. The functional abilities of the patient should always be addressed and any improvement should be documented, so that progress can be tracked.

When treating pain in this patient population, improved quality of life should also be monitored. Can the patient do more on their own than before the opioids were initiated? What is the goal that the patient has selected as appropriate and how is the progress toward that goal? Is the patient able to go to church or shop for groceries, if that is what is important for the patient? Some direction may be needed here. The goal that the patient selects should be appropriate and achievable. No pain is rarely achievable with a patient who has chronic pain. Helping the patient understand what is achievable will make setting a goal an easier and more satisfying process.

Using physical therapy, exercise, massage, relaxation, acupuncture, and behavioral methods, such as mindful meditation, can help reduce anxiety and increase functionality. The patient will need to understand that a medication alone will not take the pain away and they will need to use a number of techniques to help reduce the pain to a reasonable level.

And finally, an important piece of using opioids and chronic pain in the elderly in general involves assessing the patient for depression and anxiety. Chronic pain is very wearing and older patients begin to doubt whether they will ever again be able to do some of the things they value.

Sleep can be impacted as well, making it more difficult for the patient to function during the day. Anxiety is common, and the primary care provider should discuss this with the patient and develop techniques to address the anxiety that do not involve using anxiolytic medications, which can increase sedation when used with opioids. Addressing sleep and anxiety using integrative and lifestyle changes can be very effective adjuncts to the pain-management plan.

CHILDREN

Pain is fairly common in children. They can suffer from headaches, falls and fractures, and chronic diseases such as sickle cell anemia. Approximately 5% to 28% of children suffer from chronic pain (Practical Pain Management [PPM], 2019). Approximately 73% of these children and adolescents will continue to have pain into adulthood and have the potential to develop new pain conditions (PPM, 2019). Chronic pain in children can have an impact on many of the aspects of the child's life. School attendance and peer relationships can be negatively affected. Children with chronic pain can also have comorbid anxiety and depression.

Acute pain is also common in children of all ages. Using a multimodal approach to treating the pain is recommended (Verghese & Raafat, 2010). Treatment with mild analgesics and topical anesthetics is usually the first approach to the pain. Medications for pediatric use are usually weight based and the doses increase as the child's weight increases.

As with adults, starting pain treatment with nonopioids and nonpharmacologic types of treatment is recommended. Some children do very well with imagery if they can create the image needed for the technique. Acetaminophen and NSAIDs are commonly used to treat acute pain, but the ceiling effect can limit the dose and efficacy of the medications (Verghese & Raafat, 2010). Remember that organs used to clear medications are not fully developed in children, so careful dosing and monitoring are required.

CLINICAL PEARL

Parents may think that using over-the-counter pain medications is safe for children. Education about toxicities and dose limits should be provided to the parents so that the children are not overdosed.

For more severe pain, adding an opioid is recommended only if the risks outweigh the benefits (PPM, 2019). In the past, the use of opioids in children was fairly limited to those patients with cancer, conditions such as sickle cell disease, or heavy trauma. Today, opioid use is more common. Each year from 1999 to 2014, about 20% of children with chronic musculoskeletal pain received opioids and 15% of children with minor conditions received an opioid prescription(PPM, 2019). Extreme care needs to be exercised with opioid use in infants and neonates because of the high potential for oversedation and respiratory arrest. Older children can use codeine, oxycodone, and hydrocodone in appropriate doses. The danger is highest immediately after the child ingests the opioid. These opioids have 60% bioavailability and analgesic effects begin within 20 minutes and can reach their maximum within 60 to 120 minutes (Verghese & Raafat, 2010).

When children are hospitalized for surgery and cannot take oral medications or have severe pain, a patient-controlled analgesia (PCA) pump can be used. For most children, the pump is used as a family-activated system, meaning the child does not use the activation button but the parent can activate the pump as programmed when needed. Educating parents is extremely important when a family-activated system is being used. Parents do not want to see their child in pain; so there is the potential for overuse and subsequent oversedation. Parent education and careful monitoring by the hospital staff can help maintain patient safety.

Children suffer from many of the same challengess as do older adults: communication difficulties, metabolic changes, and a high risk for adverse events. Assessment issues are similar to the older patient in that children often have trouble expressing their pain and conveying the extent of the functional impairment caused by the pain. The age span of this population ranges from newborn to teenager, making it difficult to determine a hard-and-fast rule for opioid use and dosing.

For younger children who cannot communicate pain well, an assessment tool, such as the Wong–Baker FACES Pain Rating Scale, can help the child describe the impact that the pain is having on him or her. There are also specialized tools available for use with infants that rely on examining activity to determine whether pain is present. For the older child, using the Numeric Pain Intensity (NPI) Scale can provide a good measure of the intensity of the pain and how it changes after medication administration.

Using opioids in infants younger than 6 months is problematic due to the physiologic immaturity of their livers and reduced metabolic capacity (Oakes, 2011). For children who can tolerate opioids, weight-based dosing is used until a mature weight is reached.

Fear of addiction is very real to a parent whose child is using opioids for pain relief. One issue that complicates the situation is the lack of research on the use of opioids for children. Both the FDA Blueprint (Haegerich & Chou, 2016) and the CDC Guidelines for Opioid Use suggest that there are some indications for opioid use in children, but that research is scant and national guidelines are rare. Children deserve adequate analgesia when they have pain. However, there seems to be more support for a multimodal approach using nonopioids and nonpharmacologic management, with opioid use reserved for severe pain.

OPIOID USE IN PREGNANT WOMEN AND WOMEN OF CHILDBEARING AGE

Women who are of childbearing age and have chronic pain may be using opioids, other medications, and supplements for pain relief. For these women, there is a significant risk to the fetus if an accidental pregnancy occurs while they are on opioids or if they are using opioids for pain relief while pregnant. In accidental pregnancies, it may take a few months to determine whether the woman is pregnant. Unfortunately, all the while, the fetus is being exposed to opioids on a daily basis. In this patient population, you have the risk for not one patient, but two patients to consider.

CLINICAL PEARL

Women of childbearing age should be educated on birth control and also on the effect of opioids on developing fetuses and newborns. The risks of using opioids while pregnant should be clearly explained to the patient, and, if an opioid-dependent patient desires to become pregnant, opioids should be decreased to the lowest possible dose and, ideally, discontinued.

Pregnant women do have pain. The prevalence of low-back and pelvic pain is between 68% and 72% (Yazdy, Desai, & Brogly, 2015). Opioid use in pregnancy is higher than one might expect. In a Tennessee Medicaid study, 29% of pregnant women filled a prescription for an opioid from 1995 to 2009. In a larger study, in 47 states with Medicaid-enrolled women, 21.6% filled an opioid prescription during pregnancy (Yazdy et al., 2015). Data suggest that opioids are being prescribed for acute pain, whereas data on chronic opioid use in pregnant patients show that the percentage of chronic opioid use ranges from <1% to 2.5% (Yazdy et al., 2015).

What effect do opioids taken by the mother have on the fetus? Ethically, studies cannot be performed using opioids in pregnant women who do not have pain to compare them with pregnant women on opioids. The pertinent data are collected from pregnant women who were given opioids or were on chronic opioids while pregnant.

Babies born to mothers who used opioids compared to mothers who did not use opioids demonstrated no difference in head size or body length. The results are mixed when weight at birth is compared between nonopioid users and opioid users, with some studies showing a negative effect, causing low birth weights. Data on preterm births are more consistent and show an impact on babies of opioid users; babies are born prematurely in 8.2% of opioid users versus 2.3% of nonopioid users (Yazdy et al., 2015).

Cardiac defects in newborns were positively correlated with codeine use in the first trimester of pregnancy, specifically atrioventricular septal defects, left ventricular outflow tract obstruction defects, and hypoplastic left heart syndrome. Other opioids, such as oxycodone and hydrocodone, caused cardiac effects and different defects in infants. Additional defects included cleft palate, pulmonary valve stenosis, and spina bifida (Yazdy et al., 2015).

After birth, a baby whose mother used opioids while pregnant is dependent on opioids. The infant will go through opioid withdrawal in the first days of life. This is called *neonatal abstinence syndrome (NAS)*. In the United States, between 2000 and 2009, the incidence of NAS increased from 1.20 to 3.39 per 1,000 live births (Volkow, 2016). Infants with NAS are usually admitted to the NICU for observation and treatment as needed. The infant will experience the same type of withdrawal as adults who stop using opioids. Crying, abdominal pain, diarrhea, difficulty nursing, and, in some cases, seizures can occur. It takes several days for the opioids to clear. Because these infants can also have cardiac issues, the newborns who have been exposed to opioids before birth are likely to experience a longer stay in the hospital with time spent in the NICU.

Given the serious nature of the potential for preterm births and cardiac defects, using other means of pain control in pregnant women is highly recommended. The American College of Obstetricians and Gynecologists (ACOG; 2017) has a practice statement that recommends universal screening for opioid and substance abuse for all new obstetrical patients at the first prenatal visit. ACOG also recommends a coordinated multidisciplinary approach for patients who use opioids during pregnancy, so that all needs can be met. Using buprenorphine over methadone for maintenance treatment is favored in patients with opioid use disorder (OUD; ACOG, 2017).

ACOG (2017) recommends nonopioids, exercise, behavioral approaches, and physical therapy as the first options for pain relief. When using nonmedication therapies, for better compliance, ask the patient what type of exercise therapy works best for her. Some patients prefer pool therapy, whereas others prefer yoga or walking. Because these patients are younger, there may be time constraints or an inability to travel distances or support additional costs. Choosing a therapy that the patient feels will work for her should provide greater compliance.

The ACOG (2017) recommendations for caring for patients on opioids or with an OUD are as follows:

- Screen for substance abuse with all new patients at the first prenatal visit.
- For obstetric patients with chronic pain, avoid or minimize opioid use, replacing them with other options such as nonopioids, exercise, physical therapy, and behavioral approaches.
- Refer patients with an OUD, for opioid antagonist therapy (buprenorphine).
- Assess whether opioids are indicated, if they are being considered. Use the state prescription monitoring program to review patient prescription history for opioid use.
- Discuss the risks and benefits of opioids thoroughly with the patient and document all conversations with the patient.
- A patient on opioids may require more frequent ultrasounds to determine whether fetal weights are in the normal range.

TREATING A PATIENT WITH A HISTORY OF OUD FOR PAIN

Patients with a history of opioid abuse can experience healthcare providers who have a bias about treating their pain. Some providers feel that the prior opioid abuse caused the increased pain these patients feel, so the patients have caused their own problems. However, the truth is that the patient with a history of opioid abuse deserves pain management as much as any other patient. But some providers are afraid of prescribing opioids for an addict in recovery for fear of creating a relapse.

This group of patients has additional concerns that complicate the use of opioids, but a patient with a history of opioid abuse can be treated effectively for pain. Truthfully, these patients do experience higher levels of pain because of the physiologic changes that occurred when they were abusing opioids, for example, taking high doses daily. Over time, the patient becomes more sensitive to pain, but less responsive to medications used for pain (D'Arcy, 2011).

For patients with a substance abuse history, it is even more important to make sure that pain management follows recommended guidelines and the information and interactions are completely documented. Items that will need full documentations are as follows:

- Use of a pain tool, such as the Brief Pain Inventory (BPI) indicating the pain levels, source of pain, and efficacy of current medications
- Use of an opioid screen, such as the Opioid Risk Tool (ORT), with any follow-up screenings and record the score and the decision for treatment that was made based on the score

- If opioids are to be tried, a completed patient–provider agreement (PPA) is needed, with all expectations clearly outlined
- A complete review is needed of prior opioid misuse or abuse, such as medications, amount used daily, any relapses, any arrests for illicit substance use, any convictions for theft or prescription forging
- How long the patient has been in recovery and any participation in a 12-step program
- A clear understanding that the patient could become readdicted and the steps that will be followed if opioid abuse takes place

For some patients with a history of substance abuse, the fear of readdiction is so significant that they forgo the use of opioids, even for surgery. For these patients, a discussion of alternate means of pain relief, such as nerve blocks and local anesthetics, topical pain medications, intravenous (IV) medications, or oral medications, such as NSAIDs or acetaminophen, is needed. Although acetaminophen can be given IV and Toradol can be used, they are used very rarely. It is important to the patient relationship that support for the decision continues even if the decision seems to be counter to the usual course of postoperative pain relief.

For patients with a history of opioid abuse, chronic pain can be a challenge. With these patients, a multimodal approach using steroid blocks and injection, local anesthetics, topical analgesics, nonopioid medications, and the lowest possible dose of opioids is taken. Integrative techniques, such as relaxation, physical therapy, massage, and biofeedback, can provide additional relief. Careful monitoring and reviews of the PPA for compliance and the state Prescription Drug Monitoring Program (PDMP) database need to occur more frequently.

Primary care providers may not have the time required to do the comprehensive follow-up that is needed. Referral to pain management or a pain specialist can help reduce this burden. In the end, some patients cannot be managed in primary care. High opioid screening scores, complicated medication management, and noncompliance with required follow-ups, such as urine screens and follow-up appointments, make these patients inappropriate for primary care.

SUMMARY

There are groups of patients who are considered specialty groups, for example, the elderly, pediatric patients, and so forth. The FDA Blueprint (2012) recognizes these patients and offers recommendations for treating their pain. Primary care practitioners need to recognize when patients fall into one of the specialty groups and use the recommendations to provide high-quality, effective pain management.

TRENDING IN PAIN MANAGEMENT

- Look for the development of alternate types of pain medications that use targeted molecules rather than opioids.
- Look for continued development of programs for treating infants with NAS.
- Look for developing guidelines on pain and the use of opioids in children.

CASE STUDY

Carlos is a 73-year-old retired attorney. He likes to walk several miles daily to stay in shape and he also plays golf two or three times a week. He enjoys the company of his golfing partners and likes the exercise. Recently, he has been having a deep pain in his lower back and pain going down both legs.The pain has caused him to cut back on his activities dramatically. Now he spends a lot of time watching TV and reading. He would much rater be walking and golfing. He has taken NSAIDS and used over-the-counter analgesic creams and patches with little relief. He rates his pain as 3/10 at rest and 8/10 when trying to walk any distance.

When he sees his primary care provider, he is diagnosed with spinal stenosis, a narrowing of the spinal canal caused by arthritis. The condition is a normal part of aging that can be very debilitating and decreases quality of life dramatically. The healthcare provider sends Carlos to physical therapy for reconditioning and strengthening. He is also given a prescription for a stronger NSAID. Carlos is instructed to use ice and heat for added pain relief.

In 2 weeks, Carlos returns to the clinic and tells the provider that the physical therapy is painful, the NSAID is really not helping his pain, and the ice and heat help for short periods of time.

Given the minimal improvement in Carlos's pain and activity, the provider considers trying an opioid to see whether it would increase Carlos's tolerance for physical therapy and provide better overall pain relief. The healthcare provider reviews the state prescribing program for the records of prescription medication use by Carlos. He also has Carlos complete a screening tool for opioid risk.

Carlos has no record of prior opioid use and screens in the low level for risk if opioids are used. A discussion about the risks and potential benefits of using opioids takes place and the healthcare provider documents the discussion. A PPA is signed and placed into the patient's record.

(continued)

CASE STUDY (*continued*)

Carlos agrees to a trial of a low-dose opioid hydrocodone 5 mg/325 acetaminophen. He can take up to three tablets per day. Carlos is also told to report any side effects like sedation, confusion, or nausea.

In 2 weeks, Carlos returns to the clinic. He has had no side effects from the opioids and his pain is reduced. He is doing better with his physical therapy and is sleeping better. He has been gradually increasing the distances he can walk. His short-term goal is to keep increasing the distance he can walk and his long-term goal is to return to golfing at least once per week. He will continue the opioids for now and will also continue reassessment and monitoring to make sure the opioids are providing adequate pain relief with minimal risk.

- Spinal stenosis is common condition in older patients. Dealing with the intense back pain that radiates down one or both legs can be difficult. Opioids are an option, but not the first line. Once a patient fails in the earlier attempts at pain relief, a consideration of opioids is justified.
- Patients with spinal stenosis need to be involved in their treatment and they also need to understand that physical therapy and exercise are needed to return to a better level of function.
- Patients who are older can tolerate opioids in reduced dosages. However, the prescriber needs to reassess and monitor the patient at regular intervals to ensure that there are no adverse effects taking place.
- A referral to an anesthesia-based pain clinic for a spinal injection is an option for Carlos.
- Focusing on functional improvements and quality of life for older patients is a key element of any plan of care.

REFERENCES

American College of Obstetrics and Gynecology. (2017). *Opioid use and OUD in pregnancy. Committee Opinion 711*. Retrieved from ACOG.org/media/committeeopinions

Cavalieri, T. (2007). Managing pain in geriatric patients. *JAQA Supplement, 107*(6), ES10–ES16.

Center for Drug Evaluation and Research. U. S. Food and Drug Administration. (2102). Blueprint for prescriber continuing education program. *Journal of Pain and Palliative Care Pharmacotherapy, 26*(2), 127–130. doi: 10.3109/15360288.2012.680013

D'Arcy, Y. (2010). *How to manage pain in the elderly*. Indianapolis, IN: Sigma Theta Tau International.

D'Arcy, Y. (2011). *A compact clinical guide to chronic pain management*. New York, NY: Springer Publishing Company.

Haegerich, D., & Chou, R. (2016). CDC guideline for prescribing opioids for chronic pain United States, 2016. *Morbidity and Mortality Weekly Reports, 65*(1), 1–49.

Kaye, A., Baluch, A., & Scott, J. (2010). Pain management in the elderly population: A review. *Ochsner Journal, 10*(3), 179–187.

Lavan, A., Gallagher, P., & O'Mahoney, D. (2016). Methods to reduce prescribing errors in elderly patient with multimorbidity. *Clinical Interventions in Aging, 11*, 857–866. doi:10.2147/cia.s80280

Oakes, L. (2011). *A compact clinical guide to infant and child pain management*. New York, NY: Springer Publishing Company.

Periyakoil, V. (2018). *Pain Management Geriatrics Review Syllabus*. Retrieved from https://geriatricscareonline.org/FullText/B023/B023_VOL001_PART001_SEC002_CH015

Practical Pain Management. (2019). Children, opioids and pain: The stats and clinical guidelines. *Practical Pain Management, 18*(9), 1–6.

Quinlan-Colwell, A. (2012). *Geriatric pain management*. New York, NY: Springer Publishing Company.

Verghese, S., & Raafat, H. (2010). Acute pain management in children. *Journal of Pain Research, 3*, 105–123. doi:10.2147/jpr.s4554

Volkow, N. (2016). Opioids in pregnancy. *BMJ, 352*, 119. doi:10.1136/bmj.i19

Yazdy, M., Desai, R., & Brogly, S. (2015). Prescription opioids in pregnancy and birth outcomes: A review of the literature. *Journal of Pediatric Genetics, 4*, 56–70. doi:10.1055/s-0035-1556740

ADDITIONAL RESOURCES

American Geriatrics Society Beers Criteria Update Expert Panel. (2019). American Geriatrics Society 2019 updated AGS Beers criteria for potentially inappropriate medication use in older adults. *Journal of the American Geriatrics Society, 67*(4), 674–694. doi:10.1111/jgs.15767

D'Arcy, Y. (2014). *A compact clinical guide to women's pain management*. New York, NY: Springer Publishing Company.

Hulla, R., Vanzzini, N., Salas, N., Bevers, K., Gatner, T., & Gatchel, R. (2019). Pain management in the elderly. *Practical Pain Management, 17*(1), 1–9.

Levy, H. B. (2017). Polypharmacy reduction strategies: Tips on incorporating American Geriatrics Society Beers and Screening tool of older people's prescriptions criteria. *Clinics in Geriatric Medicine, 33*(2), 177–187. doi:10.1016/j.cger.2017.01.007

PART IV

Integrative and Interventional Treatment Therapies

CHAPTER 18

MOVEMENT AND HANDS-ON THERAPIES

INTRODUCTION

Efforts to curb the opioid epidemic have moved pain-management goals from complete pain relief to improved function and moderated pain. Pain-management guidelines recommend nonopioid medications and nonpharmaceutical methods as first-line treatments (Chou et al., 2017). It is important for primary care clinicians to discuss the value of these therapies with patients and to use these therapies as a first-line therapy or as a complement to other therapies.

GUIDELINES FOR USE OF HANDS-ON THERAPY

There are several guidelines published to inform pain management. Most address back pain, which can be used as a proxy for pain. It is useful to understand the limitations of these documents. Guidelines are generally based on meta-analysis, which may not recognize the effectiveness in individual studies. Though there are differences among guidelines regarding the strength of evidence and recommendations, they consistently support patient-centered care, focus not only on the pain level but also on function, and increasingly support nontraditional therapies such as acupuncture and other hands-on therapies as well as mind–body interventions.

Department of Veterans Affairs and the Department of Defense Guidelines for Diagnosis and Treatment of Low-Back Pain

In 2016, the Department of Veterans Affairs and the Department of Defense (VA/DoD) reviewed and amended the 2007 guidelines for diagnosis and treatment of low-back pain. New guidelines added a recommendation of education for patients with chronic low- back pain, including self-management strategies for pain, offering an exercise program guided by a clinician or in the community, and several integrative therapies, including acupuncture and mind–body therapies. Spinal mobilization/manipulation is recommended as part of a multidisciplinary program; insufficient evidence was found for use of transcutaneous electrical nerve stimulation (TENS; Department of Veterans Affairs, 2017).

American College of Physicians' Chronic Back Pain Guidelines

The 2017 American College of Physicians (ACP) guidelines reviewed new evidence to determine what has emerged since publication of the 2007 ACP/American Pain Society (APS)guidelines (Chou & Huffman, 2007) for treatment of chronic back pain. Limitations of the review include reviewing only English-language publications and meta-analyses. They acknowledge that not including individual studies is a limitation of the review. They found that based on new evidence, the 2007 ACP/APS guidelines are still applicable for the effectiveness of exercise, massage, acupuncture, spinal manipulation, as well as psychological therapies and multidisciplinary rehabilitation with the addition of mind–body therapies. They continued to find that passive physical therapy (PT) interventions are not useful (Chou et al., 2017).

CLINICAL PEARL

Guidelines provide guidance to inform clinical judgment. Guidelines evolve to reflect results of new research. There is emerging evidence on the effectiveness of mind–body therapies that was not acknowledged in previous guidelines. Each patient requires individual assessment and a treatment plan based on best current evidence and his or her biopsychosocial situation.

In 2011, the Bravewell Collaborative commissioned a survey of 29 integrative medicine centers and programs to explore how integrative medicine is used in the United States. Seventy-five percent of the centers listed chronic pain as the condition they treated with the most success. The next four most commonly treated conditions, gastrointestinal disorders, depression, anxiety, and stress, are commonly experienced by patients with chronic pain. Therapies frequently used include yoga, massage, supplements, pharmaceuticals, meditation, Traditional Chinese Medicine (TCM)/acupuncture, PT and exercise/fitness, and chiropractic care (Horrigan, Lewis, Abrams, & Pechura, 2012).

There is an overlap in therapies offered by various disciplines. PT and chiropractors may offer massage therapy; in some states, massage therapists may practice and bill independently. Acupuncture and dry needling both use fine filament needles based on different scientific rationales.

Walking with an altered gait due to chronic joint pain or poor core integration may increase joint or back pain; these can be addressed in PT. When patients do not have access to PT, a community program, such as group exercise, walking, or swimming, can be useful. Exercise has been demonstrated to impact anxiety and depression in patients with arthritis, and community-based programs can be effective in promoting exercise (Kelley, Kelley, & Callahan, 2018).

The effectiveness of hands-on interventions, whether acupuncture, PT, massage therapy, chiropractic care, myofascial release, or injections, can be impacted by the relationship between the clinician and the patient and the skill and experience of the clinician. If a patient does not respond to one clinician, it may be useful to try the therapy again with a different provider. If the patient does not respond to one type of therapy, a trial with a similar discipline may provide better results.

CLINICAL PEARL

Always weigh the potential risks and benefits of using or omitting a treatment approach based on the individual patient.

It is useful for the primary care clinician to reinforce personal responsibility and the patient's ability to impact his or her pain. Discuss the importance of making and keeping therapy appointments a priority. Explain that it is important for the patient's health to keep these appointments and they should also be kept out of respect for the therapist's time; also emphasize the importance of following through with a home exercise program (HEP) for sustained progress.

CLINICAL PEARL

Outcomes with hands-on therapies are impacted by the approach and skill of the individual clinician. Know the skill levels of clinicians in your area.

PHYSICAL THERAPY

PT is a key component of pain management. Physical therapists are skilled clinicians who use history and physical examination to evaluate and identify mechanical issues; they can also assist with identifying pain generators. They create treatment plans that may include manual therapy or massage, as well as exercise and other therapies and modalities, including dry needling. A doctor of physical therapy (DPT) degree is required for entry into practice as a physical therapist.

These programs generally take 3 years to complete and follow 3 to 4 years of undergraduate study.

A skilled physical therapist provides vital support to a pain-management plan. Patients with musculoskeletal pain who receive early PT will have decreased long-term opioid use and a lower intensity of opioid use (Sun et al., 2018). For acute injuries, PT can be the factor that keeps an injury from becoming a lifelong burden, providing the patient with tools to manage his or her function avoiding the adverse effects of inactivity and altered biomechanics. In a review of Medicare claims of over 439,000 patients with acute low-back pain, patients who had early PT had a lower risk of use of subsequent services (Gellhorn, Chan, Martin, & Friedly, 2012). In a 2-year study of patients presenting to military health service with new-onset back pain, 24% of patients who received early PT had lower utilization of other therapies, including surgery, injections, and opioid use as well as 60% lower costs. The authors postulate that one reason for this lower use is that PT avoids creating dependency and fosters self-efficacy (Childs et al., 2015).

Physical therapists may be generalists or specialize in specific diagnoses or patient populations, such as spine, joint, neurology, rehabilitation, pediatrics, sports medicine, and others. They are expert in identifying appropriate durable medical equipment (DME) such as joint and back braces, sacroiliac (SI) belts, or assistive devices for ambulation such as canes or walkers. Physical therapists play a key role in management of pain secondary to work-related injuries, including therapy and, when needed, work hardening and/or a functional capacity evaluation when the treatment is completed. Some physical therapists have special skills in working with patients with chronic pain or specific populations such as children, the elderly, or athletes. Find therapists with expertise that complements your patient population. Perhaps a consultant is needed who can increase patients' endurance or impact a specific pathology, such as osteoarthritis, joint injury, or spinal pathologies, including stenosis, disc disease, and spondylopathies.

When referring a patient for PT, consider the following:

- What third-party payments does the provider accept? Are they in network for the patient?
- How long does it take to get an appointment? Is there a way to expedite this if the need is urgent?
- At what times are appointments available? Some patients need early, late, or weekend appointments.
- What is the location of therapy office: Ask your patient whether he or she needs appointments that are near work or home.
- Do the therapists respond to your concerns? Do they communicate patient progress or problems?
- Do they empower patients with effective HEPs?

CLINICAL PEARL

Patients frequently need to go to PT several times a week for many weeks. Location can have a big impact on patients' ability to consistently attend therapy.

Role of Exercise

It can be useful to explain to patients that procedures, medications, and interventions can positively impact pain, which may motivate them to move and exercise, including attending PT, which can improve long-term function. PT provides a safe environment that supports and encourages patients as they increase movement. It can be useful to explain that interventions and medications can decrease pain to allow them to participate in PT, which can support enduring relief.

CLINICAL PEARL

When prescribing PT, include an HEP from the beginning, to promote the idea that the patient is an integral part of the pain-management team.

HEPs and core stability are key components in pain management for many pain syndromes, including back pain (Chang, Lin, & Lai, 2015) and patellofemoral syndrome (Chevidikunnan, Saif, Gaowgzeh, & Mamdouh, 2016). When someone is having a flareup of pain or difficulty managing pain, ask whether he or she is doing his or her HEP. It is not unusual for adherence to any exercise regimen to decrease over time; this includes prescribed exercise. A return to PT for re-evaluation, perhaps new therapies and a refresher of previously recommended HEP may be helpful.

Physical therapists have special techniques they use for common pain complaints, such as back pain and osteoarthritis, which are also effective in addressing complex refractory problems like chronic regional pain syndrome (CRPS), phantom pain, and fibromyalgia. Dry needling and guided motor imagery are two approaches that can be very helpful for some patients. Dry needling is used for musculoskeletal pain, and graded motor imagery therapy is used for phantom pain and CRPS.

Graded Motor Imagery

Graded motor imagery (GMI) is a specialized therapy for refractory pain syndromes, including hand injuries, phantom limb pain, and CRPS. GMI is a sequential therapy that moves from the central nervous system (CNS) to the peripheral nervous system, using three sequential phases: laterality training (left–right discrimination), motor imagery, and mirror visual feedback (Mannino, n.d.). A physical therapist with expertise in this technique may provide life-changing intervention for a patient suffering from severe persistent pain.

Dry Needling

Dry needling is a technique that uses a fine filiform needle to stimulate underlying myofascial trigger points and tissue; it is used as part of a broader PT program in appropriate patients (American Physical Therapy Association, n.d.). Studies are conflicting regarding the long-term efficacy of dry needling. Kietrys et al. (2013) found dry needling to be effective for patients with upper quarter myofascial pain. Dry needling regulations vary from state to state. It is currently permitted in 34 states and Washington, DC (McCorkle et al., 2019).

CLINICAL PEARL

There is disagreement among acupuncturists and physical therapists about the use of dry needling. Both techniques use fine needles to address pain. Dry needling involves inserting the needle into trigger points, whereas acupuncture is an ancient therapy that places needles at appropriate points along meridians, which may be distant from the complaint. Acupuncture is also used to treat musculoskeletal pain.

ACUPUNCTURE

Acupuncture is a technique in which practitioners stimulate specific points on the body—most often by inserting thin needles through the skin. It is one of the practices used in traditional Chinese medicine (National Center for Complementary and Integrative Health [NCCIH], 2017). It is regarded as safe when performed by skilled practitioners using sterile needles. Adverse effects can result from use of unsterile needles or poor technique (NCCIH, 2017).

To become a licensed acupuncturist requires completion of 3 to 4 years of formal master's level education and a certifying examination (NCCAOM, n.d.). This is distinct from postgraduate programs generally limited to attendance by physicians and dentists who want to attain certification in acupuncture.

Acupuncture is an ancient therapy that has been practiced in China and Japan for 3,000 years. It was introduced in Europe around 1680 by a physician who saw its use in Japan. Acupuncture has been studied in the United States for the past 40 years (Hao & Mittelman, 2014).

Classical acupuncture is a whole-body system, addressing balance among organ systems, including the parasympathetic and sympathetic nervous systems. Practitioners take a history using an Eastern medicine approach, and use combinations of acupuncture points to address patient problems; they may use additional TCM therapies.

Functional MRI and positron emission tomography have demonstrated the response of the central nervous system (CNS) to acupuncture; in addition, acupuncture impacts afferent nerve fibers and neurotransmitters (King et al., 2015).

Acupuncture had once been dismissed as ineffective in the United States, but slowly gained acceptance, and in 1997, a National Institutes of Health (NIH) consensus document described acupuncture as effective in treating migraine, arthritis, and chronic pain (Hao & Mittelman, 2014). The impact of skilled use of acupuncture continues to be demonstrated. The use of auricular or battlefield acupuncture by the Veterans Health Administration (VHA) to impact posttraumatic stress disorder (PTSD) and pain has stimulated additional interest in acupuncture.

As with any clinician, it is important to know the education, qualifications, and experience of an acupuncturist. Identify the types of practitioners available in your community. These could include licensed acupuncturists and physicians who have had postgraduate acupuncture training. It may be useful to know the style of acupuncture they use and the auxiliary techniques they use, such as moxibustion, electric current, magnets, cupping, heat, and other traditional tools, as well as how they interact with patients. What is their experience? What conditions have they treated, and how willing are they to discuss their approaches with you or your patients?

Auricular and Battlefield Acupuncture

In addition to the traditionally used Chinese and Japanese acupuncture, there is emerging use of battlefield acupuncture, which focuses on pain, and is being studied for use in PTSD (King et al., 2015; Liebell, 2019). Auricular acupuncture was developed in France by neurologist Dr. Paul Nogier in 1957 (About Auricular Acupuncture, n.d.).

Based on earlier descriptions of auricular acupuncture, in 2001, Dr. Richard Niemtzow developed battlefield acupuncture, a variation of auricular acupuncture that can be rapidly deployed. Unlike traditional acupuncture, which uses meridians across the body, battlefield acupuncture only uses specific points on the ear (Niemtzow, n.d.). It was named *battlefield acupuncture* because of its potential benefit for military use. The procedure is done quickly, achieving pain relief without sedation, using the ear—which is easily accessed. Training clinicians to use the technique can be done quickly; this technique may show results in seconds and allow the military to offer pain relief without opioids, thus allowing personnel to work on continuous duty, which would not be possible with opioid sedation.

- Battlefield acupuncture uses up to five needles in each ear.
- It is usually done with small Aiguille d'Acupuncture Semipermanente (ASP) needles that remain in place for 3 to 4 days before they fall out.
- Pain relief can be instant or occur over minutes, lasting for hours to months (Niemtzow, n.d.).

Battlefield acupuncture has been used in Iraq and Afghanistan, and in the Veterans Affairs system in the United States. It is also used in community acupuncture clinics. A systematic review of Chinese and English studies of acupuncture using sham controls examined auricular acupressure and acupuncture and found that the auricular therapy demonstrated effectiveness and use as an adjunct in decreasing the need for medication (Yeh et al., 2014).

Some third-party payers cover acupuncture sessions, and some plans specifically exclude it. Acupuncture is one of the top three integrative health services requested by veterans. In 2018, the VHA recognized acupuncture as a standalone profession (Olson, 2018).

MASSAGE

There are many types of massage and massage therapists. Many massage therapists are employed in chiropractic, PT, and medical offices. Regulations for therapists vary from state to state. In some states, they may practice independently. The American Massage Therapy Association website has links to state regulations (American Massage Therapy Association, n.d.).

A systematic review of the effectiveness of massage for nonspecific low-back pain by Kumar et al. found a small emerging body of evidence that massage is effective for managing pain, citing weak studies and recommending further research (Kumar, Beaton, & Hughes, 2013). Massage is generally considered to be low risk.

Specialized techniques include myofascial trigger point therapy, myofascial release, and active- release technique. These may be performed by massage therapists, physical therapists, or chiropractors. Some patients find massage very helpful; however, evidence is not compelling that massage works better than other therapies.

TRANSCUTANEOUS ELECTRICAL NERVE STIMULATION

TENS uses electrical current transmitted through electrodes placed on the skin to impact pain. It has both central and peripheral modes of action (DeSantana, Walsh, Vance, Rakel, & Sluka, 2008). Because they were introduced prior to 1976,

TENS units were grandfathered rather than approved by the U.S. Food and Drug Administration (FDA) and have therefore not been found by the FDA to be effective or to have clinical benefit. In 2012, the Centers for Medicare & Medicaid Services (CMS) determined that TENS "is not reasonable and necessary for the treatment of CLBP [chronic low back pain]" (CMS, 2012).

Research results on the efficacy of TENS are mixed. Efficacy disparity may be due to lead placement or patient variability. When discussing TENS, encourage patients to try various combinations of intensity and frequency and lead placement. When used at appropriate intensity and frequency, TENS can provide effective analgesia and can be effective for many different pain conditions (Vance, Dailey, Rakel, & Sluka, 2014).

CLINICAL PEARL

The use of TENS for pain management is controversial. Many patients find that TENS therapy relieves their pain, whereas others do not find it helpful. Studies are conflicting, with some finding efficacy and others no benefit.

Physical therapists use various types of electrical stimulation. If they have a unit in the clinic that mimics a home TENS unit, you can request that the physical therapist apply TENS during a session. If it is helpful in impacting pain, the patient can then make the purchase. TENS units are available without prescription, online or in various retail outlets; effective units are available for less than $40. Very few third-party payers will cover the cost of TENS units.

Special Considerations

- *Do not use* TENS for patients with *epilepsy, implanted internal defibrillators, or pacemakers.*
- *Consult with an obstetrician or certified nurse midwife* before recommending to a pregnant woman.
- *Consult with an oncologist* when offering to a patient with cancer.
    - TENS needs further study in treating cancer pain; only a few randomized controlled studies have been done.
    - Loh and Gulati (2015) state that it is safe to use high-frequency units (above 80 Hz) for cancer patients and that TENS is an effective therapy when administered appropriately.

- They found that TENS proved beneficial in 69.7% of patients over the course of 2 months (Loh & Gulati, 2015).
- The initial cost of TENS may be prohibitive for some patients; for others, it can be a worthwhile investment.

CLINICAL PEARL

TENS is a tool that a patient can access without calling for a prescription and it may be useful for managing exacerbations. It also provides patient control and the peace of mind that goes with it.

LOW-LEVEL LIGHT THERAPY, OR PHOTOBIOMODULATION

In 2014, a consensus meeting determined that *photobiomodulation (PBM)* therapy is the preferred term for low-level light therapy (LLLT) or red and near-infrared light therapy or cold laser therapy. The term *LLLT* continues to also be used because of scientific database labels and its familiarity in scientific and patient communities (Anders, Lanzafame, & Arany, 2015).

LLLT is recommended in the 2017 ACP guidelines (Chou et al., 2017). *LLLT* or *PBM* is defined as "the use of red and near-infrared light to stimulate healing, relieve pain, and reduce inflammation" (Hamblin, 2017, p. 337). Emerging evidence regarding the efficacy of PBM in pain management and antiaging, use of more cost-effective light-emitting diode (LED) arrays, and consumer advertising for red- light units has increased interest in PBM for both personal and medical prescriptive use.

Red and near-infrared light has been studied for multiple conditions since 1967. It has been studied for years by Dr. Michael Hamlin at the Massachusetts General Hospital and found to have efficacy in pain management. There is emerging research that PBM has pronounced local and systemic anti-inflammatory effects with nearly no adverse effects if appropriate protocols are followed (Hamblin, 2017).

Mechanism of Action

The effect of the light is cellular, not thermal; "unlike other medical laser procedures, LLLT is not an ablative or thermal mechanism, but rather a photochemical effect comparable to photosynthesis in plants, whereby the light is absorbed and exerts a chemical change" (Huang, Chen, Carroll, & Hamblin, 2009, p. 359). Wavelength is measured in nanometers. Effective wavelengths are red (600–700 nm) and near infrared (770–1,200 nm). The biphasic dose response of light results in suboptimal results if the incorrect wavelength is applied (Hamblin, 2017). This and other complex variables involved in delivering this therapy contribute to challenges in delivery and evaluation of treatment.

LED arrays have made PBM more accessible, and some patients have purchased them for home use for antiaging therapy or pain management. They are also used in professional offices. PBM is used to enhance healing and relieve pain and inflammation in a wide array of conditions. A systematic review of PBM for relief of postsurgical pain demonstrated that the study results were impacted by key therapeutic parameters such as wavelength, duration, energy density, number of sessions, and others. Positive outcome is dependent on appropriate protocols and more research is needed (Ezzati, Fekrazad, & Raoufi, 2019).

CLINICAL PEARL

With technology as interesting and potentially lucrative as PBM, it is important to research products for FDA approval, safety, and effectiveness, as well as appropriate indications for both professional and home units.

Third-party payers generally classify LLLT as investigational or not medically necessary.

CHIROPRACTIC

The NCCIH at the NIH describes chiropractic as a treatment that often includes manual therapy, including spinal manipulation, and emphasizes the body's ability to heal itself (NCCIH, 2019). Licensure requirements and scope of practice for chiropractors vary from state to state.

The ACP guidelines state that spinal manipulation is moderately effective for subacute or chronic low-back pain (Chou et al., 2017). In a study of 750 U.S. military service members with low-back pain, addition of chiropractic care to usual medical care resulted in decreased pain and decreased perception of disability at 12 weeks. This study included a variety of other treatments in addition to chiropractic manipulation for some patients, including therapeutic exercise, traction, and so forth (Goertz et al., 2018).

LeFebrve describes back pain, neck pain, and headache as the conditions most often treated by chiropractors, with the best available evidence supporting spinal manipulation; he also emphasizes that chiropractic care includes other evidence-based strategies, including massage, exercise therapy, and advice regarding activity (LeFebvre, Peterson, & Haas, 2012).

SUMMARY

There are many hands-on therapy options available to provide pain management in lieu of pharmacology or as adjuncts to other therapies. Exercise, acupuncture, and spinal manipulation were added to the 2017 VA/DoD Low Back Pain Guidelines (Department of Veterans Affairs, 2017). Determining which therapy to choose depends on patient preference, diagnosis, physical findings, availability of skilled clinicians, and payment resources. It is important for primary care clinicians to be familiar with the mechanisms and safety profiles of these therapies to assist patients in choosing them. Many patients may self-refer and self-pay to use these therapies and others may only be able or willing to access those covered by third-party payers. Research continues into the effectiveness of therapies, which is required for approval by regulatory agencies and payment by third-party payers. If therapy has been found to be possibly helpful, with minimal potential for adverse effect, it could be offered to patients to try if the risk/benefit ratio is appropriate.

TRENDING IN PAIN MANAGEMENT

- Continued study of effectiveness of acupuncture and acupressure in acute and chronic situations
- Research in new techniques using mirror therapy
- Increased emphasis on hands-on therapies to avoid opioid use
- Expanded use of PBM
- Ongoing evaluation and modifications of pain-management guidelines
- Continued study of expanded use of all modalities, including TENS, to decrease opioid use

CASE STUDY

Fred is a 40-year-old warehouse manager. He comes to the office requesting assistance with increased low-back pain. He is 40 pounds overweight, with mild hypertension; otherwise he is in good health. He had a lumbar laminectomy in his early 30s following an injury. Fred had good recovery with surgery and PT. He has noted the pain increasing over the past few months; he used to play basketball twice per week, but needed to stop because of discomfort and a busy schedule. He spends 4 hours/day working on a computer and 4 hours/day working on a concrete floor in

(*continued*)

CASE STUDY (*continued*)

warehouse. His only exercise is walking the family dog a few times a week. Physical exam is consistent with degenerative disc disease with no acute neurological findings. He would like to pursue nonpharmaceutical options.

- You prescribe PT with therapeutic exercise and instruct him in the importance of core stability and HEP.
- You discuss the importance of a regular HEP for ongoing function and explain it is common for people to slip from HEP when feeling well; a return to PT can be useful to help get back on track.
- You advise him to shop online for a TENS unit that he can use at home and at work. You explain it is important to try different frequency and intensity settings and lead placement. He can take his unit to PT and enlist their assistance with the TENS.
- He requests massage, which you order once a week for 4 to 6 weeks, reminding him the massage is to help him feel more comfortable so as to participate in therapeutic exercise.
- You discuss the potential benefit of acupuncture, which is not covered by his insurance. He wants to wait and see whether he responds to therapies covered by insurance; he is willing to self-pay if needed.
- You schedule follow-up in a month; if symptoms are not improving, you plan to send him to an acupuncturist who specializes in musculoskeletal conditions.

REFERENCES

About Auricular Acupuncture. (n.d.). Retrieved from https://www.thecollegeofauricularacupuncture.com/about-auricular-acupuncture

American Massage Therapy Association. (n.d.). *Massage practice laws by state*. Retrieved from https://www.amtamassage.org/about/lawstate.html

American Physical Therapy Association. (n.d.). *Description of dry needling in clinical practice*. Retrieved from http://www.apta.org/StateIssues/DryNeedling/ClinicalPracticeResourcePaper

Anders, J. J., Lanzafame, R. J., & Arany, P. R. (2015). Low-level light/laser therapy versus photobiomodulation therapy. *Photomedicine and Laser Surgery, 33*(4), 183–184. doi:10.1089/pho.2015.9848

Chang, W.-D., Lin, H.-Y., & Lai, P.-T. (2015). Core strength training for patients with chronic low back pain. *Journal of Physical Therapy Science, 27*(3), 619–622. doi:10.1589/jpts.27.619

Centers for Medicare & Medicaid Services. (2012). Decision memofor transcutaneous electrical nerve stimulation for chronic low back pain (CAG-00429N). Retrieved from https://www.cms.gov/medicare-coverage-database/details/nca-decision-memo.aspx?NCAId=256

Chevidikunnan, M. F., Saif, A. A., Gaowgzeh, R. A., & Mamdouh, K. A. (2016). Effectiveness of core muscle strengthening for improving pain and dynamic balance among female patients with patellofemoral pain syndrome. *Journal of Physical Therapy Science, 28*(5), 1518–1523. doi:10.1589/jpts.28.1518

Childs, J. D., Fritz, J. M., Wu, S. S., Flynn, T. W., Wainner, R. S., Robertson, E. K., . . . George, S. Z. (2015). Implications of early and guideline adherent physical therapy for low back pain on utilization and costs. *BMC Health Services Research, 15*(1), 150. doi:10.1186/s12913-015-0830-3

Chou, R., Deyo, R., Friedly, J., Skelly, A., Hashimoto, R., Weimer, M., . . . Brodt, E. D. (2017). Nonpharmacologic therapies for low back pain: A systematic review for an American College of Physicians Clinical Practice Guideline. *Annals of Internal Medicine, 166*(7), 493. doi:10.7326/m16-2459

Chou, R., & Huffman, L. H. (2007). Nonpharmacologic therapies for acute and chronic low back pain: A review of the evidence for an American Pain Society/American College of Physicians Clinical Practice Guideline. *Annals of Internal Medicine, 147*(7), 492. doi:10.7326/0003-4819-147-7-200710020-00007

Department of Veterans Affairs. (2017). *VA/DoD clinical practice guideline for diagnosis and treatment of low back pain*. Washington, DC: Author.

Desantana, J. M., Walsh, D. M., Vance, C., Rakel, B. A., & Sluka, K. A. (2008). Effectiveness of transcutaneous electrical nerve stimulation for treatment of hyperalgesia and pain. *Current Rheumatology Reports, 10*(6), 492–499. doi:10.1007/s11926-008-0080-z

Ezzati, K., Fekrazad, R., & Raoufi, Z. (2019). The effects of photobiomodulation therapy on post-surgical pain. *Journal of Lasers in Medical Sciences, 10*(2), 79–85. doi:10.15171/jlms.2019.13

Gellhorn, A. C., Chan, L., Martin, B., & Friedly, J. (2012). Management patterns in acute low back pain. *Spine, 37*(9), 775–782. doi:10.1097/brs.0b013e3181d79a09

Goertz, C. M., Long, C. R., Vining, R. D., Pohlman, K. A., Walter, J., & Coulter, I. (2018). Effect of usual medical care plus chiropractic care vs usual medical care alone on pain and disability among US service members with low back pain. *JAMA Network Open, 1*(1), e180105. doi:10.1001/jamanetworkopen.2018.0105

Hamblin, M. R. (2017). Mechanisms and applications of the anti-inflammatory effects of photobiomodulation. *AIMS Biophysics, 4*(3), 337–361. doi:10.3934/biophy.2017.3.337

Hao, J. J., & Mittelman, M. (2014). Acupuncture: past, present, and future. *Global Advances in Health and Medicine, 3*(4), 6–8. doi:10.7453/gahmj.2014.042

Horrigan, B., Lewis, S., Abrams, D. I., & Pechura, C. (2012). Integrative medicine in America—How integrative medicine is being practiced in clinical centers across the United States. *Global Advances in Health and Medicine, 1*(3), 18–52. doi:10.7453/gahmj.2012.1.3.006

Huang, Y. Y., Chen, A. C., Carroll, J. D., & Hamblin, M. R. (2009). Biphasic dose response in low level light therapy. *Dose-Response: A Publication of International Hormesis Society, 7*(4), 358–383. doi:10.2203/dose-response.09-027.Hamblin

Kelley, G. A., Kelley, K. S., & Callahan, L. F. (2018). Community-deliverable exercise and anxiety in adults with arthritis and other rheumatic diseases: A systematic review with meta-analysis of randomized controlled trials. *BMJ Open, 8*(2), e019138. doi:10.1136/bmjopen-2017-019138

Kietrys, D. M., Palombaro, K. M., Azzaretto, E., Hubler, R., Schaller, B., Schlussel, J. M., & Tucker, M. (2013). Effectiveness of dry needling for upper-quarter myofascial pain: A systematic review and meta-analysis. *Journal of Orthopaedic & Sports Physical Therapy, 43*(9), 620–634. doi:10.2519/jospt.2013.4668

King, H. C., Spence, D. L., Hickey, A. H., Sargent, P., Elesh, R., & Connelly, C. D. (2015). Auricular acupuncture for sleep disturbance in veterans with post-traumatic stress disorder: A feasibility study. *Military Medicine, 180*(5), 582–590. doi:10.7205/milmed-d-14-00451

Kumar, S., Beaton, K., & Hughes, T. (2013). The effectiveness of massage therapy for the treatment of nonspecific low back pain: a systematic review of systematic reviews. *International Journal of General Medicine, 6*, 733–741. doi:10.2147/IJGM.S50243

LeFebvre, R., Peterson, D., & Haas, M. (2012). Evidence-based practice and chiropractic care. *Journal of Evidence-Based Complementary & Alternative Medicine, 18*(1), 75–79. doi:10.1177/2156587212458435

Liebell, D. (2019). The science of auricular microsystem acupuncture: Amygdala function in psychiatric, neuromusculoskeletal, and functional disorders. *Medical Acupuncture, 31*(3), 157–163. doi:10.1089/acu.2019.1339

Loh, J., & Gulati, A. (2015). The use of transcutaneous electrical nerve stimulation (TENS) in a major cancer center for the treatment of severe cancer-related pain and associated disability. *Pain Medicine, 16*(6), 1204–1210. doi:10.1111/pme.12038

Mannino, R. (n.d.). *Reestablishing the connection: Using mirror therapy to reduce pain and improve movement.* Retrieved from https://www.hss.edu/conditions_using-mirror-therapy-to-reduce-pain-and-improve-movement.asp

McCorkle, K., Griffith, J., Flaming, G., Baczewski, C., Weber, C., Hsiao, A., . . . Yoon, M. (2019, November 10). *Dry needling scope of practice—Integrative dry needling.* Retrieved from https://integrativedryneedling.com/dry-needling-training/scope-of-practice

National Center for Complementary and Integrative Health. (2017, September 24). *Acupuncture.* Retrieved from https://nccih.nih.gov/health/acupuncture

National Center for Complementary and Integrative Health. (2019, April 30). *Chiropractic.* Retrieved from https://nccih.nih.gov/health/chiropractic

National Certification Commission for Acupuncture and Oriental Medicine. (n.d.). *The NCCAOM certification in Acupuncture.* Retrieved from https://www.nccaom.org/wp-content/uploads/pdf/NCCAOM Acupuncture Certification Fact Sheet060318.pdf

Niemtzow, R. (n.d.). *Battlefield acupuncture.* Retrieved from https://www.isla-laser.org/wp-content/uploads/Niemtzow-Battlefield-Acupuncture.pdf

Olson, J. L. (2018). Licensed acupuncturists join the Veterans Health Administration. *Medical Acupuncture, 30*(5), 248–251. doi: 10.1089/acu.2018.1298

Sun, E., Moshfegh, J., Rishel, C. A., Cook, C. E., Goode, A. P., & George, S. Z. (2018). Association of early physical therapy with long-term opioid use among opioid-naive patients with musculoskeletal pain. *JAMA Network Open, 1*(8), e185909. doi:10.1001/jamanetworkopen.2018.5909

Vance, C. G., Dailey, D. L., Rakel, B. A., & Sluka, K. A. (2014). Using TENS for pain control: the state of the evidence. *Pain Management, 4*(3), 197–209. doi:10.2217/pmt.14.13

Yeh, C. H., Chiang, Y. C., Hoffman, S. L., Liang, Z., Klem, M. L., Tam, W. W., . . . Suen, L. K. (2014). Efficacy of auricular therapy for pain management: a systematic review and meta-analysis. *Evidence-Based Complementary and Alternative Medicine: eCAM, 2014*, 934670. doi:10.1155/2014/934670

ADDITIONAL RESOURCE

Hamblin, M. (n.d.). *Mechanisms of Low Level Light Therapy*. Retrieved from http://photobiology.info/Hamblin.html

CHAPTER 19

MIND–BODY THERAPIES

INTRODUCTION

The combination of general interest in mind–body therapies and the urgency of the opioid epidemic has resulted in increasing interest and research on the application of mind–body therapies to impact chronic pain. This is reflected in strategies that the patients choose for themselves and for therapies included in treatment guidelines. As Memorial Sloan Kettering Cancer Center describes, “Mind–body therapies are a group of healing techniques that enhance the mind’s interactions with bodily function, to induce relaxation and to improve overall health and well-being” (Memorial Sloan Kettering Cancer Center, n.d.). Mind–body therapies include movement therapies (such as yoga and tai chi), breathing, imagery, meditation, mindfulness, and therapies that require professional clinician guidance (such as hypnosis and biofeedback).

In 2017, the National Health Interview Survey found that yoga is the most commonly used complementary therapy by U.S. adults, increasing from 9.5% in 2012 to 14.3% in 2017 (Clarke, Barnes, Black, Stussman, & Nahin, 2018). As patients embrace mind–body therapy in their lives, they may look to primary care clinicians for information on efficacy and access to these therapies.

Mind–body therapies are gaining in popularity among patients and clinicians, including in academic centers. Many academic centers have centers for integrative medicine and offer therapies or information on websites. The National Center for Complementary and Integrative Health (NCCIH) website has information on therapies and research.

The 2017 American College of Physicians guidelines for treatment of low-back pain include recommendations for complementary therapies, including mind–body therapies tai chi, yoga, progressive relaxation, mindfulness-based stress reduction (MBSR), and cognitive behavioral therapy (CBT) as the options for initial treatment (Qaseem, Wilt, McLean, Forciea, & Clinical Guidelines Committee of the American College of Physicians, 2017). A review funded by the National Center for Integrative and Complementary Care (NCCAM), describes evidence that chronic pain can change the brain, decreasing its ability to impact pain. It also found evidence that mind–body practices may reduce acute and chronic pain and help reverse the changes in the brain that are caused by chronic pain (NCCAM, 2017). Although research continues, mind–body therapies are generally found to have minimal adverse effects and provide a path to improvement for patients with pain.

CLINICAL PEARL

Ask patients whether they have ever done yoga, meditation, or hypnosis; their response can set the tone for a discussion on the impact of stress on pain, the value of addressing stress, and the benefit of mind–body therapies.

The focus of pain management has progressed from decreasing pain as measured on the Visual Analogue Scale (VAS) to a focus on improved function and quality of life. Mind–body therapies provide tools for patients to use that can support their personal sense of managing pain, and, as research is demonstrating, impact the brain's ability to respond to pain (NCCAM, 2017).

Mind–body therapies are being recognized as effective in pain management and are included in recent pain-management guidelines. However, mind–body therapies have limited guideline recommendations due to challenges of performing randomized controlled blinded studies in these therapies, which are frequently delivered in combination. There are rare reports of adverse effects of these therapies, and frequently it is not clear how closely they are tracked in studies. Recommendations following reviews nearly universally call for further studies and more evaluation. Pain-management research uses low-back pain, osteoarthritis, fibromyalgia, and cancer as exemplars; studies and guidelines that reference these conditions are used to inform general pain-management practice.

Mind–body therapies are frequently practiced together, creating synergies that also make it difficult to conduct controlled studies. This lack of controlled studies is cited as a factor in the limited recommendations for these therapies in systematic reviews and guidelines. For example, MBSR usually incorporates breathing and yoga techniques, meditation includes imagery and mindfulness, and relaxation, meditation, and mindfulness techniques all incorporate breathing patterns. These combination approaches make it difficult to rate their effectiveness using the usual review guidelines.

The challenge with evaluating effectiveness of mind–body therapies is the difficulty in isolating one variable and performing blinded studies. When reviews are contingent on the impact of one isolated variable, with a double-blind study, mind–body therapies are generally considered to have inadequate evidence.

CLINICAL PEARL

When evaluating potential benefit of a therapy, consider the potential for benefit and the risk of harm.

The VA map on biofeedback, imagery, and hypnosis states that there is little data regarding harm done by these interventions in reviews, but it is unlikely that they have clinically significant risk. Like most reviews, they recommend further studies with patient blinding (Freeman et al., 2019).

CLINICAL PEARL

Learning simple breathing patterns, like 4–7–8 or box breath, can be an easy introduction for patients who have difficulty beginning meditation or mindfulness practice (Exhibit 19.1).

EXHIBIT 19.1

BREATHING TECHNIQUE EXAMPLES

Breathing techniques are simple practices that can be demonstrated during an office visit. Different breathing patterns will appeal to different patients. You may offer them in an order that you think the patient will like, moving to another if the first one is not embraced. Focused breathing can provide calm and focus and these exercises are learned more quickly than meditation.

- Box breathing is attributed by many to the Navy Seals. It describes a pattern of focused breathing that is easy to remember and implement. Each cycle of breath has a count of four: inhale, hold, exhale, hold; repeat for multiple cycles.
- 4–7–8 breathing is a yoga technique popularized by Dr. Andrew Weil. In this practice, you inhale for count of 4, hold breath for a count of 7, and exhale for a count of 8 for four cycles (Malkin, 2020).
- Cardiac coherence smartphone app (iOS)/my cardiac coherence app (Android): App provides visual cues to inhale and exhale using a 5-minute timer.
- Many smartwatches have breathing apps or reminders.

Synergies occur among mind–body therapies, and combining them can have positive long-lasting impact on pain and function for patients with chronic pain. A study of group treatment of patients aged 20 to 70 with chronic low-back pain, with a mean duration of pain of 7.3 years, compared mindfulness (MBSR) versus CBT or usual care. Groups were conducted weekly for 8 weeks. Patients who received MBSR also received practice in meditation, yoga, and breathing awareness. Patients in the CBT group received CBT with training in setting goals, pacing activity, relaxation practice, and pain coping skills. There was no overlap in the auxiliary skills taught to the two groups. MBSR and CBT resulted in more improvement in back pain and decrease in functional limitations at 26 weeks than usual care, with no significant difference between CBT and MBSR (Cherkin et al., 2016).

YOGA AND TAI CHI

Both yoga and tai chi include basic movement and breathing sequences. Each rewards consistent practice with increased mind–body connection and health benefits.

Each practice has compelling evidence supporting its effectiveness in managing chronic pain, while also having other health benefits on mood, hypertension, and so forth. Yoga classes are available in many communities, either in private businesses, community centers, or gyms.

Yoga

Yoga is the most commonly used complementary therapy in the United States; participation showed an increase from 9.5% of U.S. adults practicing it in 2012 to 14.3% in 2017 (Centers for Disease Control and Prevention [CDC], 2018).

Chang describes yoga as a "process of physical and mental training towards self-realization, the process of which has 8 components (Chang, Holt, Sklar, & Groessl, 2016). Although yoga is a complex system, in general use, it frequently is misunderstood to be only a form of exercise with extreme postures, and sometimes extreme heat, that may include breathing and meditation components. Although some people fully embrace the discipline of yoga as a lifestyle, learning to use the three components outlined here can provide access to the healing benefits of the practice and reduce pain.

Yoga combines

- Meditative exercise
- Rhythmic breathing
- Physical postures (Gothe, Khan, Hayes, Erlenbach, & Damoiseaux, 2019)

When discussing yoga as a therapy, it is useful to explain the extensive evidence of the effectiveness of yoga not only for improving quality of life for people with pain, but also for comorbidities such as hypertension. People frequently have the misperception that yoga is focused on achieving very flexible postures. Research has demonstrated that the most powerful impact of yoga is on the nervous system. In a review of MRI, functional MRI, and single-photon emission computed tomography (SPECT) scan studies of the impact of yoga on brain structures and flow, Gothe et al. (2019) found positive impacts on the amygdala, hippocampus, prefrontal cortex, cingulate cortex, and brain networks. This study focused on the potential impact of yoga on a problem frequently encountered in primary care: the neurodegenerative changes of aging. Mind–body connection can be beneficial with both pain and aging. In a systematic review, Chang et al. (2016) found that yoga can be safely practiced to reduce pain and disability.

Yoga has many health benefits, including stress and pain reduction, improved sleep, and other factors that improve quality of life. "Therapeutic yoga is defined as the application of yoga postures and practice to the treatment of health conditions and involves instruction in yogic practices and teachings to prevent reduce or alleviate structural, physiological, emotional and spiritual pain, suffering or limitations" (Woodyard, 2011).

Research continues to add to the extensive data on the effectiveness of yoga in managing many types of chronic disease, including hypertension, anxiety, osteoarthritis (OA), and so forth, which are commonly present in patients with chronic pain. A pilot randomized controlled trial (RCT) of yoga for treatment of OA used an integrated therapeutic approach of yoga therapy (IAYT) program that included meditation; yogic breathing; yogic lifestyle, including cleanses; and doing yoga postures for 7 days. At the end of the study, patients had improved quality-of-life measures and improved functional performance, including sit to stand (Deepeshwar, Tanwar, Kavuri, & Budhi, 2018). In keeping with these findings, yoga is recommended as a nonpharmacologic therapy for chronic low- back pain in the 2017 American College of Physicians (ACP) guidelines (Chou et al., 2017).

Yoga instructors are trained, but not licensed. The Yoga Alliance (YA) is an organization that mandates and documents training, but does not certify individuals. It is important to know the skills of any yoga teacher you will refer a patient to, especially if you are referring a patient with physical limitations. Because yoga is potentially very valuable for your patients, and training and approaches are so variable, it is important for clinicians to take the time to research local yoga teachers in order to identify those with the skills and ability to work with patients with pain or physical limitations. In addition to providing movement, core integration, stability, and flexibility, a skilled yoga teacher provides a mindful/meditative environment, which can be very therapeutic. Table 19.1 lists some criteria to assist you in evaluating a yoga instructor. Creating your personal rubric based

TABLE 19.1 How to Choose a Yoga Instructor

Training	Multiple levels available (minimum to maximum: 200-hr, 500-hr, Master Teacher, yogi raj)
Credentials	YA is a registry of qualified schools that acknowledges levels of training. It is not a licensing group "IYT" denotes specific advanced training
Specialties	Anatomy; restorative yoga; prenatal yoga; condition-specific yoga, such as for osteoporosis, cancer, trauma; yoga for teens; IYT
Experience	Years of teaching and populations served: studio classes, private classes, community classes
Presence	Does the teacher present as calm, balanced, vital?
Motivation	What is the teacher's passion? Understand the teacher's purpose in teaching
Cost	Community or group programs vary (private fees $80–200/hr)
Style	• Hatha: Most common style taught; movement is linked with breath • ISHTA • Iyengar: Focus is on alignment, with props used for support • Ashtanga: Demands strength • Yin and restorative: Slow, gentle movements • Kundalini: Emphasis is on increasing breath capacity and absorption of breath (not appropriate for chronic or acute illness) • Power or hot: High level of fitness required
Choosing a yoga approach	**Beginner or individual with health conditions:** ISHTA, Yin, Restorative, Gentle, Chair, Therapeutic **Fitness/mobility needed:** Ashtanga, Iyengar, Vinyasa, Power/hot, Kundalini

ISHTA, Integrative Science of Hatha, Tantra, and Ayurveda; IYT, Integrated Yoga Therapy; YA, Yoga Alliance.

Source: Used with permission from Deirdre Breen, Master Yoga Teacher–ISHTA lineage, AHC, NBC-HWC.

on this table can be useful when evaluating a clinician when considering referral for any therapy. An excellent way to evaluate a yoga studio is to use these criteria to form an opinion as you take a class, speak with the instructor, and view the experience through the eyes of a patient with pain.

Tai Chi

Tai chi is a mind–body practice that originated in China as a martial art in the 12th century A.D., using the philosophy of balance of yin (water) and yang (fire). The three basic components of tai chi are movement, meditation, and deep breathing done together (Supreme Chi Living, n.d.).

Tai chi is more accessible than yoga for people with limited mobility due to age or pain, because it is done standing and does not include getting up and down from the floor. When practicing tai chi, the practitioners feel their feet on the ground and purposefully shift their weight while controlling their breath.

Tai chi is not regulated and there is no standard training for teachers. The American Tai Chi and Qigong Association offers practitioner and instructor certification (Supreme Chi Living, n.d.).

A 52-week, single-blind randomized control study comparing tai chi and aerobic exercise for fibromyalgia found more or similar benefits from tai chi (Wang et al., 2018). This could be useful for patients who find aerobic exercise daunting, as the slower pace of tai chi could offer anl alternative. A systematic review and meta-analysis of tai chi for chronic pain demonstrated positive evidence for chronic OA pain and some benefit for low-back pain and osteoporosis. The minimal duration of effectiveness of practice is 6 weeks and longer duration of exercise may increase gains (Kong et al., 2016).

Tai chi is recommended in the both the 2017 ACP (Chou et al., 2017) and Veterans Affairs/Department of Defense (VA/DoD; Veterans Affairs, 2017) guidelines for managing back pain.

Tai Chi Versus Qigong

- *Chi* and *Qi* are both terms for *energy* or *life force*.
- Both tai chi and qigong are practices that are thousands of years old and use movement, meditation, and breathing to support health.
- Tai chi has more defined forms, with movements that could be described as useful for self-defense.
- Qigong is more fluid and adaptable. In China, qigong is practiced more widely than any other martial art.

The goal of both tai chi and qigong is improved wellness; these practices could be useful for all primary care patients. "You need not be strong, flexible, or balanced to engage in the exercises. The overall goal of the arts is to make you more flexible, strong, and balanced" (Mohoric, 2019). Access to instructors and classes and personal preference impact the choice of yoga, tai chi, or qigong. There are minimal adverse effects reported for each, and of course, careful selection of an instructor can impact the risk and benefit of the therapies. They each emphasize and improve the mind–body connection using mindful breath and movement, which impacts the balance of the sympathetic and parasympathetic nervous systems to improve wellness. If patients have interest in these therapies, they could benefit from integrating one or more of these practices into their pain-management or overall wellness program.

The VA/DoD clinical practice guideline for diagnosis and treatment of low-back pain recommends exercise, including yoga, Pilates, and tai chi to treat low-back pain, based on weak evidence (Veterans Affairs, 2017).

CLINICAL PEARL

Mind–body therapies can be very personal. Clinicians and patients may have beliefs or misconceptions about them. It is important for primary care clinicians to respect patient philosophy and perspectives when offering any treatment options, especially with mind–body therapies.

RELAXATION AND IMAGERY

Relaxation

Relaxation techniques include progressive relaxation, guided imagery, self-hypnosis, and deep- breathing exercise with the goal of lowering blood pressure, slowing breathing, and improving the patient's sense of well-being; they are generally described as safe. Relaxation, imagery, biofeedback, meditation, and hypnosis overlap as strategies to calm the nervous system; this overlap results in frequent reluctance of reviews to recommend the therapies due to inability to separate the unique factor of impact that creates benefit. Because each of these therapies is generally considered safe and several have minimal cost, it is worthwhile to offer them to patients as adjuncts to other pain-management strategies.

Initial identification of the benefits of progressive relaxation is attributed to Dr. Edmund Jacobson in the 1920s (Gessel, n.d.). Dr. Herbert Benson pioneered the use of relaxation practice in 1974 with his book *The Relaxation Response*. His approach to using mind–body medicine to promote health and decrease disease was revolutionary in 1974, and is the foundation for many contemporary mind–body strategies. Techniques involve sitting quietly, focusing on breathing, and using repetition of a few words (Benson, n.d.).

When considering use of these techniques, *proceed cautiously in patients with psychiatric diagnoses or history of trauma or abuse*. Relaxation techniques are generally considered to be low risk, but there are rare reports of adverse effects, such as increased anxiety or other mental health adverse effects in people with psychiatric conditions or history of abuse. Patients with heart disease should consult their clinician before trying progressive relaxation, and some patients may report anxiety or fear of losing control (NCCIH, 2019).

In follow-up interviews with 26 hospitalized cancer patients who had participated in a study using progressive relaxation and guided imagery to impact cancer pain, patients reported that active involvement in the activity and distraction contributed to the positive impact of the interventions. Nearly half of the participants qualified as responders to the therapy with a 30% or greater decrease in pain scores, with a greater number of patients perceiving progressive muscle relaxation as effective (Kwekkeboom, Hau, Wanta, & Bumpus, 2008).

In progressive relaxation, the patient sequentially tightens and releases muscles of the upper and lower body. Patients may do this following a recorded script or may choose to go through the progression on their own (Morone & Greco, 2007). There are also meditation practices that incorporate progressive relaxation into the script, especially for sleep.

An RCT of the effectiveness of guided imagery and progressive relaxation for patients receiving chemotherapy resulted in improved quality-of-life scores, including improved mood and decreased pain, fatigue, nausea, and vomiting (Charalambous et al., 2016).

CLINICAL PEARL

Mind–body therapies can provide immediate positive effects on mood or offer a sense of peace, but require practice to achieve the full benefit of improving overall quality of life. Inform and remind patients to keep practicing and to try different styles to find what works best for them (Box 19.1).

Imagery

"Guided imagery involves the use of one's imagination to create mental images that distract attention away from pain or that alter the pain sensation itself"

BOX 19.1

MIND–BODY THERAPIES

Mind–body therapies provide pain-management tools that can be offered to most patients with acute or chronic pain. Some therapies may not be covered by third-party payers and may be cost prohibitive for some patients. Breathing and meditation techniques are available to all patients regardless of financial resources. Including mind–body therapies as part of pain-management plans provides access to therapies that are affordable and improve self-efficacy. They are generally regarded as safe. See Additional Resources at the end of this chapter.

(Kwekkeboom et al., 2008, p. 2). In a review of RCTs of guided imagery, Giacobbi et al. (2015) found that guided imagery is used alone or in combination with other treatments and is a scalable, potentially cost-effective treatment that is useful for arthritis and other rheumatic diseases. All studies reviewed delivered the guided-imagery scripts using audio technology. They also recommend further research. In practice, they recommend using guided imagery with various technologies (Giacobbi et al., 2015). There are many online resources for guided imagery; several are listed in Additional Resources at the end of this chapter.

MINDFULNESS AND MEDITATION

Meditation and mindfulness are similar, but these different practices frequently are referred to interchangeably. Meditation includes four elements: being quiet without distractions, a comfortable position, focus, and an open attitude (National Center for Complementary and Integrative Health, n.d.). The 2017 National Health Statistics Survey used a composite of mantra meditation, mindfulness, and spiritual meditation, including centering prayer. In this survey, the use of meditation by adults increased from 4.1% in 2012 to 14.2% in 2017 (Clarke et al., 2018).

Mindfulness

Jon Kabat-Zinn describes mindfulness as paying attention on purpose in the moment without judging (Kabat-Zinn, 2005b, p. 4).

Mindfulness is a way to be, which can be cultivated using the techniques first described and studied by molecular biologist Jon Kabat-Zinn, at the University of Massachusetts. Many studies have demonstrated the positive benefits of mindfulness on pain and anxiety.

MBSR is a structured program with very specific training for instructors and students. It is generally the format used for research into the benefits of mindfulness practice. Formal MBSR instruction can be informative and useful, but it is not required to practice mindfulness. Being mindful includes using the seven attitudes of mindfulness, ideally with both formal and informal practice.

The seven attitudes of mindfulness are:

- Non-judging
- Patience
- Beginner's mind
- Trust
- Nonstriving

- Acceptance
- Letting go (Kabat-Zinn, 2005a)

As with any skill, mindfulness takes practice. There are two types of practice, formal practice and informal practice. Each is valuable and supports the other. A formal practice occurs when time is set aside (5–60 minutes) to practice mindfulness. During this time, the person focuses on being mindful, and noticing, without labeling anything. One of the books by Jon Kabat-Zinn is titled "*Falling Awake—How to Practice Mindfulness in Everyday Life*" (Kabat-Zinn, 2018). The phrase *falling awake* can be helpful when discussing mindfulness as something that is useful in the course of daily living, learning to be present in the moment. It is normal for the mind to wander, and students are advised to just "notice" that their mind strayed, that doing this is being mindful, and the practice continues.

In informal practice, as a student becomes more aware, the student thinks to be mindful of where they are. An example could be a mom with small children; her task list includes playing with the children, doing the laundry, and cooking dinner. If she focuses on rushing through the tasks to finish them, she feels harried. If she takes the time to enjoy being with the children while they play, and then, when it is time to do the laundry, is "present" while loading the washing machine, transferring the clothes, and folding them when they are dry, and, while cooking dinner, notices the vegetables she cleans and the protein she cooks, she can enjoy being able to provide for her family. When she is done doing these tasks this way, she is calm and less harried.

Decreasing the social isolation and loneliness that frequently accompany chronic pain can provide patients with the ability to focus on something outside their pain and improve their quality of life. Forty healthy older adults interested in mindfulness enrolled in an 8-week MBSR program, with 120-minute group sessions and 30 minutes of daily home practice. Participants were randomized to a wait list or MBSR intervention group. C-reactive protein (hs-CRP), interleukin-6 (IL-6), and loneliness were measured pre- and postintervention. At the conclusion of the study, MBSR participants had a 25% decrease in loneliness markers, a mild decrease in hs-CRP, and no significant change in IL-6, compared to wait-list participants (Creswell et al., 2012). A 2-week study of the impact of a smartphone mindfulness program on loneliness included information on acceptance and provided intrapersonal skills, but no social contact with a group. Following the program, participants reported increased social interaction in daily activities and a 22% decrease in loneliness (Lindsay, Young, Brown, Smyth, & Creswell, 2019).

Following a review of 72 studies, Khusid and Vythilingam (2016) recommend MBSR as part of an integrated pain-management approach and as a self-management strategy for insomnia as well as for relapse prevention to improve health-related quality of life in individuals with substance use disorder.

Meditation

There are many styles of meditation, including transcendental, mantra-based meditation, and others that have an internal focus. Some patients may be more willing to try mindfulness than meditation. Some patients decline to do either due to religious reasons or no interest. As always, respecting their personal choices is important.

Some people have the inaccurate perception that that meditation must be done sitting cross-legged on the floor. Meditation can be done in any position that is comfortable for the person meditating. It may be done seated in a chair, or on a cushion, or lying down. There are also walking meditation practices that can be very helpful for people who are unable to stay in one position. There are multiple online resources to guide meditation. Several are listed in the Additional Resources at the end of this chapter. The Insight Timer and Headspace apps include walking meditations. The key is that while meditating, you are comfortable enough to focus on the meditation. It is worthwhile to explore different styles and teachers to find an approach that feels doable and provides positive results such as improved mood, sense of peace or calm, and decrease in discomfort.

Prayer and contemplation provide significant benefit for some people. At an appropriate time, a trial of additional mind–body therapies, such as imagery, relaxation, or yoga, could be recommended.

The benefits of meditation have been recognized by practitioners for thousands of years. Contemporary studies identifying the areas of the brain affected by yoga practice and measuring the positive impact on brain plasticity provide data to support recommending them in clinical care. Taking time to focus thoughts and breathing can have a positive impact. There are many styles of meditation; they can be accessed virtually or in person in groups or 1:1. The process of meditation remains very personal; using the approach that works for the individual is key. For some people, this is prayer; for others, being outdoors; and for some others, sitting in meditation. It is useful to check in with patients during primary care visits and encourage them to continue with practices that are successful, and to explore other practices if what they have tried did not work or was not appealing to them (Box 19.2).

CLINICAL PEARL

Being present during daily activities with an informal MBSR practice decreases stress and tension.

BOX 19.2

MEDITATION

Advances in neuroscience and use of advanced imaging techniques are demonstrating objective results of ancient practices. Changes in key brain centers that impact pain and emotion support the use of meditation for pain. We are learning more and more about science to support mind–body therapies. The patient wants to feel better with it. In any area of primary care, a meditation practice can promote wellness. Integrate mind–body discussions, including meditation, into routine discussions of health and when addressing physical complaints. Support patient exploration, and, when ready, help to implement the practice.

BIOFEEDBACK

"Biofeedback is a process that enables an individual to learn how to change physiological activity for the purposes of improving health and performance. Precise instruments measure physiological activity such as brainwaves, heart function, breathing, muscle activity, and skin temperature" (Association for Applied Psychophysiology and Biofeedback, n.d.). Biofeedback is used for many different physiological applications; neurofeedback and pelvic floor biofeedback are gaining in popularity. Conditions treated with biofeedback include chronic pain, temperomandibular joint disease (TMJ), headache, urinary incontinence (pelvic floor), and drug addiction.

In biofeedback, the patient is an active participant in treatment. A therapist applies a measurement device and instructs the patient on techniques influencing the physiologic parameter and the patient practices in a quiet environment. Eventually, the patient is able to make changes without the feedback, incorporating the behavior into their daily life.

Certification to provide biofeedback requires specialized training in biofeedback after obtaining a healthcare degree.

Types of biofeedback:

- Electromyogram (EMG)
- Galvanic skin response (GSR)
- Skin temperature
- Neurofeedback

A comprehensive efficacy review paper by Nestoriuc and Martin (2007) found biofeedback to be useful for both migraine and tension-type headache; in this review, they found that a home program in addition to therapy sessions increased effectiveness by 20% and patients with chronic headache had more benefit from treatment. In addition to a decrease in pain from headache, the review found that biofeedback impacted self-efficacy, medication use, anxiety, and depression (Efficacy of Biofeedback for Tension Type, n.d.). Meta-analyses provide evidence of medium to large effects of biofeedback on improving migraine and tension-type headaches, including the frequency and duration of headaches, when compared with a variety of wait-list controls and placebo (Ehde, Dillworth, & Turner, 2014).

Biofeedback can be an effective treatment for a patient who is interested in the therapy. Challenges to use of biofeedback include access to certified clinicians and financial resources and variable third-party payment.

HYPNOSIS

"Clinical hypnosis is an altered state of awareness, perception or consciousness that is used by licensed trained doctors or masters prepared individuals, for treating a psychological or physical problem. It is a highly relaxed state" (American Society of Clinical Hypnosis, n.d.). Some hypnotherapists also teach self-hypnosis to the patients.

Key Concepts

- Clinical hypnosis can facilitate psychological and physiological changes in three ways:
    1. Using mental imagery
    2. Using ideas or suggestions
    3. Using unconscious exploration
- Hypnosis is most effective when a patient is highly motivated to change.
- A skilled hypnotherapist who is also familiar with the treatment of the patient's individual problem is important for success (American Society of Clinical Hypnosis, n.d.).

CLINICAL PEARL

Look for a hypnotherapist who is a member of the American Society of Clinical Hypnosis (ASCH) or the Society for Clinical and Experimental Hypnosis.

A 2-year study of hypnosis and self-hypnosis with 50 patients in palliative care demonstrated positive impact on pain and anxiety (Brugnoli et al., 2017).

AROMATHERAPY

The National Cancer Institute PDQ website describes aromatherapy as "the therapeutic use of essential oils (also known as volatile oils) from plants (flowers, herbs, or trees) for the improvement of physical, emotional, and spiritual well-being" (National Cancer Institute, n.d.). Widely used for their multiple anti-inflammatory, anti-infective, and mood effects by the general population and having been used in traditional medicine for thousands of years, folklore and science are entwined in the use of essential oils. Today, scientists are studying the actions of essential oils with objective screening using the electroencephalogram to evaluate the effect of essential oils and sophisticated chemical analysis to determine the molecular components of essential oils. Contemporary research demonstrates efficacy, and there are endless anecdotal stories about the benefits people have attained with aromatherapy. Used appropriately, they have very low risk of adverse effects and provide an avenue for people to self-manage their pain. There is minimal research on the analgesic effects of aromatherapy, but there are multiple studies on the positive effects of aromatherapy on mood and sleep.

Essential oils have been used for thousands of years and have gained popularity in recent decades. Science is evolving, and research on the biochemistry of various essential oils is providing information on the action of these ancient treatments. Su et al. (2015) studied the impact of frankincense and myrrh on adjuvant-induced arthritis (AIA) in rats and found treatment with this combination decreased inflammatory cytokines, explaining the anti-inflammatory effects of this combination.

Plant selection, use of the appropriate part of the plant, such as leaves, bark, stem, or flower, and correct distillation technique are key components in producing quality essential oils. It is important to use essential oils from quality suppliers to ensure potency and purity.

A review of 12 studies demonstrated that aromatherapy is more consistently effective for nociceptive and inflammatory pain as well as acute pain, including postoperative pain and painful obstetric and gynecologic conditions, and less effective for chronic pain. Many of the studies in this review included massage that included essential oils, and authors postulate that some of the benefits may be from the massage. They found that aromatherapy is a useful adjunct to other pain-management protocols and recommend continued research (Lakhan, Sheafer, & Tepper, 2016).

CLINICAL PEARL

Before considering aromatherapy, talk with the patient; you may find the patient is an expert, has extensive experience, or has strong feelings regarding use. Discuss the cost. It is worthwhile to purchase oils of good quality to ensure they contain true fragrance.

Examples of Essential Oils Used for Pain

Frankincense, or olibanum oil, is used in traditional middle and Far-Eastern medicine as an anti-inflammatory agent for bones, joints, and respiratory system, as well as an expectorant and antiseptic. The oil is made from the resin of the *Boswellia* tree. Anti-inflammatory mechanism is via inhibition of 5-lipoxygenase (5-LOX), cyclooxygenase-2 (COX-2), and nuclear factor-kB (NF-kB) (Al-Yasiry & Kiczorowska, 2016). When frankincense and myrrh are combined, each oil is transformed, with a synergistic increase in anti-inflammatory, analgesic, and antiseptic qualities (Cao et al., 2019).

Lavender has been used for thousands of years and has wide common household use today as an anti-inflammatory agent and to support sleep and mood. There is no generally accepted evidence regarding the efficacy of lavender due to wide variations in the concentration, quality, and types of oils used in studies. A review by Koulivand, Ghadiri, and Gorji (2013) found studies indicating inhaled lavender impacts the autonomic nervous system, supporting its parasympathetic activity, and the limbic system, supporting its effectiveness in sleep and mood. Although the use of lavender is of low risk, more studies are needed to document its indications and effects (Koulivand et al., 2013). Sleep can be a major challenge for patients with chronic pain. In a 12-week study of midlife women with insomnia, inhaled lavender was found to improve sleep and provide short-term increase in parasympathetic nervous system tone (Chien, Cheng, & Liu, 2012).

Inhaling *peppermint* prior to intravenous cardiac catheterization decreased pain and anxiety (Akbari, Rezaei, & Khatony, 2019).

Inhalation of *eucalyptus* oil decreased blood pressure and Visual Analogue Scale (VAS) scores in postoperative knee replacements (Jun et al., 2013). See Box 19.3 for more information about essential oils.

The International Alliance of Aromatherapists has a defined curriculum and standards of practice for aromatherapists. Basic qualifications for an aromatherapist include a minimum of 200 approved aromatherapy contact hours or certification (Hall, n.d.).

Although many people use aromatherapy in their homes for self-care, its use is complex. It is important to use prudence and follow recognized standards when using essential oils in clinical practice and evaluating the positive and negative

BOX 19.3

USING ESSENTIAL OILS

Use pure, authentic essential oils sourced from a reliable supplier.

Some oils may cause skin reactions and should not be applied directly to the skin.

Know the safety profile of the essential oil.

Know patient's allergenic tendencies.

- Methods of use: Topical, inhaled, diffused, or internal; oil may be used in a cream; avoid application of undiluted oil
- Do not use on damaged, diseased, or inflamed skin
- Children and elderly are more sensitive; follow constituent-specific guidance when using
- Special populations: Essential oils *can trigger an asthma attack* or may cause contact dermatitis in a sensitive patient (National Association for Holistic Aromatherapy, n.d.)

effects for each patient and each product. Aromatherapy involves a multifaceted intervention with multiple essential oil options and potential benefits from the synergy created by combining two or more oils. Some oils can be irritating and some patients may be sensitive to them. If you want to add advanced aromatherapy to your treatment plans, consult with an aromatherapist for guidance on strategies and precautions.

COGNITIVE BEHAVIORAL THERAPY

"CBT describes a category of therapies that address the effect that thoughts have on behavior, emotions, and symptoms. It is more focused on the present situation rather than the influence of the past on your current experience" (Hanscom, Brox, & Bunnage, 2015). Formal CBT is provided by behavioral health clinicians. Other clinicians, including physical therapists, nurses, and primary care clinicians, can integrate the CBT approach in their care to improve the outcomes of pain-management plans.

Multiple RCTs have demonstrated the efficacy of CBT across diverse chronic pain syndromes. CBT outcomes are improved when patients are engaged and do assignments outside sessions (Ehde et al., 2014).

The gate theory, presented in 1965 by Melzack and Wall, transformed pain management and was the foundation for the use of CBT in pain management,

BOX 19.4

MIND–BODY INTERVENTIONS FOR PAIN MANAGEMENT

It is essential that each plan for pain management be individualized. Mind–body interventions can impact pain and also support many aspects of health. They provide adjunctive support for some conditions; in some circumstances, mind–body therapy will be more useful than medication or procedures. Treatment selection depends on the pain generator and patient's perspective and situation.

including recognition of the cognitive and affective components of pain. Before this, only sensory inputs had been considered (Ehde et al., 2014).

The CDC guideline for prescribing opioids for chronic pain recommends integrating a cognitive behavioral approach to care, with consideration of multimodal therapies when a single therapy is not effective. It recommends options, such as education on relaxation and coping strategies, and access to stress reduction and other mental benefits, with referral for professional therapy (CBT) for patients with significant psychological distress (Dowell, Haegerich, & Chou, 2016).

Primary care clinicians can integrate a cognitive behavioral approach when working with patients with pain by encouraging participation in normal activities, including recreation, working with them to focus on what they can do, and setting goals for improving function to be able to do more (Box 19.4).

SUMMARY

It is important to use all available tools to improve quality of life for patients with pain. Mind–body therapies, in general, have the potential to positively impact quality of life for all patients in primary care, especially for patients with chronic pain. There are many free resources available online for guided imagery, meditation, and mindfulness (see Additional Resources at the end of this chapter). It is useful to be familiar with the content and perspective of these sites, so that you can effectively describe them and how to access them to your patients.

Mind–body techniques can improve personal awareness of the body and the impact of the mind on the sense of well-being and comfort. This provides patients with tools they can use whenever they wish to reduce their pain. This can be very comforting. They also impact the autonomic nervous system, decreasing the sympathetic tone, which can decrease pain sensation or intensity. Many patients in primary care could benefit from incorporation of one or more mind–body techniques in their treatment plans for wellness or chronic disease management.

Trying various therapies is helpful to find the best fit for the patient. When patients find the therapy that resonates for them and they experience the benefit of the feeling of well-being attained through mind–body connection, their quality of life increases and suffering decreases.

Ideally, mind–body approaches are combined with physical therapy or a self-directed plan to increase movement, which is also essential for sustained pain relief. Yoga or tai chi can provide physical activity, and group classes may be an option for patients who cannot afford physical therapy. It may require discussion over multiple visits to find an approach acceptable or appealing to a patient.

TRENDING IN PAIN MANAGEMENT

- Development of additional apps for meditation and imagery teaching and practice
- Increasing access to mindfulness and other mind–body information and programs on healthcare websites
- Use of technology, including virtual reality, to support mind–body therapies
- Research on the impact of the microbiome on the nervous system, inflammation, and mood
- Research into effectiveness of groups for movement therapies, CBT, and meditation
- Use of technology to enable patients to access hypnotherapy via smartphone or computer

CASE STUDY

Cindy is 54 years old with chronic back pain and headaches. She is mildly depressed, hypertensive, and slightly obese. Her exercise is walking her large dog for 20 minutes three to four times per week. She has been attending physical therapy (PT), with an improvement in her back pain as she has increased her core stability and is doing a home exercise program four times per week. She acknowledges the improvement and wants to know what else she can do to improve her pain and wellness. She mentions that sleep has improved since her back pain has improved, and she is feeling better, but feels sleep could still be better.

(*continued*)

CASE STUDY (*continued*)

- What mind–body techniques would be most useful?

  Yoga has the dual benefit of improving hypertension and pain. You suggest she visit two yoga studios you have identified as having restorative programs that would be welcoming to her. There is one tai chi program at the community center that meets once per week and is based on donations. You recommend she investigate each program and try them, giving them two to three sessions to decide whether she likes the class and teacher.

- What can you recommend for sleep?

  1. You offer the lifestyle changes that can be useful for most people: sleep hygiene, including a bedtime routine, stopping screen/monitor use 2 to 3 hours before bedtime, magnesium and meditation at bedtime
  2. You recommend she use lavender essential oil, which she can put in an infuser or a pillow sachet. You also suggest a few minutes of focused breathing when settling in for sleep: 4–7–8 or box breathing to calm the sympathetic nervous system.

REFERENCES

Akbari, F., Rezaei, M., & Khatony, A. (2019). Effect of peppermint essence on the pain and anxiety caused by intravenous catheterization in cardiac patients: A randomized controlled trial. *Journal of Pain Research, 12*, 2933–2939. doi:10.2147/JPR.S226312

Al-Yasiry, A. R., & Kiczorowska, B. (2016). Frankincense–Therapeutic properties. *Postepy Higieny i Medycyny Doswiadczalnej (Online), 70*, 380–391. doi:10.5604/17322693.1200553

American Society of Clinical Hypnosis. (n.d.). *When will hypnosis be beneficial.* Retrieved from https://www.asch.net/Public/GeneralInfoonHypnosis/WhenWillHypnosisbeBeneficial.aspx

Association for Applied Psychophysiology and Biofeedback. (n.d.). *About biofeedback.* Retrieved from https://www.aapb.org/i4a/pages/index.cfm?pageid=3441

Benson. (n.d.). *Steps to elicit the relaxation response.* Retrieved from http://relaxationresponse.org/steps

Brugnoli, M., Pesce, G., Pasin, E., Basile, M., Tamburin, S., & Polati, E. (2017). The role of clinical hypnosis and self-hypnosis to relief pain and anxiety in severe chronic diseases in palliative care: A 2-year long- term follow-up of treatment in a nonrandomized clinical trial. *Annals of Palliative Medicine, 7*(1), 17–31.

Cao, B., Wei, X. C., Xu, X. R., Zhang, H. Z., Luo, C. H., Feng, B., . . . Zhang, D. K. (2019). Seeing the unseen of the combination of two natural resins, frankincense and myrrh: Changes in chemical constituents and pharmacological activities. *Molecules (Basel, Switzerland), 24*(17), 3076. doi:10.3390/molecules24173076

Centers for Disease Control and Prevention. (2018, November 8). *Use of Yyoga and meditation becoming more popular in U.S.* Retrieved from https://www.cdc.gov/nchs/pressroom/nchs_press_releases/2018/201811_Yoga_Meditation.htm

Chang, D. G., Holt, J. A., Sklar, M., & Groessl, E. J. (2016). Yoga as a treatment for chronic low back pain: A systematic review of the literature. *Journal of Orthopedics & Rheumatology, 3*(1), 1–8.

Charalambous, A., Giannakopoulou, M., Bozas, E., Marcou, Y., Kitsios, P., & Paikousis, L. (2016). Guided imagery and progressive muscle relaxation as a cluster of symptoms management intervention in patients receiving chemotherapy: A randomized control trial. *PloS One, 11*(6), e0156911. doi:10.1371/journal.pone.0156911

Cherkin, D. C., Sherman, K. J., Balderson, B. H., Cook, A. J., Anderson, M. L., Hawkes, R. J., . . . Turner, J. A. (2016). Effect of mindfulness-based stress reduction vs Cognitive behavioral therapy or usual care on back pain and functional limitations in adults with chronic low back pain: A randomized clinical trial. *Journal of the American Medical Association, 315*(12), 1240–1249. doi:10.1001/jama.2016.2323

Chien, L. W., Cheng, S. L., & Liu, C. F. (2012). The effect of lavender aromatherapy on autonomic nervous system in midlife women with insomnia. *Evidence-Based Complementary and Alternative Medicine: eCAM, 2012*, 740813. doi:10.1155/2012/740813

Chou, R., Deyo, R., Friedly, J., Skelly, A., Hashimoto, R., Weimer, M., . . . Brodt, E. D. (2017). Nonpharmacologic therapies for low back pain: A systematic review for an American College of Physicians Clinical Practice Guideline. *Annals of Internal Medicine, 166*, 493–505. doi:10.7326/M16-2459

Clarke, T., Barnes, P., Black, L., Stussman, B., & Nahin, R. (2018, November). *Use of yoga, meditation, and chiropractors among U.S. adults aged 18 and over.* Centers for Disease Control and Prevention, NCHS Data Brief No. 325. Retrieved from https://www.cdc.gov/nchs/products/databriefs/db325.htm

Creswell, J. D., Irwin, M. R., Burklund, L. J., Lieberman, M. D., Arevalo, J. M., Ma, J., . . . Cole, S. W. (2012). Mindfulness-based stress reduction training reduces loneliness and pro-inflammatory gene expression in older adults: a small randomized controlled trial. *Brain, Behavior, and Immunity, 26*(7), 1095–1101. doi:10.1016/j.bbi.2012.07.006

Deepeshwar, S., Tanwar, M., Kavuri, V., & Budhi, R. B. (2018). Effect of yoga based lifestyle intervention on patients with knee osteoarthritis: A randomized controlled trial. *Frontiers in Psychiatry, 9*, 180. doi:10.3389/fpsyt.2018.00180

Dowell, D., Haegerich, T. M., & Chou, R. (2016). CDC guideline for prescribing opioids for chronic pain—United States, 2016. *Morbidity and Mortality Weekly Reports, 65*(1), 1–49. doi:10.15585/mmwr.rr6501e1

Ehde, D. M., Dillworth, T. M., & Turner, J. A. (2014). Cognitive-behavioral therapy for individuals with chronic pain: efficacy, innovations, and directions for research. *American Psychologist, 69*(2), 153–166. doi:10.1037/a0035747

Freeman, M., Ayers, C., Kondo, K., Noonan, K., O'Neil, M., Morasco, B., & Kansagara, D. (2019). *Guided imagery, biofeedback, and hypnosis: A map of the evidence.* Retrieved from https://www.hsrd.research.va.gov/publications/esp/guided-imagery.pdf

Gessel, A. (n.d.). *Edmund Jacobson*. Retrieved from http://www.progressiverelaxation.org

Giacobbi, P. R., Jr, Stabler, M. E., Stewart, J., Jaeschke, A. M., Siebert, J. L., & Kelley, G. A. (2015). Guided imagery for arthritis and other rheumatic diseases: A systematic review of randomized controlled trials. *Pain Management Nursing: Official Journal of the American Society of Pain Management Nurses, 16*(5), 792–803. doi:10.1016/j.pmn.2015.01.003

Gothe, N. P., Khan, I., Hayes, J., Erlenbach, E., & Damoiseaux, J. S. (2019). Yoga effects on brain health: A systematic review of the current literature. *Brain Plasticity, 5*(1), 105–122. doi:10.3233/bpl-190084

Hall, S. (n.d.). *Standards of practice*. Retrieved from https://www.alliance-aromatherapists.org/standards-of-practice

Hanscom, D. A., Brox, J. I., & Bunnage, R. (2015). Defining the role of cognitive behavioral therapy in treating chronic low back pain: An overview. *Global Spine Journal, 5*(6), 496–504. doi:10.1055/s-0035-1567836

Jun, Y. S., Kang, P., Min, S. S., Lee, J. M., Kim, H. K., & Seol, G. H. (2013). Effect of eucalyptus oil inhalation on pain and inflammatory responses after total knee replacement: A randomized clinical trial. *Evidence-Based Complementary and Alternative Medicine: eCAM, 2013*, 502727. doi:10.1155/2013/502727

Kabat-Zinn, J. (2005a). *Full catastrophe living: Using the wisdom of your body and mind to face stress, pain, and illness*. New York, NY: Delta Trade Paperbacks.

Kabat-Zinn, J. (2005b). *Wherever you go, there you are: Mindfulness meditation in everyday life*. New York, NY: Hachette Books.

Kabat-Zinn, J. (2018). *Falling awake: How to practice mindfulness in everyday life*. New York, NY: Hachette Books.

Khusid, M. A., & Vythilingam, M. (2016). The emerging role of mindfulness meditation as effective self-management strategy, Part 2: Clinical implications for chronic pain, substance misuse, and insomnia. *Military Medicine, 181*(9), 969–975. doi:10.7205/milmed-d-14-00678

Kong, L. J., Lauche, R., Klose, P., Bu, J. H., Yang, X. C., Guo, C. Q., . . . Cheng, Y. W. (2016). Tai Chi for chronic pain conditions: A systematic review and meta-analysis of randomized controlled trials. *Scientific Reports, 6*(1), 25325. doi:10.1038/srep25325

Koulivand, P. H., Ghadiri, M. K., & Gorji, A. (2013). Lavender and the nervous system. *Evidence-Based Complementary and Alternative Medicine, 2013*, 1–10. doi:10.1155/2013/681304

Kwekkeboom, K. L., Hau, H., Wanta, B., & Bumpus, M. (2008). Patients' perceptions of the effectiveness of guided imagery and progressive muscle relaxation interventions used for cancer pain. *Complementary Therapies in Clinical Practice, 14*(3), 185–194. doi:10.1016/j.ctcp.2008.04.002

Lakhan, S. E., Sheafer, H., & Tepper, D. (2016). The effectiveness of aromatherapy in reducing pain: A systematic review and meta-analysis. *Pain Research and Treatment, 2016*, 8158693. doi:10.1155/2016/8158693

Lindsay, E. K., Young, S., Brown, K. W., Smyth, J. M., & Creswell, J. D. (2019). Mindfulness training reduces loneliness and increases social contact in a randomized controlled trial. *Proceedings of the National Academy of Sciences, 116*(9), 3488–3493. doi:10.1073/pnas.1813588116

Malkin, K. (2020, February 6). *Andrew Weil, M.D. Osher Benefit 4-7-8 Breath*. Retrieved from https://vimeo.com/145943369

Memorial Sloan Kettering Cancer Center. (n.d.). *About mind-body therapies*. Retrieved from https://www.mskcc.org/cancer-care/diagnosis-treatment/symptom-management/integrative-medicine/mind-body

Mohoric, M. (2019). What are the differences between Qigong and Tai Chi? Retrieved from www.qigongenergyhealing.com/blog-qigong-energy-healing/qigong-vs-tai-chi

Morone, N. E., & Greco, C. M. (2007). Mind-body interventions for chronic pain in older adults: A structured review. *Pain Medicine*, *8*(4), 359–375. doi: 10.1111/j.1526-4637.2007.00312.x

National Association for Holistic Aromatherapy. (n.d.). *Exploring aromatherapy*. Retrieved from https://naha.org/explore-aromatherapy/safety

National Cancer Instituite. (n.d.). *Aromatherapy with essential oils (PDQ®)–Health professional version*. Retrieved from https://www.cancer.gov/about-cancer/treatment/cam/hp/aromatherapy-pdq

National Center for Complementary and Integrative Health. (2017, September 24). *NCCAM review analyzes evidence on brain fffects from chronic pain and mind and body approaches*. Retrieved from https://nccih.nih.gov/research/results/spotlight/062113

National Center for Complementary and Integrative Health. (2019, October 11). *Relaxation techniques for health*. Retrieved from https://nccih.nih.gov/health/stress/relaxation.htm

National Center for Complementary and Integrative Health. (n.d.). *Meditation: In depth*. Retrieved from https://www.nccih.nih.gov/health/meditation-in-depth

Nestoriuc, Y., & Martin, A. (2007). Efficacy of biofeedback for migraine: A meta-analysis. *Pain, 128*(1–2), 111–127. doi:10.1016/j.pain.2006.09.007

Qaseem, A., Wilt, T. J., McLean, R. M., Forciea, M. A., & Clinical Guidelines Committee of the American College of Physicians. (2017). Noninvasive treatments for acute, subacute, and chronic low back pain: A clinical practice guideline from the American College of Physicians. *Annals of Internal Medicine, 166*(7), 514. doi:10.7326/m16-2367

Su, S., Duan, J., Chen, T., Huang, X., Shang, E., Yu, L., & Tang, Y. (2015). Frankincense and myrrh suppress inflammation via regulation of the metabolic profiling and the MAPK signaling pathway. *Scientific Reports,* **5**, 13668. doi:10.1038/srep13668

Supreme Chi Living. (n.d.). Retrieved from http://www.americantaichi.net/TaiChiOverview.asp

Veterans Affairs. (2017). *Diagnosis and treatment of low back pain (LBP).* Retrieved from www.healthquality.va.gov/guidelines/Pain/lbp/.

Wang, C., Schmid, C. H., Fielding, R. A., Harvey, W. F., Reid, K. F., Price, L. L., . . . McAlindon, T. (2018). Effect of tai chi versus aerobic exercise for fibromyalgia: Comparative effectiveness randomized controlled trial. *BMJ (Clinical research ed.), 360*, k851. doi:10.1136/bmj.k851

Woodyard, C. (2011). Exploring the therapeutic effects of yoga and its ability to increase quality of life. *International Journal of Yoga*, *4*(2), 49–54. doi:10.4103/0973-6131.85485

ADDITIONAL RESOURCES

Meditation Apps

Calm
Headspace
Insight Timer

Guided Imagery

Ohio State University Wexner Medical Center MP3 files: https://wexnermedical.osu.edu/integrative-complementary-medicine/resources/guided-imagery

Psych Central Imagery written scripts: https://psychcentral.com/lib/audio-scripts-for-imagery/?li_source=LI&li_medium=popular17

VA Center for Integrated Health Care. Written guided imagery script https://www.mirecc.va.gov/cih-visn2/Documents/Patient_Education_Handouts/Visualization_Guided_Imagery_2013.pdf

Meditation

University of California Los Angeles: https://www.uclahealth.org/marc/audio

Mindfulness

UC San Diego Center for Mindfulness: https://medschool.ucsd.edu/som/fmph/research/mindfulness/programs/mindfulness-programs/MBSR-programs/Pages/audio.aspx

Relaxation

Relaxation Response: http://www.relaxationresponse.or/steps

The American Psychological Association (APA) Society of Psychological Hypnosis has a brochure that describes the process and applications that can be useful for patients to understand hypnosis (https://www.apadivisions.org/division-30/about/hypnosis-brochure.pdf).

CHAPTER 20

ENERGY THERAPY

INTRODUCTION

There are a number of integrative medicine techniques and therapies that can be used either alone or in conjunction with a medication regimen to promote health and reduce pain. One of the most interesting, less well-known approaches is the use of energy healing. This approach requires a practitioner to help the patient repattern any negative energy toward health by using their hands to channel the surrounding universal energy forces through the body of the patient.

Practitioners who use energy healing are focused on the patient's need for returning to health. They focus their intervention directly on any blocked areas impeding energy flow in the patient's body to help the patient return to a normal energy flow internally. The only patients who are not good candidates for healing touch are pregnant women, based on the idea that energy may interfere with the fetus.

Asian cultures have used energy healing for many years. The basis of the techniques is *qigong,* the idea that there is both an external and an internal energy life force. Healing can take place when a healing energy practitioner channels energy from the universal energy forces all around us to the patient (D'Arcy, 2014). This energy transfer can unblock any blocked chakras and return the patient's energy flow to normal (Box 20.1).

Healing energy is based on several key concepts.

- The human body has an energy field that is generated from within the body to the outer world. It is sometimes called an *aura* around the body that can have multiple layers.
- There is a universal energy that flows through all living things and is available to all of them.
- Self-healing is promoted through the free-flowing energy field.
- Disease and illness can be felt in the patient's energy field and can be felt and changed by the healing intent of the practitioner (Pierce, 2009).

Today there are healing energy techniques that can be used to help reduce pain and promote relaxation: therapeutic touch (TT) and Reiki. There are differences

BOX 20.1

SEVEN CHAKRAS OF THE HUMAN BODY

There are seven chakras in the human body. They are located along the spine and are centers of spiritual energy. The seven chakras are located at the crown of the head, brow—where the third eye is located, throat, heart, solar plexus, belly or sacrum, and root, which is above the pubis (Stein, 1995).

in the two techniques. In TT, the practitioner does not touch the patient's body, but places hands above the blocked areas and focuses the energy onto that area. In Reiki, the practitioner will divide the patient's body into sections and channel energy into the chakras to open up energy flow. In both TT and Reiki, practitioners take coursework to help them learn how to channel external energy to effect change in the patient's internal energy flow.

CLINICAL PEARL

When considering referring a patient for healing therapies, make sure that the TT or Reiki practitioner has been formally trained and is qualified to see and treat patients.

THERAPEUTIC TOUCH

TT is defined as "a holistic, evidence-based practice that incorporates the intentional and compassionate use of universal energy to promote balance and well-being in all aspects of the individual's body, mind, and spirit" (Therapeutic Touch International Association [TTIA], n.d.).

TT originated in the 1970s as a collaboration between two nurses, Dolores Krieger and Dora Kunz. They originally had a clinic where nurses could provide TT to patients with a variety of health issues. They also used the technique with the infants to calm them down. It is interesting to note that tapes showed infants who were crying calm down and stop crying when TT was used. This calming effect was beneficial to providing care to the infants. As infants, they also had no knowledge of what was providing the calming effect.

In the early days, Krieger and Kunz hoped that TT would become a part of general patient care. Unfortunately, the technique has suffered from a lack of clinical trials to provide evidentiary support. It is difficult to format a study using blinded cohorts because the patient can see whether they are getting real TT versus a sham treatment if the patient is placed in the placebo arm of the study. Because testing the technique is so difficult, researchers turned instead to looking at results and outcomes with the use of TT.

There are a few studies that demonstrate greater pain relief in patients with fibromyalgia and chronic pain (Pierce, 2009). A group of 90 patients with cancer demonstrated pain relief with the use of TT (TTIA, n.d.). Other types of conditions that have shown some benefit with TT are stress in patients with dementia, headache, postoperative pain, phantom pain, and multiple sclerosis (Weintraub, Mamtani, & Micozzi, 2008).

A 2008 Cochrane review evaluating 24 studies including 1,153 patients found that touch therapies had a modest effect on reducing pain. It also found that Reiki had a greater effect and studies with more experienced Reiki practitioners provided better results (So, Jiang, & Qin, 2008). A small meta-analysis with four Reiki studies and 212 patients found that Reiki is an effective means of reducing pain (Demir, 2008).

There have been questions related to the interpretation of these results. It should be noted that the Cochrane review only allowed studies in which a sham therapy was used as a control. As always, using the patient's report of pain is a subjective means of measuring pain. But given these issues, there was still an indication that touch therapies could affect pain.

Burn patients suffer from pain, anxiety, and an altered immune function. In a study using 5 days of TT treatment, pain levels and anxiety ratings were both decreased. There was an impact on immune function, but the positive change was difficult to extrapolate (Weintraub et al., 2008).

Touch therapies are a noninvasive method of helping to reduce pain. They may or may not work. We may not fully understand why they do work. But if there is a chance that the patient can benefit from the therapy and is willing to try it, practitioners should be willing to refer the patient for a trial to see what benefit ensues.

Standards for TT Practice

The guidelines for TT practice have been developed by the TTIA. At minimum, they include the following:

- Completion of a 12-contact-hour basic-level workshop taught by a Therapeutic Touch Practitioner (TTP)
- Practitioner who meets the identified criteria of a qualified teacher
- Commitment to a minimum of 1-year mentoring opportunity under the support of a Qualified Therapeutic Touch Teacher (TTQT); this mentoring involves regular contact, consistent practice of TT (at least twice per week) with journaling, a biannual knowledge-and-skills update with a qualified teacher.

- It is the responsibility of the mentee to clarify their scope-of-practice parameters with the state regulatory board or an attorney
- To advance to the intermediate level of TT, requires 14 contact hours of additional coursework taught by a TTQT
- The intermediate class can be taken approximately 6 months after the basic class with mentorship beginning any time after completion of the basic course
- After the completion of the two courses and the mentorship, the TT practitioner can practice independently (TTIA, n.d.)

In addition, the TT practitioner should have intent and traits that make the practitioner a good TT practitioner. These include:

- Adherence to the TTIA Code of Ethics
- Demonstrating compassion and the desire to help another person
- Regular participation in meditation, mindfulness, or centering practices (TTIA, n.d.)

TT can be used in hospitals, especially with postoperative patients and palliative care or hospice patients. The use of TT can have a calming effect and provide the patient with additional pain relief. Because The Joint Commission has a guideline that promotes using nonpharmacologic therapies, implementing TT in a hospital setting is a good way to address this requirement.

TT practitioners are caring, compassionate, and interested in helping patients achieve a better quality of life. They provide a positive environment for patients who need to feel that someone cares and is willing to help them.

The only negative issue with TT is that many insurance companies will not pay for TT sessions. Fortunately, TT does not require expensive testing or medical equipment. For patients who can afford the cost of the TT sessions, it is a noninvasive, holistic means of decreasing pain and providing positive support for patients in need.

REIKI

Reiki is a healing energy therapy that uses hand placement on specific areas of the body to open blocked chakras and promote normal energy flow (Stein, 1995). The term *Reiki* means *universal life force energy* (Stein, 1995). The Reiki practitioner accesses the Reiki universal energy and passes it into the body of the patient. The patient may feel warmth in the area being treated and the practitioner's hands will be warm as well. The patient may also feel a sense of well-being and relaxation.

Reiki was developed as a formal therapy in 1914 by a Buddhist monk from Japan, Mikao Usui (Pierce, 2009). Hands-on healing was known much earlier in Asian and Indian cultures, and some equate it with the laying on of hands that Jesus and Buddha practiced.

Usui sought ways to heal using the laying on of hands and found that Buddhist teachings provided the information he was searching for. He retreated to a mountain and prayed and fasted for 21 days. At the end of the 21 days, he saw and felt a light energy enter him and his hands became very warm. After that, he was able to heal people using his hands, which would become warm during the treatment.

Reiki is based on three pillars: *Gassho*, *Reiji-Ho*, and *Chiryo*. Each concept addresses an aspect of Reiki practice.

Gassho means *two hands coming together*. It is meditation that is done in the morning or in the evening before sleep. The practitioner places his or her two hands together in a steepled or prayer position in front of the body, with the focus on the two middle fingers of each hand. The effect of the meditation is meant to help the practitioner deidentify him- or herself from his or her thoughts and feelings during meditation.

Reiji-Ho: *Reiji* means *indication of the Reiki power* and *Ho* means *methods*. There are three rituals that are done before each Reiki session. Reiji-Ho describes how to connect to the Reiki power.

1. Assume the Gassho position and connect with the Reiki power by asking the Reiki power to flow through you.
2. Pray for the health and recovery of the patient on all levels.
3. Hold your folded hands in front of your third eye (located on the forehead) and ask the Reiki power to guide your hands to where the energy is needed. The healing is performed through the Reiki practitioner who offers to perform the therapy.

Chiryo means *treatment*. The person doing the treatment places his or her dominant hand on the crown of the patient's head. The practitioner's hands are then directed to the areas needing healing. The practitioner places his or her hands on the painful areas until they no longer hurt and normal energy flow is restored (Usui & Petter, 2011).

A Reiki session is performed by placing the practitioner's hands in 12 positions along the patient's body. The process begins at the crown of the head and moves down the body progressively. Eventually, it covers all of the endocrine glands and organs of the body. The hand positions are meant to energize the patient:

- On the physical level through the warmth of the hands—Reiki level 1
- On the mental level through the thoughts or Reiki symbols—Reiki level 2

- On the emotional level through the love that flows with them—Reiki level 2
- On the energetic level, through the presence of an initiated person, as well as the Reiki power itself (Usui & Petter, 2011)

The intent of Reiki is to heal and is based on love and compassion. The healing is promoted by the desire to help the patient by using the universal energy. The result should be an overall healing that promotes health and wellness in the patient.

CLINICAL PEARL

Performing a Reiki treatment can affect the patient on many levels. Patients can feel warm in the area being treated. They may also experience a sense of peace and relaxation that can promote sleep. Some patients may experience a period of sleep after a Reiki treatment that is particularly restful.

Levels of Reiki Practice

There are three levels of Reiki practice. At the basic level, hand placements are performed. At the second level, more advanced training takes place and Reiki symbols are learned. At level three—Reiki master and teacher—advanced techniques, such as sending healing energy over distance, are practiced (Usui & Petter, 2011).

To practice Reiki, three levels of training are offered. The basic level requires taking coursework from a recognized Reiki teacher. The basic level can be used for self Reiki, in which the practitioner uses the Reiki treatment on him- or herself. The basic session takes about 8 hours. During this session, the hand placements are practiced and performed on other students and the teacher.

In the second level of Reiki training, the Reiki symbols are learned and used in therapy. These symbols are used to direct energy, so that healing can take place. Other symbols can help to promote enlightenment and peace. Which symbols are used depends on what particular area of the patient needs healing.

Reiki Master and Teacher is the third level of Reiki practice. In this level, the Reiki practitioner uses the tools of the first two levels, but adds advanced techniques to his or her practice. In addition to the lower level healing techniques, the Reiki master uses absentee healing, often called *distance healing*.

Distance healing involves sending of healing energy to someone who is not present. The distance can be long or short. To perform distance healing, the practitioners visualize the person or a representation of the person. They then direct healing energy to the person in the area that needs it. One special technique for distance healing is visualization: "Use energy healing for distance healing by visualizing roses. Make a rose in any color and give it the name of the person who will receive the energy. Send Reiki to the rose and watch it bloom, and then let the rose dissolve" (Wallace & Henkin in Stein, 1995, p. 12). Reiki masters typically use meditation and a quiet place for sending distance healing.

HELPING A PATIENT DECIDE ON HEALING-TOUCH THERAPIES

Some patients are open to unusual therapies, like touch therapy, and others are very resistant to such ideas. Primary care providers are in an ideal situation to suggest a therapy like healing touch. They have a relationship with their patients and understand what they may be open to trying. In offering healing-touch therapies, it is important to explain that they are not intended to remove all the pain, but to help relieve the pain and provide relaxation, which may also reduce pain. Patients can also be offered healing-touch therapy on a trial basis. If they try it and like it, they can continue. If they try it and do not feel it is helping, they can simply stop going to the healing-touch practitioner.

To locate a healing-touch practitioner, you can contact your local healing-touch community, which will be listed on the Internet. Before sending a patient to a specific healing-touch practitioner, review his or her qualifications, training, and fee schedules to determine whether he or she would be a good fit for the patient. There are also ratings listed on the Internet that will give an idea of patient satisfaction with the therapy provided.

SUMMARY

Healing-touch therapies can be a perfect adjunct to standard pain management such as medication management. For a patient who is interested in trying another approach to pain management, the meditation and relaxation offered through healing-touch therapies can be highly effective.

TRENDING IN PAIN MANAGEMENT

- More research is needed to support the use of healing-energy therapies for patients of all types.
- Watch for efforts to get insurance reimbursement for healing-touch therapies.

CASE STUDY

Sandra is a 37-year-old patient who was burned severely in a house fire 2 years ago. She lost several family members in the fire and mourns their loss. She has significant scarring over her lower body and has difficulty walking because her legs do not bend and flex normally. She also has daily pain and is depressed and anxious. She has difficulty sleeping because she is afraid there will be another fire. She is taking a neuropathic pain medication that helps relieve some of the pain, but she still rates the pain at 5/10. She is seeing a psychologist for her depression and anxiety, but she cannot get past her grief and fear of another fire occurring while she is sleeping.

Her primary care provider thinks she might benefit from healing-energy therapy to help her relax, sleep better, and decrease her pain. Because she has sensitive scarred areas on her body, Sandra goes to see a TT practitioner who does not have to touch her during treatment.

When her primary care practitioner sees her next, Sandra is more relaxed, rates her pain at 3, and says she is sleeping better. She can at least get several hours of uninterrupted sleep . She says she is feeling much better overall and is doing better with her depression since the psychologist adjusted her medications for depression. Sandra says she likes the TT and will continue with it to help maintain her increased well-being. The TT practitioner has taught Sandra some relaxation methods to help her sleep that seem to be working. Overall, Sandra seems less anxious and has better pain relief.

- Using healing energy can help a patient relax and provide a better level of pain relief. Sandra is a good candidate because she had several causes of residual pain that could be treated with a healing-energy technique.
- The resulting feelings of well-being that can result from a TT treatment can help Sandra with her depression and sleep as well.
- When making a referral for TT, it is important to know what type of training the practitioner has had and what kinds of patients he or she sees. Each practitioner should have a fee schedule that he or she uses to determine the fees for treatment. Unfortunately, most healing-energy treatments are not reimbursed by insurance.

REFERENCES

Brennan, B. A. (1987). *Hands of light: A guide to healing through the human energy field.* New York, NY: Bantam Books.

D'Arcy, Y. (2014). *A compact clinical guide to women's pain management.* New York, NY: Springer Publishing Company.

Demir, D. (2018). The effect of reiki on pain: a meta-analysis. *Complementary Therapies in Clinical Practice, 31*, 384–387. doi:10.1016/j.ctcp.2018.02.020

Pierce, B. (2009). A non-pharmacologic adjunct for pain management. *Nurse Practitoner, 34*(2), 10–13. doi:10.1097/01.npr.0000345262.11633.5e

So, P. S., Jiang, Y., & Qin, Y. (2008). Touch therapies for pain relief in adults. *Cochrane Database of Systematic Reviews, 8*(4).

Stein, D. (1995). *Essential Reiki.* New York, NY: Berkley Press-Random House.

Therapeutic Touch International Association. (n.d.). *About TTIA.* Retrieved from www.therapeutictouch.org

Usui, M., & Petter, F. (2011). *The original Reiki handbook.* Twin Lakes, WI: Lotus Press.

Weintraub, M., Mamtani, R., & Micozzi, M. (2008). *Complementary and integrative medicine in pain management.* New York, NY: Springer Publishing Company.

ADDITIONAL RESOURCE

Brennan, B. A. (1987). *Hands of light: A guide to healing through the human energy field.* New York, NY: Bantam Books.

CHAPTER 21

INTERVENTIONAL OPTIONS FOR PAIN MANAGEMENT

INTRODUCTION

When conservative treatment is not affecting pain, interventional procedures may provide temporary or long-lasting relief. Some procedures can be done in the primary care setting, whereas others require referral to an interventionist who may do the procedure in their office or a surgery setting. As with any pain treatment, identifying the pain generator is key to determining effective treatment. It is useful to have relationships with skilled interventionists who perform the procedures that your patient population needs. Many interventionists are skilled in the identification and diagnosis of pain generators and can assist with this when it has been elusive. Interventions include nerve and musculoskeletal injections, including trigger point and joint injections and various types of spinal injections. Injections can be administered using local anesthetic or corticosteroids alone or together. Platelet-rich plasma injections are also being used in multiple applications. Implantable devices and pumps use technology to address intractable pain. There is increasing use of infusions of ketamine and lidocaine to manage pain without using opioids.

Interventions are included as one of the five approaches to pain management described in the U.S. Department of Health and Human Services Pain Management Inter-Agency Best Practices Task Force Report (U.S. Department of Health and Human Services, 2019, p. 19). The other four approaches are opioid and nonopioid medications, restorative therapies, behavioral health, and complementary and integrative health.

> The risk of interventional therapies varies by procedure. Interventional treatments have some associated risk (e.g., small risk of infection or nerve injury), but the overall safety and efficacy of interventional therapies make them attractive alternatives to long-term opioid therapy when performed by properly trained and certified clinicians. (U.S. Department of Health and Human Services, 2019, p. 19).

INJECTIONS

Injections range from simple, which can be performed in an exam room, to complex, which require an equipped procedure room. Administration of specialized blocks and spinal injections are performed by specialists, such as interventional pain specialists, and interventional radiologists using fluoroscopic or ultrasound guidance. Techniques and practices of specialists vary. Some use conscious sedation, whereas others use only local anesthetic. Collaborative care improves pain-management outcomes; follow your patients' outcomes after procedures and discuss any questions or concerns with the interventionist.

It is important to establish relationships with interventionists who meet the needs of your patients: What is the wait time for appointments? What procedures do they perform most often? Does their preferred sedation policy meet individual patient's needs?

Because of their personal relationship with the patient, the primary care clinician has the responsibility of providing information on risks and benefits and what having the procedure will be like for the patient. Recommend that patients pace activity following a procedure. It can be tempting to overdo activity when pain is significantly decreased; it can be helpful to say, "Enjoy feeling good, move around, but don't overdo, ease into increased activity."

CLINICAL PEARL

Trigger point and some joint injections can be performed in the primary care setting if the clinician has had the requisite education and clinical training. Clinicians seeking additional experience can attend courses at national conferences and those offered through continuing education.

Trigger Point Injections

"Myofascial Trigger Points (MTrPs) are hard, discrete, palpable nodules in a taut band of skeletal muscle that may be spontaneously painful (i.e. active), or painful only on compression (i.e. latent)" (Shah et al., 2015, p. 746). Accurate identification of the trigger points is key to effective relief with injections; it takes time and practice to quickly and accurately locate MTrPs. The increased availability of ultrasound may improve visualization and decrease complications (Wong & Wong, 2012). The efficacy of trigger point injections depends on presence of twitch response, accuracy of locating the trigger point, and the skill of the injector (O'Neill, 2016).

Trigger point injections can be a useful part of addressing MTrPs, but will be most effective if they are part of multimodal treatment that includes exercise and appropriate posture. Patients may be more comfortable and able to participate in therapy following trigger point injections. Trigger point injections can be done with dry needles or local anesthetic. Some clinicians use ultrasound to guide the injection, whereas others do not.

In the appropriate setting and with the proper expertise, trigger point injections may be helpful as an adjunctive treatment of the most common headache disorders (Robbins et al., 2014).

Joints and Bursa

As with any procedure, a good history and physical examination are needed to identify the target for the procedure to be able to formulate a treatment plan with imaging as indicated to rule out infection.

Image guidance (fluoroscopy or ultrasound) is recommended for some joint injections and required for others. The trend is for more image-guided interventions, with ultrasound enjoying increased use.

Corticosteroids have risks and benefits; used wisely for joint injections, they are useful for pain management. Corticosteroids have a "time- and dose-dependent effect on articular cartilage, with beneficial effects occurring at low doses and durations and detrimental effects at high doses and durations" (Wernecke, Braun, & Dragoo, 2015, p. 1).

Sterile technique is essential to prevent infection. Combine with physical therapy (PT) as indicated; sometimes a patient is able to use the relief obtained from an injection to be able to participate in therapy. Choice of local anesthetic and corticosteroid depends on the site of injection, the desired effect, and clinician preference. Ultrasound guidance is being used increasingly for injections. Injections may be helpful for osteoarthritis, tendinitis, and rheumatoid arthritis (Salinas & Rosenberg, 2020).

Trochanteric Bursa Injection

Trochanteric bursitis is a clinical diagnosis that is a common cause of leg pain. A systematic review of the efficacy of treatment of trochanteric bursitis was limited by inconsistencies in diagnosis before treatment. Reviewers found that treatment of trochanteric bursitis with injection was effective in most patients; many improved with only one injection, whereas others benefited from repeat injections. There was no improvement of efficacy if injection was done with fluoroscopic guidance (Lustenberger, Ng, Best, & Ellis, 2011). In a randomized controlled trial (RCT) Cohen et al. (2009) found no difference between bedside and fluoroscopically guided injection.

Sacroiliac Joint Injection

Sacroiliac joint pathology is a frequent cause of back pain. The Spine Intervention Society Panel recommends injection with a local anesthetic and steroid in the presence of a positive exam if pain is greater than 4/10 and causing loss of function (Macvicar, Kreiner, Duszynski, & Kennedy, 2017).

Joint Injections

Joint injections and trigger point injections may be given by a specialist or in a primary care office. If you plan to do injections, as always, it is essential to complete and document appropriate education and training for the procedures and to comply with your state scope of practice. Be sure you documented your education, approved scope in your state, and proficiency. The shoulder, hip, knee, and wrist are joints that are commonly injected.

Nerve Blocks

Primary care consultation with pain management as part of early management of pain following injury can provide relief and decrease the need for systemic medication. Nerve blocks may also be beneficial for pain that is difficult to localize. Interventional pain specialists have expertise in identifying and accessing nerves that may be causing refractory pain throughout the body; with consultation, they may offer an approach that provides relief.

Stellate Ganglion Block

Stellate ganglion block (SGB) has been used for refractory upper extremity pain for many years and is being studied by the Department of Veterans Affairs (VA) as a treatment for posttraumatic stress disorder (PTSD). Located near C7, the stellate ganglion is part of the sympathetic nervous system and is also known as the *cervicothoracic ganglion*.

For managing pain, SGB is an outpatient procedure done by a specialist using ultrasound or fluoroscopic guidance. It is important that patients be prepared for the short-term effects of sympathetic blockade on the injected side. These include drooping eyelid and/or bloodshot eye, stuffy nose, and increase in temperature; transient hoarseness may also be experienced. These side effects subside in 4 to 6 hours (Brigham and Women's Hospital, n.d.).

Pain relief following SGB is variable; it may only last a few hours or it may last for days or weeks. The procedure can be repeated and it is not unusual for relief to be longer with successive treatments (Cleveland Clinic, n.d.).

The SGB has been used by anesthesiologists and pain specialists for years to block the sympathetic nervous system so as to relieve upper extremity chronic regional pain syndrome (CRPS) and some types of intractable facial pain (Jeon, 2016). Research is underway at the Long Beach VA, evaluating the impact of SGB on PTSD in veterans.

Spinal Injections

Guidelines and reviews of spinal injections provide conflicting recommendations. Indications and outcomes are influenced by many factors, including patient selection, diagnostic accuracy, and skill of the interventionist. Pain specialists will provide guidance regarding required imaging, an appropriate procedure, and potential risk and benefit for patients referred for evaluation and treatment. Spinal injections are performed using fluoroscopy and can be given in the cervical, thoracic, or lumbar spine.

There are multiple approaches to performing spinal injections. The pain specialist will determine the appropriate therapy based on patient history and exam and imaging as indicated.

Spinal injections include epidural injections, which may be given as *caudal, transforaminal,* or *interlaminar* and facet procedures, which include *facet blocks, medial branch blocks,* and *radiofrequency ablation (RFA).* Spinal injections are done with fluoroscopic guidance. Medial branch blocks are done using a local anesthetic; therefore, pain relief following a medial branch block is rapid and short acting. For epidural injections, typically 1% lidocaine is injected to anesthetize the skin and a steroid is injected; most epidural steroid injections take several days to show their full effect (Chen, Mehnert, Stitik, & Foye, 2018).

Epidural injections are included in the Centers for Disease Control (CDC) guidelines for prescribing opioids for chronic pain to provide short-term improvement in pain secondary to lumbar radiculopathy. The guidelines also note that rare but serious adverse events that can occur with epidural spinal injections are loss of vision, stroke, paralysis, and death (Dowell, Haegerich, & Chou, 2016).

CLINICAL PEARL

The efficacy of the injection is dependent on correct diagnosis and skill of the injector in placing the steroid where it will be most effective; this may explain variations in reported efficacy.

Patients are seen in follow-up around 2 weeks following the procedure to evaluate the immediate impact of the injection and persistence of relief. If pain is not improved or improved insufficiently, the injection may be repeated. Generally, a series of up to three epidural injections may be offered to patients, determined on a case-by-case basis. This general practice is not guideline driven, but anecdotally effective.

Interlaminar, caudal, or transforaminal epidural steroid injections under fluoroscopic guidance are suggested to provide short-term symptomatic relief (2 weeks to 6 months) for lumbar stenosis, but there is conflicting evidence regarding efficacy (Nance, n.d.).

CLINICAL PEARL

Facets are also known as *z-joints* or *zygapophyseal joints.*

Blocking the medial branch nerves can be diagnostic and therapeutic. For a medial branch block, a local anesthetic is injected into the medial branches that enervate the suspected facet; this procedure is used to confirm the location and diagnosis of facet disease. Two separate blocks that relieve 50% to 90% of pain is diagnostic (Nance & Adcock, 2017). Two effective blocks are frequently required for third-party payment for radiofrequency ablation (RFA), which can provide longer term relief.

The American Academy of Physical Medicine and Rehabilitation supports physical therapy and activity as the necessary treatment components before and after injection therapy.

CLINICAL PEARL

It is understandable that patients might overdo activity if they get profound relief from an injection; caution them to take the time to enjoy feeling good and not to overdo physical activity, or they may find the relief short lived.

RADIOFREQUENCY ABLATION

Prior to performing RFA, medial branch blocks are performed to identify specific pain generators. Third-party payers generally require two effective medial branch blocks before authorizing RFA.

> "During RFA, a high-frequency electrical current runs through an insulated needle. At the tip of the needle, the electric field causes molecule movement which, in turn, produces thermal energy. The heat from the tip of the RFA device is targeted to create a small lesion within a nerve, which disrupts the pain signal." (Leggett et al., 2014, p. e148)

The U.S. Department of Health and Human Services (HHS) Best Practices Task Force endorses conventional and pulse radiofrequency waves to ablate nerves that are contributing to chronic pain, while acknowledging that more research is needed on pulse radio frequency (U.S. Department of Health and Human Services, 2019). A systematic review by Leggett et al. (2014) found RFA to be an effective treatment for lumbar facet joint and sacroiliac joint pain.

IMPLANTABLES

Spinal Cord and Peripheral Nerve Stimulators

The first spinal cord stimulator (SCS) was implanted in 1967 in a patient with cancer by a neurosurgeon, Dr. C. Norman Shealy, who also invented the transcutaneous electrical nerve stimulation (TENS) unit and founded the American Holistic Medicine Association (Realholisticdoc, n.d.). The mechanism of action of SCS is the gate theory, which suggests there are cognitive as well as sensory components to pain. This premise supports the use of psychological evaluation prior to implantation.

"SCS is expected to reduce pain by blocking the conduction of primary nerve pathway. Spinal cord stimulators have reported success rates ranging from 20-70%" (Campbell, Jamison, & Edwards, 2013, p. 1). For patients with severe chronic pain, it is tempting to believe efficacy claims for new therapies. It is helpful for primary care providers and specialists to give evidence-based, balanced risk-and-benefit information.

CRPS, postherpetic neuralgia, traumatic nerve injury, failed back surgery syndrome, and visceral pain may be indications for SCS in the appropriate patient. In a review of randomized controlled studies and cohort studies of SCS for failed back surgery syndrome, Palmer, Guan, and Chai (2019) found short-term relief (2 years) with no evidence regarding longer term efficacy and concerns regarding study bias due to study funding. Pain relief is more likely with predominantly leg pain rather than axial pain; psychological testing before implantation is the standard of care. The failure rate of implanted SCS is up to 50% 1 to 2 years after implantation (Doleys, 2006).

Before implanting a stimulator, the patient undergoes a psychological evaluation. If the psychological evaluation indicates the patient is an appropriate candidate for SCS, a trial is done. The psychological evaluation is performed by a behavioral health clinician familiar with pain and implanted devices to evaluate psychosocial factors that could impact patient tolerance to having an implanted device and the potential success of the SCS. In some communities, it is difficult to find a behavioral health clinician skilled in this complex evaluation; sometimes there are challenges with third-party payment for the psychological evaluation. If the patient is deemed to be an appropriate candidate for the stimulator, the interventional pain physician will do a stimulator trial.

During the trial, the leads are inserted percutaneously and attached to an external power source. Pain coverage is established in the procedure room, and the patient then spends a few days with the stimulator to evaluate effectiveness and tolerance; after the trial, the leads are removed and the results are reviewed with the patient. If the trial is successful, the patient is scheduled to have a permanent system implanted.

Several large companies manufacture and support SCSs; there are also smaller companies researching new technologies. The system consists of a generator implanted subcutaneously to either percutaneous wire leads or paddle leads (Pinzon & Killeffer, 2015).

Implanted devices have wireless external controllers that allow the patient to control the spread/location of coverage and also the intensity of the SCS. They may have more than one program to allow flexibility in addressing their personal needs.

Research and development continue to improve pulse generator size and longevity, to improve therapeutic waveforms, and lead performance.

CLINICAL PEARL

An implanted defibrillator or pacemaker may damage an SCS, and the electrical pulses from the SCS may result in malfunction of the implanted cardiac device.

Eldabe, Buchser, and Duarte (2016) reviewed published complication rates of SCSs and peripheral nerve stimulators. They found that most complications of SCS and peripheral nerve stimulators (PNS) were equipment related, with lead migration being the most common and severe complications of neurological damage are rare.

Pollard et al. (2019) performed a systematic review of randomized controlled trials of SCSs and found that although the odds of decreasing medication use increased with implantation of the SCS, data were limited and further study is needed. Technology continues to evolve for spinal cord stimulation, including dorsal root ganglion SCS, high-frequency SCS, and burst SCS. Efficacy of the stimulator system is dependent on many factors such as the implanter, comorbidities, including mental health, pain generator, and smoking status (Verrills, Sinclair, & Barnard, 2016). "New SCS technologies are being used increasingly in the clinical environment, but often there is a lag period between the clinical application and the publishing of high-quality evidence on safety and efficacy" (Verrills et al., 2016, p. 481).

Implanted Pumps for Intrathecal Medication Delivery

Implanted pumps deliver medication via the intrathecal route for patients with intractable pain. They are used for cancer pain and chronic noncancer pain. Intrathecal pumps require a specialist to implant and to manage ongoing use of the pump, including monitoring and refilling it.

Intrathecal medication is indicated by the U.S. Food and Drug Administration (FDA) for severe and retractable pain, including neck and back pain, abdominal pain, CRPS, postherpetic neuralgia, and cancer pain. Guidelines for use of intrathecal pumps were updated in 2017 at the Polyanalgesic Consensus Conference (PACC). Multiple clinical factors that need to be considered before pursuing this option are listed in the guidelines, including patient-expected survival time, and the psychological status of patients with chronic pain (International Neuromodulation Society, 2017).

The FDA has issued two warnings regarding these pumps:

- January 11, 2017, warning regarding possible pump malfunctions as a result of MRI, including over- or underinfusions or not functioning after MRI. Detailed recommendations are included at the FDA site (Center for Devices and Radiological Health, 2017).
- November 14, 2018, warning that only Infumorph (morphine sulfate) and Prialt (zicotinide) be used in intrathecal pumps. Both of these medications are branded and preservative free. Use of any other medication, concentration, or compounded medication increases the risk of adverse effects secondary to pump malfunction (Center for Devices and Radiological Health, 2018).

CLINICAL PEARL

If you have a patient with an implanted pump, flag his or her chart for special precautions when considering an MRI.

INFUSIONS

Intravenous (IV) infusions of ketamine and lidocaine are being used to manage refractory neuropathic pain. Although these medications can be effective in impacting pain, they carry risks and must be administered in appropriately monitored environments, with careful patient selection and use of protocols.

Ketamine

IV ketamine is FDA approved for anesthesia, and in March 2019, nasal spray ketamine was approved for in-office treatment of depression via the FDA Fast-Track Approval; it is under a restricted distribution system per the Risk Evaluation and Mitigation Strategy (REMS; FDA, 2019). IV ketamine for pain management is used off label. It is available through specialty infusion centers.

Ketamine is an *N*-methyl-D-aspartate (NMDA) antagonist, with demonstrated anti-inflammatory effects. It is used off label to treat central and peripheral neuropathic pain (Kurdi, Theerth, & Deva, 2014).

Because of the increase in need for and use of ketamine, the American Society of Regional Anesthesia and Pain Medicine, the American Academy of Pain Medicine, and the American Society of Anesthesiologists published the Consensus Guidelines on the Use of Intravenous Ketamine Infusions for Chronic Pain in 2018 (Cohen et al., 2018). The 2017 Consensus Guideline group found that most studies were small and poorly blinded with the risk of adverse effects similar to placebo. Multiple contraindications are included in the guidelines, with recommendations for preinfusion testing. They state that further studies are needed to refine the therapeutic dose and determine the long-term risks of repeated infusions.

Guideline recommendations: There is low-grade evidence for the use of ketamine infusion except for CRPS. Relative contraindications to ketamine infusion, including active psychosis or substance abuse and others, are listed in the Guidelines. Guidelines recommend that for a ketamine infusion, the supervising clinician be experienced with ketamine infusion, such as an anesthesiologist, a critical care physician, or a pain physician; the administering clinician has to be an RN or physician assistant (PA) with formal training in safe administration of moderate sedation; and, depending on the dosage used, the infusion should be administered in a setting with resuscitation equipment. Further studies are recommended (Cohen et al., 2018).

CLINICAL PEARL

Ketamine is being used in outpatient infusion centers with claims that it is life-changing for people with chronic pain and depression. The evidence for effectiveness and long-term safety is scant.

Ketamine is an NMDA receptor antagonist that acts on the brain and spinal cord. It also has anti-inflammatory effects. It has many adverse effects, including hallucination, dysphoria, anxiety, nausea, sedation, tachycardia, and others; adverse effects are dose dependent. There is limited evidence for the use of ketamine for chronic noncancer pain. A trial of low-dose ketamine may be worthwhile in refractory cancer pain (Bell & Kalso, 2018).

Lidocaine

IV lidocaine infusions are being used off label to treat neuropathic pain and fibromyalgia. "Lidocaine as an infusion has opioid sparing effects, blocks sodium channels, uncouples G protein, blocks NMDA receptor, reduces circulating inflammatory cytokines, and prevents secondary hyperalgesia and central sensitization" (Kandil, Melikman, & Adinoff, 2017). These actions hold promise, but randomized controls are lacking.

To evaluate the effectiveness of IV lidocaine, the Canadian Agency for Drugs and Technologies in Health did a review of available literature and found evidence for effectiveness of IV lidocaine in chronic pain to be lacking in quality and quantity (Mayhew, 2018).

The safe and effective dosage for IV lidocaine has not been established. Zhu et al. (2019) did a systematic review and meta-analysis of research on the use of IV lidocaine. Studies have been small with inconsistent results. Because lidocaine can cause cardiac arrhythmia, patients are monitored during studies for possible adverse reactions; no serious reactions occurred in any of the trials reviewed. Although lidocaine was found to relieve pain in the immediate infusion period, long-lasting effects were not demonstrated. Well-designed RCTs are needed to establish its efficacy and dosing.

SUMMARY

Interventions performed by skilled clinicians can provide pain relief by delivering the steroid to a target, avoiding the adverse effects of systemic use, decreasing inflammation and pain, and improving function. There are risks to interventions, including potential infection and complications of procedures. Used judiciously, they can positively impact the quality of life for a patient with persistent pain.

Know the resources available in your local area. Interventional pain physicians and interventional radiologists perform spinal injections. They can assist in identifying pain generators and creating treatment plans. Knowing when to use interventions, not too soon and not too late, is an art and a science. Use the least invasive, safest therapy first. Consider whether injections are needed before, after, or while doing physical therapy . Some patients get permanent relief from one injection, whereas others require repeat injections to maintain function. Remind patients not to wait until pain is unbearable to discuss options; frequently, better relief is obtained if the pain has not been long-standing. Timing and frequency of spinal injections are different from those of joint injections. Joint injections with corticosteroids are not repeated more than every 6 weeks or more than three to four per year. There are no official guidelines, but this is good practice based on concerns that steroids can damage cartilage. Sophisticated technology and newer medication protocols can be life changing for some patients, but they are not without risk. Consult a pain specialist to explore options, weighing the risks and benefits for each patient individually. New technology and procedure approaches hold hope for patients with intractable pain; collaboration between primary care and specialists is essential.

TRENDING IN PAIN MANAGEMENT

- Continued research on the benefits of platelet-rich plasma and stem cells
- Continued evaluation via ultrasound and fluoroscopy to guide injections
- Risks and benefits with protocols for ketamine and lidocaine infusion

CASE STUDY

Myrtle is an 82-year-old patient with chronic back and leg pain secondary to lumbar stenosis. She does not want to take pain medication except for an occasional Tylenol. She lives alone and is very independent. She drives to her office visits and loves to travel. She plans to go on a cruise in 3 months and is concerned that her pain will limit her. The leg pain is disrupting her routines and making it difficult for her to practice tai chi; she wants to know what she can do.

- You discuss the multimodal approach to spinal stenosis and the importance of physical therapy with interventions.
- You refer her to a pain specialist for evaluation for epidural steroid injection.
- She returns 2 weeks later, reporting that she is delighted her pain is 50% better.
- You refer her to PT and advise her to share her tai chi practice and travel plans with her physical therapist, so that her exercise regimen can be tailored to support Myrtle's activities.
- She returns in 1 month, reporting that she feels great—stronger and with less pain. She is following a home exercise program and will check in with PT every few weeks until she leaves on her cruise and again when she returns.
- You congratulate her on her progress and remind her of the importance of continuing the home program while she is traveling, and make appointment for follow-up when she returns.

REFERENCES

Bell, R. F., & Kalso, E. A. (2018). Ketamine for pain management. *PAIN Reports*, *3*(5), e674. doi:10.1097/pr9.0000000000000674

Brigham and Women's Hospital. (n.d.). *Stellate ganglion blocks*. Retrieved from https://www.brighamandwomens.org/anesthesiology-and-pain-medicine/pain-management-center/stellate-ganglion-blocks

Campbell, C. M., Jamison, R. N., & Edwards, R. R. (2013). Psychological screening/phenotyping as predictors for spinal cord stimulation. *Current Pain and Headache Reports, 17*(1), 307. doi:10.1007/s11916-012-0307-6

Center for Devices and Radiological Health. (January 11, 2017). *Safety concerns with implantable infusion pumps in the MR environment.* Retrieved from https://www.fda.gov/medical-devices/safety-communications/safety-concerns-implantable-infusion-pumps-magnetic-resonance-mr-environment-fda-safety

Center for Devices and Radiological Health. (2018). *Implanted pumps for intrathecal medicines safety communication.* Retrieved from https://www.fda.gov/medical-devices/safety-communications/use-caution-implanted-pumps-intrathecal-administration-medicines-pain-management-fda-safety

Chen, B., Mehnert, M., Stitik, T., & Foye, P. (2018, August). *Epidural steroid injections.* Retrieved from https://emedicine.medscape.com/article/325733-overview

Cleveland Clinic. (n.d.). *Stellate ganglion block.* Retrieved from https://my.clevelandclinic.org/health/treatments/17507-stellate-ganglion-block

Cohen, S. P., Bhatia, A., Buvanendran, A., Schwenk, E. S., Wasan, A. D., Hurley, R. W., . . . Hooten, W. M. (2018). Consensus guidelines on the use of intravenous ketamine infusions for chronic pain from the American Society of Regional Anesthesia and Pain Medicine, the American Academy of Pain Medicine, and the American Society of Anesthesiologists. *Regional Anesthesia and Pain Medicine, 43*(5), 521–546. doi: 10.1097/AAP.0000000000000808

Cohen, S. P., Strassels, S. A., Foster, L., Marvel, J., Williams, K., Crooks, M., . . . Williams, N. (2009). Comparison of fluoroscopically guided and blind corticosteroid injections for greater trochanteric pain syndrome: multicentre randomised controlled trial. *BMJ (Clinical research ed.), 338,* b1088. doi:10.1136/bmj.b1088

Doleys, D. M. (2006). Psychological factors in spinal cord stimulation therapy: Brief review and discussion. *Neurosurgical Focus, 21*(6), 1–6. doi:10.3171/foc.2006.21.6.4

Dowell, D., Haegerich, T. M., & Chou, R. (2016). CDC guideline for prescribing opioids for chronic pain—United States, 2016. *Morbidity and Mortality Weekly Reports, 65*(1), 1–49. doi:10.15585/mmwr.rr6501e1

Eldabe, S., Buchser, E., & Duarte, R. V. (2016). Complications of spinal cord stimulation and peripheral nerve stimulation techniques: A review of the literature. *Pain Medicine, 17*(2), 325–336. doi:10.1093/pm/pnv025

INS Guidelines for Intrathecal Drug Delivery. (2017). *Overview.* Retrieved from http://paccguidelines.cmeoutfitters.com/

Jeon, Y. (2016). Therapeutic potential of stellate ganglion block in orofacial pain: a mini review. *Journal of Dental Anesthesia and Pain Medicine, 16*(3), 159–163. doi:10.17245/jdapm.2016.16.3.159

Kandil, E., Melikman, E., & Adinoff, B. (2017). Lidocaine infusion: A promising therapeutic approach for chronic pain. *Journal of Anesthesia & Clinical Research, 8*(1), 697. doi:10.4172/2155-6148.1000697

Kurdi, M. S., Theerth, K. A., & Deva, R. S. (2014). Ketamine: Current applications in anesthesia, pain, and critical care. *Anesthesia, essays and researches, 8*(3), 283–290. doi:10.4103/0259-1162.143110

Leggett, L. E., Soril, L. J., Lorenzetti, D. L., Noseworthy, T., Steadman, R., Tiwana, S., & Clement, F. (2014). Radiofrequency ablation for chronic low back pain: A systematic review of randomized controlled trials. *Pain Research & Management, 19*(5), e146–e153. doi:10.1155/2014/834369

Lustenberger, D. P., Ng, V. Y., Best, T. M., & Ellis, T. J. (2011). Efficacy of treatment of trochanteric bursitis: A systematic review. *Clinical Journal of Sport Medicine: Official Journal of the Canadian Academy of Sport Medicine, 21*(5), 447–453. doi:10.1097/JSM.0b013e318221299c

Macvicar, J., Kreiner, D. S., Duszynski, B., & Kennedy, D. J. (2017). Appropriate use criteria for fluoroscopically guided diagnostic and therapeutic sacroiliac interventions: Results from the Spine Intervention Society Convened Multispecialty Collaborative. *Pain Medicine, 18*(11), 2081–2095. doi:10.1093/pm/pnx253

Mayhew, A. (2018, January 26). *Intravenous lidocaine for chronic pain: A review of the clinical effectiveness and guidelines.* Retrieved from https://www.ncbi.nlm.nih.gov/books/NBK531808

Nance, P. (n.d.). *Lumbar stenosis.* Retrieved from https://now.aapmr.org/lumbar-stenosis/#references

Nance, P., & Adcock, E. (2017, March). *Facet mediated pain.* Retrieved from https://now.aapmr.org/facet-mediated-pain/

O'Neill, B. (2016, August). *Myofascial pain.* Retrieved from https://now.aapmr.org/myofascial-pain/

Palmer, N., Guan, Z., & Chai, N. C. (2019). Spinal cord stimulation for failed back surgery syndrome—Patient selection considerations. *Translational Perioperative and Pain Medicine, 6*(3), 81–90.

Pinzon, E. G., & Killeffer, J. A. (2015). Spinal cord stimulation: Fundamentals. *Practical Pain Management, 13*(2). https://www.practicalpainmanagement.com/treatments/interventional/stimulators/spinal-cord-stimulation-fundamentals

Pollard, E. M., Lamer, T. J., Moeschler, S. M., Gazelka, H. M., Hooten, W. M., Bendel, M. A., . . . Murad, M. H. (2019). The effect of spinal cord stimulation on pain medication reduction in intractable spine and limb pain: A systematic review of randomized controlled trials and meta-analysis. *Journal of Pain Research, 12*, 1311–1324. doi:10.2147/JPR.S186662

Realholisticdoc. (n.d.). *C. Norman Shealy, M.D., PH.D.* Retrieved from https://realholisticdoc.com/dr-c-norman-shealy-energy-medicine/

Robbins, M. S., Kuruvilla, D., Blumenfeld, A., Charleston, L., Sorrell, M., Robertson, C. E., . . . Ashkenazi, A. (2014). Trigger point injections for headache disorders: Expert consensus methodology and narrative review. *Headache: The Journal of Head and Face Pain, 54*(9), 1441–1459. doi:10.1111/head.12442

Salinas, J. D., & Rosenberg, J. N. (2020, January 15). *Which joint and soft tissue conditions may benefit from treatment with corticosteroid injection?* Medscape. Retrieved from https://www.medscape.com/answers/325370-155837/which-joint-and-soft-tissue-conditions-may-benefit-from-treatment-with-corticosteroid-injection

Shah, J. P., Thaker, N., Heimur, J., Aredo, J. V., Sikdar, S., & Gerber, L. (2015). Myofascial trigger points then and now: A historical and scientific perspective. *PM & R : The Journal of Injury, Function, and Rehabilitation, 7*(7), 746–761. doi:10.1016/j.pmrj.2015.01.024

U.S. Department of Health and Human Services. (2019, May). *Pain Management Best Practices Inter-Agency Task Force Report: Updates, gaps, inconsistencies, and recommendations*. Retrieved from https://www.hhs.gov/ash/advisory-committees/pain/reports/index.html

U.S. Food and Drug Administration. (2019, March). *FDA approves new nasal spray medication for treatment-resistant depression; available only at a certified doctor's office or clinic*. Retrieved from https://www.fda.gov/news-events/press-announcements/fda-approves-new-nasal-spray-medication-treatment-resistant-depression-available-only-certified

Verrills, P., Sinclair, C., & Barnard, A. (2016). A review of spinal cord stimulation systems for chronic pain. *Journal of Pain Research*, *9*, 481–492. doi:10.2147/JPR.S108884

Wernecke, C., Braun, H. J., & Dragoo, J. L. (2015). The effect of intra-articular corticosteroids on articular cartilage: A systematic review. *Orthopaedic Journal of Sports Medicine*, *3*(5), 2325967115581163. doi:10.1177/2325967115581163

Wong, C. S., & Wong, S. H. (2012). A new look at trigger point injections. *Anesthesiology Research and Practice*, *2012*, 492452. doi:10.1155/2012/492452

Zhu, B., Zhou, X., Zhou, Q., Wang, H., Wang, S., & Luo, K. (2019). Intra-venous lidocaine to relieve neuropathic pain: A systematic review and meta-analysis. *Frontiers in Neurology*, *10*, 954. doi:10.3389/fneur.2019.00954

INDEX

Printed in the United States
by Baker & Taylor Publisher Services